Practical Andrology

Practical Andrology

Editor: Maisie Ellis

FOSTER
ACADEMICS

www.fosteracademics.com

www.fosteracademics.com

FOSTER ACADEMICS

Cataloging-in-Publication Data

Practical andrology / edited by Maisie Ellis.
p. cm.
Includes bibliographical references and index.
ISBN 978-1-63242-962-9
1. Andrology. 2. Generative organs, Male. 3. Male reproductive health.
4. Human reproduction--Endocrine aspects. 5. Men--Physiology. I. Ellis, Maisie.
RC875 .P73 2020
612.6--dc23

Foster Academics,
118-35 Queens Blvd., Suite 400,
Forest Hills, NY 11375, USA

ISBN 978-1-63242-962-9 (Hardback)

Contents

Preface

Every book is initially just a concept; it takes months of research and hard work to give it the final shape in which the readers receive it. In its early stages, this book also went through rigorous reviewing. The notable contributions made by experts from across the globe were first molded into patterned chapters and then arranged in a sensibly sequential manner to bring out the best results.

The understanding of the male reproductive system, its physiology and pathophysiology is vital to addressing the various issues related to male sexual health. The clinical discipline of andrology involves a holistic study of the disorders of the male reproductive system and other pathologies, including the common issue of infertility. Infertility in men is an extremely common medical problem and a major cause of childlessness. It can arise due to genetic abnormalities, cancer, endocrine disorders, as well as a consequence of various medical procedures. The management of sexual dysfunction, prostatic disease, penile disease and genital tract cancer are also under the scope of andrology. Certain procedures are helpful in the diagnostic process, such as vasography, digital rectal examination, collection of sperm, surgical exploration of the genital tract, biopsy, etc. This book is compiled in such a manner, that it will provide in-depth knowledge about the theory and practice of andrology. The topics covered in this extensive book deal with andrological conditions, and their therapeutic interventions. It will prove to be immensely beneficial to students and researchers in andrology.

It has been my immense pleasure to be a part of this project and to contribute my years of learning in such a meaningful form. I would like to take this opportunity to thank all the people who have been associated with the completion of this book at any step.

Editor

1

Intermittent versus continuous androgen deprivation for locally advanced, recurrent or metastatic prostate cancer

Tobias Engel Ayer Botrel[1,2*], Otávio Clark[1,2], Rodolfo Borges dos Reis[2], Antônio Carlos Lima Pompeo[2], Ubirajara Ferreira[2], Marcus Vinicius Sadi[2] and Francisco Flávio Horta Bretas[2]

Abstract

Background: Prostate cancer is the most common cancer in older men in the United States (USA) and Western Europe. Androgen deprivation (AD) constitutes, in most cases, the first-line of treatment for these cases. The negative impact of CAD in quality of life, secondary to the adverse events of sustained hormone deprivation, plus the costs of this therapy, motivated the intermittent treatment approach. The objective of this study is to to perform a systematic review and meta-analysis of all randomized controlled trials that compared the efficacy and adverse events profile of intermittent versus continuous androgen deprivation for locally advanced, recurrent or metastatic hormone-sensitive prostate cancer.

Methods: Several databases were searched, including MEDLINE, EMBASE, LILACS, and CENTRAL. The endpoints were overall survival (OS), cancer-specific survival (CSS), time to progression (TTP) and adverse events. We performed a meta-analysis (MA) of the published data. The results were expressed as Hazard Ratio (HR) or Risk Ratio (RR), with their corresponding 95% Confidence Intervals (CI 95%).

Results: The final analysis included 13 trials comprising 6,419 patients with hormone-sensitive prostate cancer. TTP was similar in patients who received intermittent androgen deprivation (IAD) or continuous androgen deprivation (CAD) (fixed effect: HR = 1.04; CI 95% = 0.96 to 1.14; p = 0.3). OS and CSS were also similar in patients treated with IAD or CAD (OS: fixed effect: HR = 1.02; CI 95% = 0.95 to 1.09; p = 0.56 and CSS: fixed effect: HR = 1.06; CI 95% = 0.96 to 1.18; p = 0.26).

Conclusion: Overall survival was similar between IAD and CAD in patients with locally advanced, recurrent or metastatic hormone-sensitive prostate cancer. Data on CSS are weak and the benefits of IAD on this outcome remain uncertain. Impact in QoL was similar for both groups, however, sexual activity scores were higher and the incidence of hot flushes was lower in patients treated with IAD.

Keywords: Androgen deprivation, Prostate cancer, Systematic review

* Correspondence: tobias.engel@evidencias.com.br
[1]Evidencias Scientific Credibility, Campinas, São Paulo, Brazil
[2]Comitê Brasileiro de Estudos em Uro-Oncologia (CoBEU), São Paulo, Brazil

Background

Prostate cancer is the most common cancer in older men in the United Kingdom (UK), United States (USA) and Western Europe [1]. Despite its high incidence, the disease is often responsive to treatment even when metastatic and may be cured when localized. In patients with locally advanced tumors, recurrent or metastatic, the goals of therapy are to prolong survival, slow the progression of disease and preserve the quality of life [2].

Androgen deprivation (AD) constitutes, in most cases, the first-line of treatment for these cases. However, the deleterious effects of continuous androgen deprivation (CAD) are widely known and are related to some degree of deterioration in the quality of life. The most frequent symptoms resulting from AD include sexual dysfunction, fatigue, anemia, reduced muscle and bone mass, depression, abnormal lipid metabolism, cognitive dysfunction and development or worsening of metabolic syndrome [3,4]. The negative impact of CAD in quality of life, secondary to the adverse events of sustained hormone deprivation, plus the costs of this therapy, motivated the intermittent treatment approach.

In recent years, non-randomized studies (most of them with heterogeneous criteria for selection and clinical assessment) were performed to confirm the effectiveness of intermittent androgen deprivation (IAD) in patients with prostate cancer. Two systematic reviews [5,6] previously published analyzed the results of these non-randomized studies and the authors suggested that the best candidates for intermittent androgen deprivation are patients with biochemical progression after prostatectomy or radiation, with no evidence of metastases and with mildly aggressive tumors. On the other hand, patients with large tumor volumes, positive lymph nodes and bone metastases, PSA >100 ng/ml or short PSA doubling time, would be best treated with continuous deprivation.

Irrespective of official guideline recommendations, IAD is a treatment option used worldwide by both urologists and oncologists even outside of clinical trials [5].

The 2008 UK National Institute for Health and Clinical Excellence (NICE) recommends that IAD may be offered to men with metastatic prostate cancer providing they are informed that there is no long-term evidence of its effectiveness [7].

The results of some randomized controlled trials (RCT) were statistically inconclusive [8] or controversial. Crook et al. [9,10] analyzed IAD versus CAD for prostate-specific antigen (PSA) elevation after radiotherapy, assessing overall survival (OS) in a non-inferiority randomized trial with 1,386. The results demonstrated that IAD was non-inferior to CAD in regard to OS (8.8 years versus 9.1 years respectively - hazard ratio for death, 1.02; CI 95% 0.86 to 1.21, p for non-inferiority = 0.009), besides providing potential benefits in aspects such as physical function, fatigue, urinary problems, hot flashes, libido, and erectile function. Furthermore, the authors pointed that time to hormone resistance was statistically significantly improved on the IAD arm (HR 0.80, 95% CI 0.67-0.98; p = 0.024).

Regarding time-to-progression or castration-resistant disease, however, Crook et al. [9,10] showed better results in favor of CAD, while the results of Salonen et al. [11,12] were favorable to IAD. Such contradictory results make it difficult to emit a strong scientific-based recommendation for or against IAD.

The objective of this study is to analyze all published randomized controlled trials (RCTs) that compared the efficacy and adverse events profile of IAD versus CAD for locally advanced, recurrent or metastatic hormone-sensitive prostate cancer.

Methods

Study selection criteria

Types of studies

We included RCTs with parallel design that compared the use of intermittent versus continuous androgen deprivation.

Types of participants

The selected studies included patients with locally advanced, recurrent or metastatic hormone-sensitive prostate cancer.

Search strategy for identification of studies

A wide search on the main computerized databases was conducted, including EMBASE, LILACS, MEDLINE, SCI, CENTRAL, The National Cancer Institute Clinical Trials service and The Clinical Trials Register of Trials Central. In addition, the abstracts published in the proceedings of the American Society of Clinical Oncology (ASCO), American Society of Radiation Oncology (ASTRO), the European Society of Medical Oncology (ESMO), Society of Urologic Oncology (SUO), European Society for Radiotherapy and Oncology (ESTRO) and American Urological Association (AUA) were also searched.

For MEDLINE, we used the search strategy methodology for randomized controlled trials [13] recommended by the Cochrane Collaboration [14]. For EMBASE, adaptations of this same strategy were used [13], and for LILACS, we used the search strategy methodology reported by Castro et al. [15]. An additional search on the SCI database was also performed to retrieve articles that were cited on the included studies. The specific terms relevant to this review were added to the overall search strategy methodology for each database.

The overall search strategy was: #1: prostate cancer, #2: intermittent, #3: androgen deprivation and #4: Randomized Controlled Trial. Searches in electronic databases combined the terms: #1 AND #2 AND #3 AND #4.

The search was not limited by date, language or specific outcome.

Critical evaluation of the selected studies

All the references retrieved by the search strategies had their title and abstract evaluated by two of the researchers. Every reference with the least indication of fulfilling the inclusion criteria was listed as pre-selected. The complete article of all pre-selected references was retrieved. The articles were analyzed by two different researchers and included or excluded according to the previously reported criteria. The excluded trials and the reason of their exclusion are listed in this article. Data was extracted from all the included trials.

Details regarding the main methodology characteristics empirically linked to bias [16] were extracted with the methodological validity of each selected trial assessed by two reviewers (T.E.A.B and O.C). Particular attention was given to some items such as: the generation and concealment of the sequence of randomization; blinding; application of intention-to-treat analysis; sample size pre-definition; loss of follow-up description; adverse events reports; if the trial was performed in multiple center or a single center; and the sponsorship.

Data extraction

Two independent reviewers extracted the data. The name of the first author and year of publication were used to identify the study. All data were extracted directly from the text or calculated from the available information when necessary. The data of all trials were based on the intention-to-treat principle, so they compared all patients allocated in one treatment with all those allocated in the other.

The primary endpoint was overall survival (OS). The OS was calculated from the date of randomization to the date of death, with data censored at the last known date that the patient was alive.

Other clinical outcomes were also evaluated:

- Cancer-specific survival (CSS): the cancer-specific survival was calculated from the date of randomization to the date of death from prostate cancer or a complication of cancer treatment;
- Time to progression (TTP) or castration-resistant disease: defined as increases in PSA level or evidence of new clinical disease while the patient was receiving androgen-deprivation therapy and testosterone was at castration level;
- Differences in the quality of life (QoL): hot flashes, desire for sexual activity, urinary symptoms, depression and gynecomastia;
- Died because of cardiovascular events.

Analysis and presentation of results

Data analysis was performed using the Review Manager 5.1.2 statistical package (Cochrane Collaboration Software) [17].

Dichotomous clinical outcomes are reported as Risk Ratio (RR) and survival data as Hazard Ratio (HR) [18]. The corresponding 95% confidence interval (CI 95%) was calculated, considering *P* values less than 5% ($p < 0.05$). Statistic Heterogeneity was calculated through I2 method (25% was considered low-level heterogeneity, 25-50% moderate-level heterogeneity and >50% high-level heterogeneity) [19,20].

To estimate the absolute gain in OS, cancer-specific survival and time to progression, the meta-analytic survival curves were calculated as suggested by Parmar et al. [18]. A pooled estimate of the HR was computed by a fixed-effect model according to the inverse-variance method [21]. Thus, for effectiveness or adverse events, an HR or RR >1 favors the standard arm (continuous treatment) whereas an HR or RR <1 favors the intermittent treatment.

If statistic heterogeneity was found in the meta-analysis, an additional analysis was performed, using the random-effects model described by DerSimonian and Laird [22] that provides a more conservative analysis.

To assess the possibility of publication bias, the funnel plot test described by Egger et al. was performed [23]. When the pooled results were significant, the number of patients needed to treat (NNT or NNH) to cause or to prevent one event was calculated by pooling absolute risk differences in the trials included in this meta-analysis [24-26]. For all analyses, a forest plot was generated to display the results.

Results

The diagram represents the flow of identification and inclusion of trials, as recommended by the PRISMA (Preferred Reporting Items for Systematic reviews and Meta-Analyses) statement [27] (Figure 1).

Overall, 73 references were identified and screened.

Twenty-nine studies were selected and retrieved for full-text analysis. Of these studies, 16 were excluded for various reasons described on Table 1.

Characteristics of included studies

Thirteen randomized trials comprising 6,419 patients with hormone-sensitive prostate cancer were included in this analysis. More than 2,800 patients (44%) had metastatic disease and 1,595 patients (25%) had PSA progression after

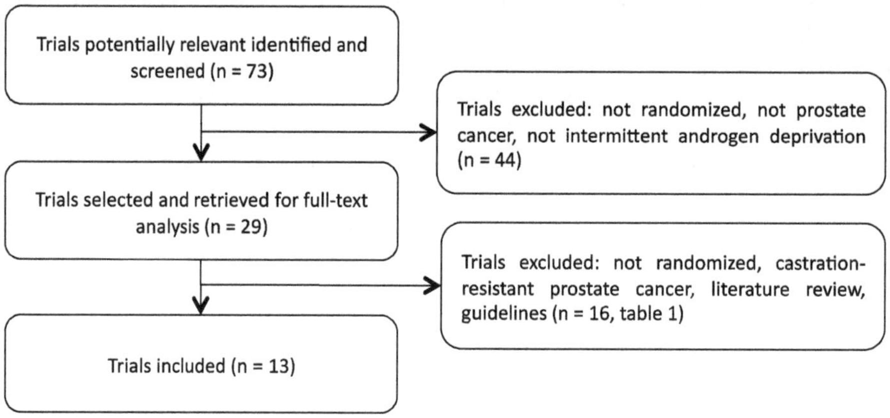

Figure 1 Trial selection flow.

prostatectomy (n = 209) or radiotherapy (n = 1,386). The number of patients in these trials varied from 43 to 1,535, but only 5 involved >500 patients. The average age of patients was 70 years.

PSA was measured every 2-3 months in most studies [1,9-12,44-54]. Only in one study [8,55] PSA levels were measured monthly.

Full details of trial design are not available for all studies: several reports are available only in abstract form [48,49,56].

The criteria for stopping and re-start of therapy in groups treated with IAD were similar, however not uniform (Table 2). Average follow-up time in these studies was of >2 years. The induction period varied, but most patients used IAD for a period of approximately 3-6 months (Table 3).

Two studies [48,49,54] did not use luteinizing hormone–releasing hormone agonist (LHRHa) or orchiectomy. These studies used cyproterone acetate (CPA) with doses between 300-400 mg/day orally. Overall, goserelin was the most used LHRHa, followed by leuprorelin (Table 3).

Evaluation of OS was the primary endpoint in 4 studies [8-10,50,55,58] and TTP or time to androgen-independent was the primary endpoint in 7 studies [1,11,12,44-47,50-54, 56,57] (Table 2). Five studies [1,8-10,44-47,55,58] were designed to evaluate the non-inferiority of IAD compared to CAD (Table 4).

More details on the treatment modality, follow-up, number of patients and primary endpoint in the 13 trials included in this analysis are summarized in Tables 2 and 3.

The efficacy analysis was summarized in Table 4.

Table 1 Characteristics of excluded studies

Study	Reason for exclusion
Klotz [28]	Not a randomized trial
Goldenberg [29]	Not a randomized trial
Higano [30]	Not a randomized trial
Oliver [31]	Not a randomized trial
Bierkens [32]	Not a randomized trial
Grossfeld [33]	Not a randomized trial
Calais da Silva Jr F [34]	Analysis of pooled data from 2 trials
De Conti P [35]	Systematic Review
Loblaw [36]	Practice guideline
Heidenreich [37]	Practice guideline
Heidenreich [38]	Not a randomized trial
Heidenreich [39]	Practice guideline
Buchan [40]	Not a randomized trial
Kelzman [41]	Not a randomized trial
Gruca [42]	Literature review
Organ [43]	Castration-resistant prostate cancer

Meta-analysis

Overall, TTP was similar in patients who received IAD or CAD (fixed effect: HR = 1.04; CI 95% = 0.96 to 1.14; p = 0.3), with high moderate heterogeneity (Chi^2 = 13.59, df = 8 [P = 0.09]; I^2 = 41%) (Figure 2).

OS and CSS were also similar in patients treated with IAD or CAD (OS: fixed effect: HR = 1.02; CI 95% = 0.95 to 1.09; p = 0.56 with moderate heterogeneity Chi^2 = 9.57, df = 7, P = 0.21, I^2 = 27% and CSS: fixed effect: HR = 1.06; CI 95% = 0.96 to 1.18; p = 0.26 also with moderate heterogeneity Chi^2 = 9.75, df = 6, P = 0.14, I^2 = 38% (Figures 3 and 4, respectively).

In order to explore this heterogeneity, the study by Salonen et al. [11,12] was removed from the survival analysis, since patients treated in the IAD arm had lower levels of baseline PSA than patients on CAD group (IAD: mean PSA 116.0 ± 173.4 ng/ml; CAD: mean PSA

Table 2 Characteristics of randomized included studies

Study	Patients with PCa	N (ITT)	PSA levels (ng/ml)		Primary endpoint	Median follow-up (years)
			Cease treatment	Restarted treatment		
Crook 2012 [9,10] *(CIC-CTG PR.7 Trial)*	Recurrent (after radiotherapy)	1386	<4 and not > 1 above the previous recorded value as monitored	>10	OS	6.9
Calais da Silva 2009/2011 [44,45] *(SEUG Trial)*	Locally advanced, metastatic	626	<4 ≤80% initial level	≥10 (symptomatic) or ≥20 (asymptomatic) ≥20% above nadir value	TTP	4.75
Hussain 2013 [8,55] *(SWOG 9346 Trial)*	Metastatic	1535	≤4	≥20 or ≥10 or symptoms	OS	9.2
Salonen 2012/2013 [11,12] *(FinnProstate Trial VII)*	Locally advanced, metastatic or recurrent (after radiotherapy or prostatectomy)	554	<10 >50% (PSA < 20)	PSA or CP	TTP	5.4
Tunn 2012 [1,46,47] *(EC507 Trial)*	Recurrent (after prostatectomy)	201	≤0.5	≥3 or when was CP	Time to androgen-independent	2.4
De Leval 2002 [51]	Locally advanced, metastatic or recurrent (after prostatectomy)	68	≤4	≥10	Time to androgen-independent	2.7
Langenhuijsen 2008/2011 [52,53] *(TULP Trial)*	Locally advanced or metastatic	193	<4	≥10 (M0) ≥20 (M1)	TTP	2.58
Miller 2007 [56]	Locally advanced or metastatic	335	<4 ≤90% initial level	-	TTP	NR
Mottet 2012 [50] *(TAP 22 Trial)*	Metastatic and PSA ≥ 20 ng/ml	173	< 4	≥10 or CP	OS	3.7
Verhagen 2008/2013 [48,49]	Asymptomatic metastatic	258	Good or moderate response	PSA or CP	Quality of life	NR
Hering 2000 [54]	Metastatic	43	0.4	≥10 (initial ≤20) ± 50% initial (initial > 20)	TTP and adverse events	4
Irani 2008 [57]	Locally advanced or metastatic	129	6 months	6 months	Quality of life and TTP	5
Silva 2013 [58] *(SEUG 9901 Trial)*	Locally advanced or metastatic	918	< 4	≥20 or CP	OS	5.5

Abbreviations: OS overall survival, *TTP* time to progression, *PCa* prostate cancer, *PSA* prostate-specific antigen, *CP* clinical progression, *NR* not reported, *ITT* intent-to-treat, *CP* clinical progression.

186.3 ± 454.4 ng/ml). Regarding OS, results remain similar between the groups (fixed effect: HR = 1.04; CI 95% = 0.96 to 1.12; p = 0.32) while there was a decrease in heterogeneity ($Chi^2 = 6.87$, df = 5, P = 0.23, $I^2 = 27\%$). Furthermore, CSS was favorable to CAD (fixed effect: HR = 1.16; CI 95% = 1.02 to 1.31; p = 0.02; NNT = 6) with no heterogeneity ($Chi^2 = 3.51$, df = 5, P = 0.62, $I^2 = 0\%$).

Four studies [8,48-50,54,55] included only patients with metastatic disease (or ≥90% metastatic). In this subgroup of patients, only 1 study [50] reported TTP data and another [54] reported cancer-specific survival data, so a meta-analysis was not feasible. Two studies [8,50,55] reported OS data, which permitted meta-analysis. OS was also similar in patients treated with IAD or CAD (fixed effect: HR = 1.10; CI 95% = 0.98 to 1.24; p = 0.11) with no heterogeneity ($Chi^2 = 0.02$, df = 1, P = 0.88, $I^2 = 0\%$).

Two studies [1,9,10,46,47] included only patients with recurrent disease after definitive local therapy (prostatectomy or radiotherapy). In this subgroup, TTP was favorable to patients who received CAD (fixed effect: HR = 1.19; CI 95% = 1.01 to 1.39; p = 0.03), with moderate heterogeneity ($Chi^2 = 1.57$, df = 1 [P = 0.21]; $I^2 = 36\%$). However, when the random-effects model analysis was performed, no significant difference was detected (random effects: HR = 1.16, CI95% = 0.92 to 1.45; p = 0.22). It was not possible to perform a meta-analysis for OS and CSS, since only Crook et al. [9,10] reported these data.

One study [58], on re-introduction of treatment in IAD group, used a hormone therapy scheme (cyproterone 300 mg/d) that was different from the one used in the CAD group (LHRHa: triptoreline 11.25 mg plus cyproterone 200 mg/d). When OS analysis was performed

Table 3 Treatment regimens in the included studies

Crook 2012 *(CIC-CTG PR.7 Trial)* [9,10]	***Intermittent:*** induction only (8 mo): LHRHa injections plus a non-steroidal antiandrogen, with the latter continued for a minimum of 4 weeks.
	Continuous: consisted of a LHRHa plus a non-steroidal antiandrogen, with the latter continued for a minimum of 4 weeks, or orchiectomy.
Calais da Silva 2009/2011 *(SEUG 9401 Trial)* [44,45]	***Intermittent:*** induction only (3 mo): CPA 200 mg for 2 weeks followed by monthly depot injections of a LHRHa plus 200 mg of CPA daily.
	Continuous: received an LHRHa plus 200 mg of CPA daily.
Hussain 2013 *(SWOG 9346 Trial)* [8,55]	***Intermittent:*** induction only (7 mo): received LHRHa (goserelin) plus bicalutamide.
	Continuous: LHRHa plus bicalutamide
Salonen 2012/2013 *(FinnProstate Study VII)* [11,12]	***Intermittent:*** induction only (6 mo): goserelin acetate (3.6 mg) SC every 28 days. The CPA was given in 100 mg twice daily during the first 12.5 days to minimize flare reaction.
	Continuous: continued with goserelin acetate or bilateral orchiectomy.
Tunn 2012 *(EC507 Trial)* [1,46,47]	***Intermittent:*** induction only (6 mo): received LHRHa (Leuprorelin acetate 11.25 mg, 3-mo depot, SC or IM) plus CPA 200 mg/day orally was administered for the first 4 weeks to prevent tumor flare.
	Continuous: LHRHa
De Leval 2002 [51]	***Intermittent:*** induction only (3-6 mo): flutamide (250 mg, 3 times, daily) for 15 days. This therapy was followed by flutamide and goserelin acetate (3.6 mg, monthly).
	Continuous: goserelin plus flutamide (250 mg orally every 8 hours) without interruption.
Langenhuijsen 2008/2011 *(TULP Trial)* [52,53]	***Intermittent:*** induction only (6 mo): Buserelin depot 6.6 mg, a 2-monthly SC plus nilutamide 300 mg (once a day for the first 4 weeks and 150 mg daily thereafter).
	Continuous: buserelin depot plus nilutamide
Miller 2007 [56]	***Intermittent:*** induction only (6 mo): goserelin plus bicalutamide
	Continuous: goserelin plus bicalutamide
Mottet 2012 *(TAP 22 Trial)* [50]	***Intermittent:*** induction only (6 mo): leuprorelin SR 3.75 mg, SC every 28 days and flutamide, one 250 mg tablet, three times daily.
	Continuous: leuprorelin and flutamide continued until disease progression or study end.
Verhagen 2008/2013 [48,49]	***Intermittent:*** induction only (3-6 mo): CPA 100 mg three times daily
	Continuous: CPA 100 mg thrice daily.
Hering 2000 [54]	***Intermittent:*** induction only (10.5 mo): CPA 200 mg/day orally
	Continuous: CPA 200 mg/day orally
Irani 2008 [57]	***Intermittent:*** induction only (6 mo): goserelin 10.8 mg 3-mo depot and flutamide 250 mg three times daily and resumed 6 mo later
	Continuous: goserelin and flutamide 250 mg three times daily continued without interruption
Silva 2013 *(SEUG 9901 Trial)* [58]	***Intermittent:*** induction only (3 mo): CPA 200 mg/d for 2 weeks followed by monthly depot injections of triptoreline plus 200 mg of CPA daily and restarted monotherapy with CPA 300 mg/d in the progression
	Continuous: CPA 200 mg/d for 2 weeks followed by monthly depot injections of triptoreline plus 200 mg of CPA daily.

Abbreviations: *Mo* months, *CPA* cyproterone acetate, *LHRHa* luteinizing hormone–releasing hormone agonist, *SC* subcutaneous, *IM* intramuscular injection.

without this study, the results remained similar between IAD and CAD (fixed effect: HR = 1.04; CI 95% = 0.97 to 1.12; p = 0.25; with no heterogeneity: $Chi^2 = 7.08$, df = 6, P = 0.31, $I^2 = 15\%$).

In most studies [8-10,44,48-50,55] baseline quality-of-life scores were similar in both groups for the majority of items, with no clinically significant differences. Sexual activity scores appeared to be favorable in the IAD group (Table 5).

The prevalence of adverse events of androgen deprivation such as hot flushes (fixed effect: RR = 0.86; CI 95% = 0.82 to 0.90; p < 0.00001), gynecomastia (fixed effect: RR = 0.72; CI 95% = 0.65 to 0.80; p < 0.00001) and headache (fixed effect: RR = 0.81; CI 95% = 0.68 to 0.97; p-0.02) were more frequent in patients treated with CAD, with high heterogeneity levels (Figure 5). As planned, a random-effects model analysis was performed to better explore this heterogeneity. In this analysis, with exception of hot flushes (RR = 0.65; CI 95% = 0.45 to 0.95; p = 0.03; NNH = 10), adverse events were similar in both groups (gynecomastia: RR = 0.66; CI 95% = 0.39 to 1.13; p = 0.13 and headache: RR = 0.68; CI 95% = 0.42 to 1.10; p = 0.11).

Mortality secondary to cardiovascular events was report in only 4 studies [9-12,44,45,58]. Results of this analysis

Table 4 Efficacy analysis in the trials included in the meta-analysis

Study	Arm	Design of study	Time to progression or time to castration-resistant disease	Cancer-specific survival	Overall survival (95% CI)
Crook 2012 [9,10] *(CIC-CTG PR.7 Trial)*	CAD	Non-inferiority	10 years	HR: 1.18 (0.90-1.55)	9.1 years
	IAD	(HR <1.25)	9.8 years	p = 0.24	8.8 years
			HR: 0.80 (0.67-0.98) p = 0.024		HR: 1.02 (0.86-1.21) for non-inferiority (IAD *vs* CAD ≥1.25) = 0.009
Calais da Silva 2009/2011 [44,45] *(SEUG Trial)*	CAD	Non-inferiority	HR: 0.81 (0.63-1.05) favoring CAD	HR: 1.27 (0.98-1.64)	HR: 0.96 (0.80-1.14) favoring CAD
	IAD	(<30%)			
Hussain 2013 [8,55] *(SWOG 9346 Trial)*	CAD	Non-inferiority	NR	NR	5.8 years
	IAD	(HR <1.20)			5.1 years
					HR: 1.10 (0.97-1.25)
Salonen 2012/2013 [11,12]	CAD	Compare the efficacy	30.2 months	44.3 months	45.7 months
(FinnProstate Trial VII)	IAD		34.5 months	45.2 months	45.2 months
			HR: 1.08 (0.90-1.29) favoring IAD	HR: 1.17 (0.91-1.51) favoring IAD	HR: 1.15 (0.94 -1.4) favoring IAD
Tunn 2012 [1,46,47] *(EC507 Trial)*	CAD	Non-inferiority	16 risk of progression	NR	NR
	IAD		37 risk of progression		
			p = 0.853		
			HR: 0.97 (0.68-1.38) &		
De Leval 2002 [51]	CAD	Compare the efficacy	14.4 months	4 (12.1%) deaths	NR
	IAD		25.7 months	2 (5.7%) deaths	
			HR: 0.57 (0.07-4.64) &	NS	
				HR: 0.46 (0.09-2.35) &	
Langenhuijsen 2008/2011 [52,53]	CAD	Compare the efficacy	24.1 months[#]	NR	NS
(TULP Trial)	IAD		18 months		
			NS		
Miller 2007 [56]	CAD	Compare the efficacy	11.5 months	NR	53.8 months
	IAD		16.6 months		51.4 months
			p = 0.1758		p = 0.658
			HR: 0.69 (0.41-1.16)[&]		HR: 1.04 (0.86-1.28)[&]

Table 4 Efficacy analysis in the trials included in the meta-analysis *(Continued)*

Mottet 2012 [50] *(TAP 22 Trial)*	CAD	Compare the efficacy	15.1 months	NR	52 months
	IAD		20.7 months		42.2 months
			p = 0.74		p = 0.75
			HR: 0.88 (0.63-1.4)[&]		HR: 1.14 (0.74-1.77)[&]
Verhagen 2008/2013 [48,49]	CAD	Compare the efficacy	NS	NS	NS
	IAD				
Hering 2000 [54]	CAD	Compare the efficacy	20.1 months	2 (11.1%) deaths	NR
	IAD		NR	2 (8%) deaths	
			NS	NS	
				HR: 0.70 (0.09-5.44) &	
Irani 2008 [5[illegible]]	CAD	Compare the efficacy	HR: 1.1 (0.6-1.8) p = 0.3 favoring IAD	HR: 0.6 (0.2–1.6) p = 0.12 favoring CAD	HR: 0.6 (0.3–1.3) p = 0.06 favoring CAD
	IAD				
Silva 2013 [53] *(SEUG 9901 Trial)*	CAD	Non-inferiority	HR: 1.16 (0.93-1.47)	HR: 1.0 (0.76-1.32)	HR: 0.90 (0.76-1.07)
	IAD	(HR < 1.20)			

Abbreviations: *ITT* intention-to-treat, *HR* Hazard ratios, *Mo* months, *NS* not significant, *IAD* intermittent androgen deprivation, *CAD* continuous androgen deprivation.
[#]No hazard ratio or *P* value reported.
[&]Calculated the meta-analytic survival curves as suggested by Parmar et al. [18].

Study or Subgroup	log[Hazard Ratio]	SE	Weight	Hazard Ratio IV, Fixed, 95% CI
Calais da Silva 2009/2011	0.21072103	0.128224	11.1%	1.23 [0.96, 1.59]
Crook 2012	0.22314355	0.0904782	22.3%	1.25 [1.05, 1.49]
De Leval 2002	-0.56211892	1.06998962	0.2%	0.57 [0.07, 4.64]
Irani 2008	-0.09531018	0.09195977	21.6%	0.91 [0.76, 1.09]
Miller 2007	-0.37106368	0.26558368	2.6%	0.69 [0.41, 1.16]
Mottet 2012	-0.12783337	0.38521043	1.2%	0.88 [0.41, 1.87]
Salonen 2012/2013	-0.07696104	0.09302291	21.1%	0.93 [0.77, 1.11]
Silva 2013	0.14842001	0.11275243	14.4%	1.16 [0.93, 1.45]
Tunn 2012	-0.03045921	0.18122949	5.6%	0.97 [0.68, 1.38]
Total (95% CI)			**100.0%**	**1.04 [0.96, 1.14]**

Heterogeneity: $Chi^2 = 13.59$, df = 8 (P = 0.09); $I^2 = 41\%$
Test for overall effect: Z = 1.03 (P = 0.30)

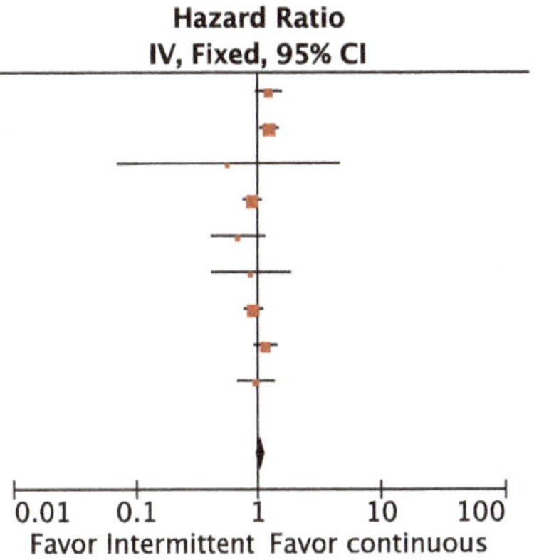

Figure 2 Time-to-progression: comparative effect of intermittent versus continuous androgen deprivation in prostate cancer.

were favorable to the group treated with IAD (fixed effect: RR = 0.80; CI 95% = 0.67 to 0.94; p = 0.007; NNH = 33) however with high heterogeneity levels ($Chi^2 = 6.67$, df = 3 [P = 0.08]; $I^2 = 55\%$).

According to funnel plot analysis [23] the possibility of publication bias was low for all of the outcomes. When funnel plot shows asymmetry, there is a possibility of bias and despite its limmitations, this method is widely used by authors.

Discussion

Currently, many oncology guidelines do not recommend the use of IAD for patients with metastatic hormone-sensitive prostate cancer [36,59]. But it is important to note that these guidelines date back to 2007. Guidelines from the European Association of Urology (EUA) state that IAD is now widely offered to patients with prostate cancer and should no longer be regarded as investigational [60,61].

Two other meta-analysis published earlier [62,63] showed that both treatments had similar results regarding OS and CSS. Analysis of OS was performed with 4 studies [8-12,44,45,55] in the Niraula et al. meta-analysis [62] and 7 studies [8-12,44,45,50,52,53,55,57] in Tsai et al. [63]. CSS analysis was performed with 3 [9-12,44,45] and 6 studies [8-12,44,45,51,55,57] respectively.

In this present meta-analysis, we included a larger number of studies. When HRs were not directly reported in the original study, they were estimated indirectly by using the reported number of events and the corresponding *P* value for the log-rank statistics, or by reading survival curves as suggested by Parmar et al. [18]. To reduce reading errors, original survival curves were digitalized and enlarged, and data extraction was based on reading electronic coordinates for each point of interest, as described by DeLaurentiis in another meta-analysis [64].

In the final OS and CSS analyses we included 8 and 7 studies respectively. The induction time of androgen deprivation was, in general, 3-6 months. Two studies were available only in abstract form [48,49,56]. Overall, goserelin was the most used LHRHa, followed by leuprorelin. Only two studies [48,49,53] did not used luteinizing hormone–releasing hormone agonist (LHRHa) or orchiectomy. These studies used cyproterone acetate (CPA).

In this meta-analysis, randomized studies included heterogeneous groups of patients (locally advanced, metastatic or recurrent). It was not possible to perform the proper

Study or Subgroup	log[Hazard Ratio]	SE	Weight	Hazard Ratio IV, Fixed, 95% CI
Calais da Silva 2009/2011	0.04082199	0.09302291	13.4%	1.04 [0.87, 1.25]
Crook 2012	0.01980263	0.08705543	15.3%	1.02 [0.86, 1.21]
Hussain 2013	0.09531018	0.06416923	28.2%	1.10 [0.97, 1.25]
Irani 2008	0.51082562	0.26909671	1.6%	1.67 [0.98, 2.82]
Miller 2007	0.03922071	0.0969628	12.4%	1.04 [0.86, 1.26]
Mottet 2012	0.13102826	0.22048025	2.4%	1.14 [0.74, 1.76]
Salonen 2012/2013	-0.13976194	0.10287809	11.0%	0.87 [0.71, 1.06]
Silva 2013	-0.10536052	0.08626502	15.6%	0.90 [0.76, 1.07]
Total (95% CI)			**100.0%**	**1.02 [0.95, 1.09]**

Heterogeneity: $Chi^2 = 9.57$, df = 7 (P = 0.21); $I^2 = 27\%$
Test for overall effect: Z = 0.58 (P = 0.56)

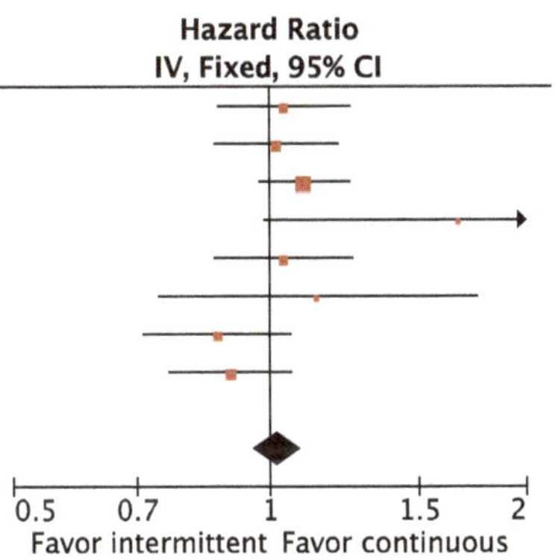

Figure 3 Overall survival. Comparative effect of intermittent versus continuous androgen deprivation in prostate cancer.

Study or Subgroup	log[Hazard Ratio]	SE	Weight	Hazard Ratio IV, Fixed, 95% CI
Calais da Silva 2009/2011	0.2390169	0.13225733	16.8%	1.27 [0.98, 1.65]
Crook 2012	0.16551444	0.08705543	38.8%	1.18 [0.99, 1.40]
De Leval 2002	−0.77652879	0.83237081	0.4%	0.46 [0.09, 2.35]
Hering 2000	−0.35667494	1.0465859	0.3%	0.70 [0.09, 5.44]
Irani 2008	0.5108	0.56053985	0.9%	1.67 [0.56, 5.00]
Salonen 2012/2013	−0.15700375	0.10287809	27.8%	0.85 [0.70, 1.05]
Silva 2013	0.0001	0.14007239	15.0%	1.00 [0.76, 1.32]
Total (95% CI)			**100.0%**	**1.06 [0.96, 1.18]**

Heterogeneity: $Chi^2 = 9.75$, df = 6 (P = 0.14); $I^2 = 38\%$
Test for overall effect: Z = 1.13 (P = 0.26)

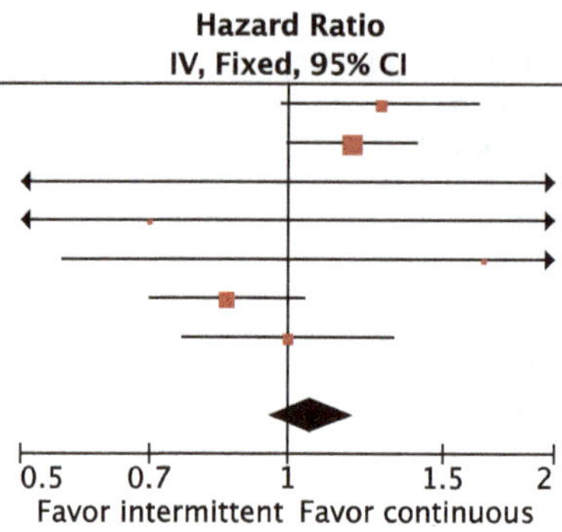

Figure 4 Cancer-specific survival. Comparative effect of intermittent versus continuous androgen deprivation in prostate cancer.

analysis of subgroups of patients (i.e. by Gleason score, initial PSA levels, minimal or extensive metastatic disease) because results for such sets were not published in the studies. As to overall survival, our results reinforce the equivalent efficacy of CAD and IAD, regardless of previous treatments.

Apropos of CSS, despite the overall analysis demonstrating only a trend towards treatment with CAD, the results must be interpreted with caution. As mentioned before, in one of the studies [11,12] the baseline PSA levels were lower on the IAD arm, suggesting that these patients had less extensive disease. Once this trial was excluded from

Table 5 Significant differences in quality of life (QoL)

Study	EORTC quality-of-life core questionnaire (QLQ-C30) and the EORTC Prostate Cancer Module
Crook 2012 [9,10] *(CIC-CTG PR.7 Trial)*	***Intermittent (better):*** hot flashes, desire for sexual activity, and urinary symptoms
	Continuous: -
Calais da Silva 2009/2011 [44,45] *(SEUG Trial)*	***Intermittent (better):*** sexual function
	Continuous (better): emotional domain, nausea and vomiting, severity of insomnia
Hussain 2013 [8,55] *(SWOG 9346 Trial)*	***Intermittent (better):*** erectile function and mental health at 3 months but not thereafter
	Continuous: -
Salonen 2012/2013 [11,12] *(FinnProstate Trial VII)*	***Intermittent (better):*** sexual function
	Continuous: -
Tunn 2012 [1,46,47] *(EC507 Trial)*	***Intermittent:*** NR
	Continuous: NR
De Leval 2002 [51]	***Intermittent:*** NR
	Continuous: NR
Langenhuijsen 2008/2013 [52,53] (*TULP Trial*)	***Intermittent:*** NS
	Continuous: NS
Miller 2007 [56]	***Intermittent (better):*** sexual activity appeared to be favorable in the intermittent
	Continuous: -
Mottet 2012 [50] *(TAP 22 Trial)*	***Intermittent:*** NS
	Continuous: NS
Verhagen 2008/2013 [48,49]	***Intermittent (better):*** symptom and potency scales
	Continuous: -
Hering 2000 [54]	***Intermittent (better):*** erectile function
	Continuous: -
Irani 2008 [57]	***Intermittent (better):*** ability to have and maintain an erection.
	Continuous: -
Silva 2013 [58] *(SEUG 9901 Trial)*	***Intermittent (better):*** sexual activity
	Continuous: -

Abbreviations: *EORTC* European Organization for Research and Treatment of Cancer, *NS* not significant, *NR* not reported.

Study or Subgroup	Intermittent Events	Intermittent Total	Continuous Events	Continuous Total	Weight	Risk Ratio M-H, Fixed, 95% CI
4.1.1 Hot flushes						
Calais da Silva 2009/2011	59	299	88	293	8.4%	0.66 [0.49, 0.88]
Hussain 2013	620	681	641	686	60.5%	0.97 [0.94, 1.00]
Langenhuijsen 2008/2011	49	97	57	96	5.4%	0.85 [0.66, 1.10]
Mottet 2012	8	86	24	83	2.3%	0.32 [0.15, 0.68]
Salonen 2012/2013	129	274	141	280	13.2%	0.93 [0.79, 1.11]
Silva 2013	36	436	105	421	10.1%	0.33 [0.23, 0.47]
Subtotal (95% CI)		**1873**		**1859**	**100.0%**	**0.86 [0.82, 0.90]**
Total events	901		1056			
Heterogeneity: $Chi^2 = 107.14$, df = 5 ($P < 0.00001$); $I^2 = 95\%$						
Test for overall effect: Z = 6.51 ($P < 0.00001$)						
4.1.2 Gynaecomastia						
Calais da Silva 2009/2011	37	299	57	293	11.0%	0.64 [0.43, 0.93]
Hussain 2013	272	681	298	686	56.6%	0.92 [0.81, 1.04]
Langenhuijsen 2008/2011	4	97	7	96	1.3%	0.57 [0.17, 1.87]
Salonen 2012/2013	5	274	3	280	0.6%	1.70 [0.41, 7.06]
Silva 2013	60	436	157	421	30.5%	0.37 [0.28, 0.48]
Subtotal (95% CI)		**1787**		**1776**	**100.0%**	**0.72 [0.65, 0.80]**
Total events	378		522			
Heterogeneity: $Chi^2 = 40.84$, df = 4 ($P < 0.00001$); $I^2 = 90\%$						
Test for overall effect: Z = 5.94 ($P < 0.00001$)						
4.1.3 Headache						
Calais da Silva 2009/2011	22	299	36	293	15.1%	0.60 [0.36, 0.99]
Hussain 2013	136	681	130	686	53.9%	1.05 [0.85, 1.31]
Mottet 2012	3	86	6	83	2.5%	0.48 [0.12, 1.87]
Silva 2013	35	436	67	421	28.4%	0.50 [0.34, 0.74]
Subtotal (95% CI)		**1502**		**1483**	**100.0%**	**0.81 [0.68, 0.97]**
Total events	196		239			
Heterogeneity: $Chi^2 = 13.39$, df = 3 ($P = 0.004$); $I^2 = 78\%$						
Test for overall effect: Z = 2.32 ($P = 0.02$)						
4.1.4 Skin complaints or rash						
Calais da Silva 2009/2011	8	299	20	293	25.5%	0.39 [0.18, 0.88]
Hussain 2013	54	681	52	686	65.5%	1.05 [0.73, 1.51]
Silva 2013	3	436	7	421	9.0%	0.41 [0.11, 1.59]
Subtotal (95% CI)		**1416**		**1400**	**100.0%**	**0.82 [0.60, 1.13]**
Total events	65		79			
Heterogeneity: $Chi^2 = 5.93$, df = 2 ($P = 0.05$); $I^2 = 66\%$						
Test for overall effect: Z = 1.21 ($P = 0.23$)						

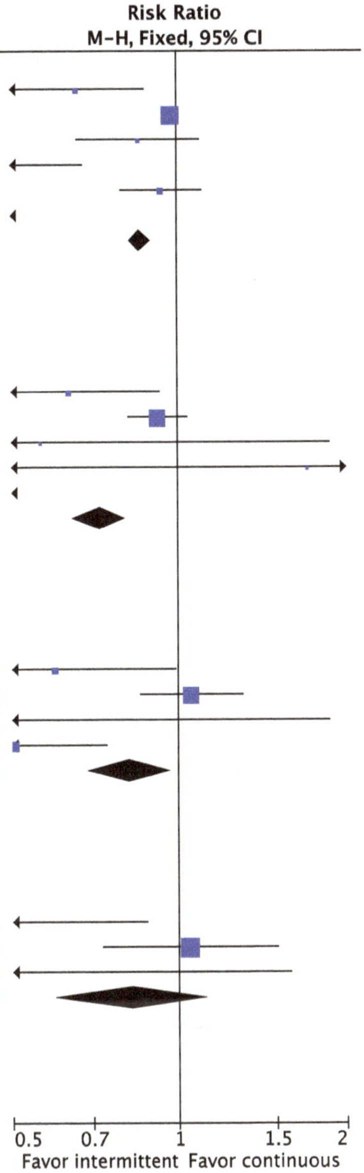

Test for subgroup differences: $Chi^2 = 8.23$, df = 3 ($P = 0.04$), $I^2 = 63.5\%$

Figure 5 Toxicities. Comparative effect of intermittent versus continuous androgen deprivation in prostate cancer.

the analysis, results favored the group treated with CAD; therefore we cannot exclude the possibility that IAD may carry a higher risk of death by cancer.

Recently, a large prospective Danish study, including over 30,000 patients, investigated the relationship between androgen deprivation therapy (ADT) and cardiovascular diseases such as myocardial infarction (MI) and stroke in men with prostate cancer [65]. The authors found that patients treated with medical endocrine therapy had an increased risk for MI and stroke with adjusted HRs of 1.31 (95% confidence interval [CI], 1.16-1.49) and 1.19 (95% CI, 1.06-1.35), respectively, compared with nonusers of ADT. However, androgen deprivation secondary to orchiectomy did no increase the risks for MI (HR: 0.90; 95% CI, 0.83-1.29) or stroke (HR: 1.11; 95% CI, 0.90-1.36). Nevertheless, the conclusions might have been affected, by the lack of information on prognostic lifestyles.

In this meta-analysis, mortality secondary to cardiovascular diseases, despite the heterogeneity found and the paucity of studies reporting this outcome, was favorable to the group treated with IAD. This aspect might have influenced the similar results achieved in OS.

In the event of biochemical recurrence after prostatectomy, when androgen deprivation is indicated, the best candidates for IAD are patients who reach PSA values <0.5 ng/mL after the induction time, according to a randomized study that was considered pure (i.e which included only patients with recurrence after prostatectomy) [1,46,47]. For biochemical recurrences after radiotherapy, the best candidates for IAD are patients who reach PSA levels <4 ng/mL after the induction time [9,10]. Only in these situations (recurrence after radiotherapy or prostatectomy), TTP seems to be favorable to patients receiving CAD. In locally advanced and/or metastatic tumors, the best candidates for IAD are patients who reach PSA values <4 ng/mL after induction time.

Although TTP analysis was performed in this meta-analysis, the results should be evaluated with caution since criteria for progression were different among the included studies.

Patients with a lower burden of disease (i.e. less extensive diseases) and without co-morbidities may be the ones achieving most benefits with IAD treatment.

The implementation of guidelines to assess, monitor and reduce known risk factors for cardiovascular disease may influence the results of overall survival in patients treated with CAD.

Regarding quality of life, differences were not clinically significant in most studies. But it was observed that sexual activity scores seemed to be higher in patients treated with IAD, and the incidence of hot flushes was lower.

Furthermore, it is important to note that IAD modality offers an economic benefit with reduction of pharmaceutical costs during "off-therapy" [62]. Economic analysis is not the aim of this investigation. The studies included failed to report the costs of both modalities (intermittent and continuous). Niraula et al. [62], analyzing only drug costs, estimated that the median cost savings with IAD would be 48%. Hering et al. [54], also based only on the average drug costs, demonstrated that the cost of treatment in IAD arm was approximately 50% lower that in the CAD, over 48 months.

Conclusions

Overall survival was similar between IAD and CAD in patients with locally advanced, recurrent or metastatic hormone-sensitive prostate cancer. Data on CSS are weak and the benefits of IAD on this outcome remain uncertain. Impact in QoL was similar for both groups, however, sexual activity scores were higher and the incidence of hot flushes was lower in patients treated with IAD.

Competing interests

The authors declare that they have no competing interests.

Authors' contributions

Systematic review and meta-analysis TEAB, OC. Identification of studies, critical evaluation and discussion. RBDR, ACLP, UF, MVS, FFHBT, TEAB. All authors read and approved the final manuscript.

References

1. Tunn U: **The current status of intermittent androgen deprivation (IAD) therapy for prostate cancer: putting IAD under the spotlight.** *BJU Int* 2007, **99**(Suppl 1):19–22. discussion 3-4.
2. National Cancer Institute: *Prostate Cancer Treatment (PDQ®). General Information About Prostate Cancer.* http://www.cancer.gov/cancertopics/pdq/treatment/prostate. Accessed on 16 December 2013.
3. Choong K, Basaria S: **Emerging cardiometabolic complications of androgen deprivation therapy.** *Aging Male* 2010, **13**(1):1–9.
4. Harle LK, Maggio M, Shahani S, Braga-Basaria M, Basaria S: **Endocrine complications of androgen-deprivation therapy in men with prostate cancer.** *Clin Adv Hematol Oncol* 2006, **4**(9):687–696.
5. Abrahamsson PA: **Potential benefits of intermittent androgen suppression therapy in the treatment of prostate cancer: a systematic review of the literature.** *Eur Urol* 2010, **57**(1):49–59.
6. Shaw GL, Wilson P, Cuzick J, Prowse DM, Goldenberg SL, Spry NA, *et al*: **International study into the use of intermittent hormone therapy in the treatment of carcinoma of the prostate: a meta-analysis of 1446 patients.** *BJU Int* 2007, **99**(5):1056–1065.
7. National Institute for Health and Clinical Excellence: *Prostate cancer: diagnosis and treatment.* February 2008. http://publications.nice.org.uk/prostate-cancer-cg58/guidance#metastatic-prostate-cancer. Accessed on 16 December 2013.
8. Hussain M, Tangen CM, Berry DL, Higano CS, Crawford ED, Liu G, *et al*: **Intermittent versus continuous androgen deprivation in prostate cancer.** *N Engl J Med* 2013, **368**(14):1314–1325.
9. Crook JM, O'Callaghan CJ, Duncan G, Dearnaley DP, Higano CS, Horwitz EM, *et al*: **Intermittent androgen suppression for rising PSA level after radiotherapy.** *N Engl J Med* 2012, **367**(10):895–903.
10. Klotz L, O' Callaghan CJ, Ding K, Dearnaley DP, Higano CS, Horwitz EM, *et al*: **A phase III randomized trial comparing intermittent versus continuous androgen suppression for patients with PSA progression after radical therapy: NCIC CTG PR.7/SWOG JPR.7/CTSU JPR.7/UK Intercontinental Trial CRUKE/01/013.** *J Clin Oncol* 2011, **2011**:4514. ASCO Annual Meeting Abstracts Vol 29, No 15_suppl (May 20 Supplement).
11. Salonen AJ, Taari K, Ala-Opas M, Viitanen J, Lundstedt S, Tammela TL: **The FinnProstate Study VII: intermittent versus continuous androgen deprivation in patients with advanced prostate cancer.** *J Urol* 2012, **187**(6):2074–2081.
12. Salonen AJ, Taari K, Ala-Opas M, Viitanen J, Lundstedt S, Tammela TL: **Advanced prostate cancer treated with intermittent or continuous androgen deprivation in the randomised FinnProstate Study VII: quality of life and adverse effects.** *Eur Urol* 2013, **63**(1):111–120.
13. Dickersin K, Scherer R, Lefebvre C: **Identifying relevant studies for systematic reviews.** *BMJ* 1994, **309**(6964):1286–1291.
14. Higgins JPT, Green S: **Cochrane Handbook for Systematic Reviews of Interventions 4.2.6 [updated September 2006].** In *The Cochrane Library, Issue 4, 2006.* Chichester, UK: John Wiley & Sons, Ltd; 2006.
15. Castro AA, Clark OA, Atallah AN: **Optimal search strategy for clinical trials in the Latin American and Caribbean Health Science Literature database (LILACS database): update.** *Sao Paulo Med J* 1999, **117**(3):138–139.
16. Egger M, Smith GD, Altman D: *Systematic Reviews in Health Care.* London: BMJ Books; 2001.
17. Review Manager (RevMan) *[Computer program]. Version 5.1.* Copenhagen: The Nordic Cochrane Centre, The Cochrane Collaboration; 2011.
18. Parmar MK, Torri V, Stewart L: **Extracting summary statistics to perform meta-analyses of the published literature for survival endpoints.** *Stat Med* 1998, **17**(24):2815–2834.
19. Higgins JP, Thompson SG, Deeks JJ, Altman DG: **Measuring inconsistency in meta-analyses.** *BMJ* 2003, **327**(7414):557–560.
20. Yang K, Wang YJ, Chen XR, Chen HN: **Effectiveness and safety of bevacizumab for unresectable non-small-cell lung cancer: a meta-analysis.** *Clin Drug Investig* 2010, **30**(4):229–241.
21. Deeks JJHJ, Altman DG: **Analysing and presenting results.** In *Cochrane Handbook for Systematic Reviews of In- terventions (ed 4.2.6 [updated September*

2006]). Edited by Higgins JP, Green S. Chichester, United Kingdom: John Wiley & Sons, Ltd; 2006.

22. DerSimonian R, Laird N: **Meta-analysis in clinical trials.** *Control Clin Trials* 1986, **7**(3):177–188.
23. Egger M, Davey Smith G, Schneider M, Minder C: **Bias in meta-analysis detected by a simple, graphical test.** *BMJ* 1997, **315**(7109):629–634.
24. McQuay HJ, Moore RA: **Using numerical results from systematic reviews in clinical practice.** *Ann Intern Med* 1997, **126**(9):712–720.
25. Smeeth L, Haines A, Ebrahim S: **Numbers needed to treat derived from meta-analyses–sometimes informative, usually misleading.** *BMJ* 1999, **318**(7197):1548–1551.
26. Altman DG, Deeks JJ: **Meta-analysis, Simpson's paradox, and the number needed to treat.** *BMC Med Res Methodol* 2002, **2:**3.
27. Liberati A, Altman DG, Tetzlaff J, Mulrow C, Gotzsche PC, Ioannidis JP, *et al*: **The PRISMA statement for reporting systematic reviews and meta-analyses of studies that evaluate health care interventions: explanation and elaboration.** *Ann Intern Med* 2009, **151**(4):W65–W94.
28. Klotz LH, Herr HW, Morse MJ, Whitmore WF Jr: **Intermittent endocrine therapy for advanced prostate cancer.** *Cancer* 1986, **58**(11):2546–2550.
29. Goldenberg SL, Bruchovsky N, Gleave ME, Sullivan LD, Akakura K: **Intermittent androgen suppression in the treatment of prostate cancer: a preliminary report.** *Urology* 1995, **45**(5):839–844. discussion 44-5.
30. Higano CS, Ellis W, Russell K, Lange PH: **Intermittent androgen suppression with leuprolide and flutamide for prostate cancer: a pilot study.** *Urology* 1996, **48**(5):800–804.
31. Oliver RT, Williams G, Paris AM, Blandy JP: **Intermittent androgen deprivation after PSA-complete response as a strategy to reduce induction of hormone-resistant prostate cancer.** *Urology* 1997, **49**(1):79–82.
32. Bierkens AF, Hendrikx AJ, De La Rosette JJ, Stultiens GN, Beerlage HP, Arends AJ, *et al*: **Treatment of mid- and lower ureteric calculi: extracorporeal shock-wave lithotripsy vs laser ureteroscopy. A comparison of costs, morbidity and effectiveness.** *Br J Urol* 1998, **81**(1):31–35.
33. Grossfeld GD, Small EJ, Carroll PR: **Intermittent androgen deprivation for clinically localized prostate cancer: initial experience.** *Urology* 1998, **51** (1):137–144.
34. da Silva Jr F C, Calais Da Silva F, Brausi M, Goncalves F, Kliment J, Queimadelos A, *et al*: *Pooled Analysis of two protocols of intermittent hormonal therapy in advanced prostatic cancer.* AUA 2013 Annual Meeting:777.
35. De Conti P, Atallah Alvaro N, Arruda Homero O, Soares Bernardo GO, El Dib Regina P, Wilt Timothy J: **Intermittent versus continuous androgen suppression for prostatic cancer.** *Cochrane Database Syst Rev* 2007(4). Available from: http://onlinelibrary.wiley.com/doi/10.1002/14651858.CD005009.pub2/abstract.
36. Loblaw DA, Virgo KS, Nam R, Somerfield MR, Ben-Josef E, Mendelson DS, *et al*: **Initial hormonal management of androgen-sensitive metastatic, recurrent, or progressive prostate cancer: 2006 update of an American Society of Clinical Oncology practice guideline.** *J Clin Oncol* 2007, **25** (12):1596–1605.
37. Heidenreich A, Aus G, Bolla M, Joniau S, Matveev VB, Schmid HP, *et al*: **EAU guidelines on prostate cancer.** *Eur Urol* 2008, **53**(1):68–80.
38. Heidenreich A, Pfister D, Ohlmann CH, Engelmann UH: **Androgen deprivation for advanced prostate cancer.** *Urologe A* 2008, **47**(3):270–283.
39. Heidenreich A, Aus G, Bolla M, Joniau S, Matveev VB, Schmid HP, *et al*: **EAU guidelines on prostate cancer.** *Actas Urol Esp* 2009, **33**(2):113–126.
40. Buchan NC, Goldenberg SL: **Intermittent versus continuous androgen suppression therapy: do we have consensus yet?** *Curr Oncol* 2010, **17**(Suppl 2):S45–S48.
41. Keizman D, Carducci MA: **Intermittent androgen deprivation–questions remain.** *Nat Rev Urol* 2009, **6**(8):412–414.
42. Gruca D, Bacher P, Tunn U: **Safety and tolerability of intermittent androgen deprivation therapy: a literature review.** *Int J Urol* 2012, **19**(7):614–625.
43. Organ M, Wood L, Wilke D, Skedgel C, Cheng T, North S, *et al*: **Intermittent LHRH therapy in the management of castrate-resistant prostate cancer (CRPCa): results of a multi-institutional randomized prospective clinical trial.** *Am J Clin Oncol* 2013, **36**(6):601–605.
44. da Silva FE C, Bono AV, Whelan P, Brausi M, Marques Queimadelos A, Martin JA, *et al*: **Intermittent androgen deprivation for locally advanced and metastatic prostate cancer: results from a randomised phase 3 study of the South European Uroncological Group.** *Eur Urol* 2009, **55** (6):1269–1277.
45. da Silva FM C, da SIlva F C, Bono A, Whelan P, Brausi M, Queimadelos A, *et al*: **Phase III study of intermittent MAB vs continuos MAB.** *J Urol* 2011, **185**(4):e288. April 2011, AUA 2011 abstract 716.
46. Tunn U, Kurek R, Keinle E, *et al*: **Intermittent is as effective as continuous androgen deprivation in patients with PSA relapse after radical prostatectomy.** *J Urol* 2004, **171**:384. Abstract 1458.
47. Tunn UW, Canepa G, Kochanowsky A, Kienle E: **Testosterone recovery in the off-treatment time in prostate cancer patients undergoing intermittent androgen deprivation therapy.** *Prostate Cancer Prostatic Dis* 2012, **15**(3):296–302.
48. Verhagen PCMS, Wissenburg LD, Wildhagen MF, *et al*: *Quality of life effects of intermittent and continuous hormonal therapy by cyproterone acetate (CPA) for metastatic prostate cancer [abstract 541].* Milan, Italy: Presented at: 23rd Annual Congress of the European Association of Urology; March 26–29, 2008; 2008.
49. Verhagen PCMS, Wildhagen MF, Verkerk A, Bolle WABM, *et al*: **Intermittent versus continuous cyproterone acetate in bone metastatic prostate cancer: Results of a randomized trial.** *Eur Urol* 2013, **12**:e680.
50. Mottet N, Van Damme J, Loulidi S, Russel C, Leitenberger A, Wolff JM: **Intermittent hormonal therapy in the treatment of metastatic prostate cancer: a randomized trial.** *BJU Int* 2012, **110**(9):1262–1269.
51. de Leval J, Boca P, Yousef E, Nicolas H, Jeukenne M, Seidel L, *et al*: **Intermittent versus continuous total androgen blockade in the treatment of patients with advanced hormone-naive prostate cancer: results of a prospective randomized multicenter trial.** *Clin Prostate Cancer* 2002, **1**(3):163–171.
52. Langenhuijsen JF, Badhauser D, Schaaf B, Kiemeney LA, Witjes JA, Mulders PF: **Continuous vs. intermittent androgen deprivation therapy for metastatic prostate cancer.** *Urol Oncol* 2011, **9**.
53. Langenhuijsen JF, Schasfoort EMC, Heathcote P, *et al*: *Intermittent androgen suppression in patients with advanced prostate cancer: an update of the TULP survival data [abstract 538].* Milan, Italy: Presented at: 23rd Annual Congress of the European Association of Urology; March 26–29, 2008; 2008.
54. Hering F, Rodrigues PRT, Lipay MA, Nesrallah L, Srougi M: **Metastatic adenocarcinoma of the prostate: comparison between continuous and intermittent hormonal treatment.** *Braz J Urol* 2000, **26:**276–282.
55. Hussain M, Tangen CM, Higano C, Schelhammer PF, Faulkner J, Crawford ED, *et al*: **Absolute prostate-specific antigen value after androgen deprivation is a strong independent predictor of survival in new metastatic prostate cancer: data from Southwest Oncology Group Trial 9346 (INT-0162).** *J Clin Oncol* 2006, **24**(24):3984–3990.
56. Miller K, Steiner U, Lingnau A, *et al*: *Randomised prospective study of intermittent versus continuous androgen suppression in advanced prostate cancer [abstract 5105].* Chicago, IL, USA: Presented at: American Society of Clinical Oncology; June 1–5; 2007.
57. Irani J, Celhay O, Hubert J, Bladou F, Ragni E, Trape G, *et al*: **Continuous versus six months a year maximal androgen blockade in the management of prostate cancer: a randomised study.** *Eur Urol* 2008, **54**(2):382–391.
58. Silva FC, Silva FM, Goncalves F, Santos A, Kliment J, Whelan P, *et al*: **Locally advanced and metastatic prostate cancer treated with intermittent androgen monotherapy or maximal androgen blockade: results from a randomised phase 3 study by the south European uroncological group.** *Eur Urol* 2013.
59. Prostate cancer: *Guideline for the management of clinically localized prostate cancer.* 2007. update. American Urological Association. Web site. http://www.auanet.org/content/guidelines-and-quality-care/clinical-guidelines/main-reports/proscan07/content.pdf.
60. Heidenreich A, Bastian PJ, Bellmunt J, *et al*: **Guidelines on prostate cancer.** *Eur Association Urol.* Web site http://wwwuroweborg/gls/pdf/08%20Prostate%20Cancer_LR%20March%2013th%202012pdf.
61. Sciarra A, Abrahamsson PA, Brausi M, Galsky M, Mottet N, Sartor O, *et al*: **Intermittent androgen-deprivation therapy in prostate cancer: a critical review focused on phase 3 trials.** *Eur Urol* 2013. **64**(5):722–730.
62. Niraula S, Le LW, Tannock IF: **Treatment of prostate cancer with intermittent versus continuous androgen deprivation: a systematic review of randomized trials.** *J Clin Oncol* 2013, **31**(16):2029–2036.
63. Tsai HT, Penson DF, Makambi KH, Lynch JH, Van Den Eeden SK, Potosky AL: **Efficacy of intermittent androgen deprivation therapy vs conventional continuous androgen deprivation therapy for advanced prostate cancer: a meta-analysis.** *Urology* 2013, **82**(2):327–334.

64. De Laurentiis M, Cancello G, D'Agostino D, Giuliano M, Giordano A, Montagna E, *et al*: **Taxane-based combinations as adjuvant chemotherapy of early breast cancer: a meta-analysis of randomized trials.** *J Clin Oncol* 2008, **26**(1):44–53.
65. Jespersen CG, Norgaard M, Borre M: **Androgen-deprivation therapy in treatment of prostate cancer and risk of myocardial infarction and stroke: a nationwide Danish population-based cohort study.** *Eur Urol* 2013.

2

A case control study of sarcosine as an early prostate cancer detection biomarker

Donna P. Ankerst[1,2,3*], Michael Liss[2], David Zapata[2], Josef Hoefler[1], Ian M. Thompson[2] and Robin J. Leach[2,4]

Abstract

Background: Sarcosine has been investigated as a prostate cancer biomarker with mixed results concerning its predictive power. We performed a case–control evaluation of the predictive value of serum sarcosine for early detection in a population-based cohort of men undergoing prostate-specific antigen (PSA) screening.

Methods: For analysis we used 251 cancer cases and 246 age-matched non-cancer cases from the San Antonio Biomarkers Of Risk (SABOR) screening study. For cancer cases, pre-diagnostic serum was utilized for sarcosine measurement. Controls were defined as men who had been followed at least for 5 years on study with no prostate cancer diagnosis; sarcosine was measured on the initial baseline serum. HPLC-electrospray ionization mass spectrometry was used for serum sarcosine quantification. The association of sarcosine with prostate cancer was assessed using area underneath the receiver-operating characteristic curve (AUC), and logistic regression adjusting for PSA, digital rectal exam, family history, age, race, and history of a prior negative biopsy. Among cancer cases, nominal logistic regression was used for the association of sarcosine with Gleason grade.

Results: Sarcosine levels were overlapping between the prostate cancer cases (median 15.8 uM, range 6.2 to 42.5 uM) and controls (median 16.2 uM, range 6.4 to 53.6 uM). The AUC of sarcosine was not statistically different from random chance either for participants with any PSA value (52.2 %) or those with PSA values in the range of 2 to 10 ng/mL (54.3 %). Sarcosine was not predictive of Gleason score and added no independent predictive power to standard prostate cancer risk factors for detection of prostate cancer (all p-values > 0.05).

Conclusions: Serum sarcosine should not be pursued further as a marker for the early detection of prostate cancer.

Keywords: Sarcosine, Prostate cancer, Prostate-specific antigen

Background

Metabolic profiling has identified sarcosine as a differential metabolite in the development and progression of prostate cancer [1]. Sarcosine, also known as N-methyglycine, is an N-methyl derivate of the amino acid glycine synthesized by glycine-N-methyltransferase (GNMT). GNMT has been implicated in methylation and prostate cancer [2]. This link led to interest in sarcosine as a prostate cancer biomarker. In the few prior studies investigating sarcosine as a biomarker of prostate cancer, results have been conflicting; some indicated higher risk associated with higher levels of sarcosine and others, a lower risk [3, 4]. The methodology of these studies has been either unclear or suboptimal, for instance by using serum samples far in advance of the time of biopsy. In order to definitively assess the potential of serum sarcosine for further study, we evaluated its operating characteristics and independent predictive value in a prospectively collected cohort of men, specifically assembled for the evaluation of prostate cancer biomarkers.

* Correspondence: ankerst@uthscsa.edu
[1]Department of Mathematics, Technische Universitaet Muenchen, Boltzmannstr 3, Garching 85748, Germany
[2]Department of Urology, University of Texas Health Science Center at San Antonio, 7703 Floyd Curl Dr, San Antonio, TX 78229, USA
Full list of author information is available at the end of the article

Methods

Serum samples were obtained spanning the years from 2001 to 2009 from men enrolled in a prospective cohort undergoing annual prostate-specific antigen (PSA) testing as part of the San Antonio Biomarkers Of Risk (SABOR) clinical validation site for the US National Cancer Institute Early Detection Research Network (EDRN). The study protocol and written consent procedures were approved by the institutional review board at the University of Texas

Health Science Center at San Antonio (UTHSCSA). Cases, controls, serum samples, and risk measures were selected as previously described [5]. Serum specimens were collected within 2.5 years prior to the prostate cancer diagnosis for cases and at the first baseline visit for controls; the majority of specimens (92.7 %) were within 1 year. Controls included cancer-free men with a minimum of 5 years follow-up after serum collection, a group selected to minimize the risk of assigning as a control a subject who harbored a tumor that would be discovered within the intermediate term. The risk factors measured included PSA (measured from the same serum sample as used for sarcosine), digital rectal exam (DRE, result used from the same patient visit as that for serum measurement of PSA), age, race, family history of prostate cancer in a first-degree relative, and history of a prior negative biopsy.

Serum sarcosine was measured using the UTHSCSA and Cancer Center Mass Spectrometry Core Facility. Serum (20 μl) was combined with stable isotope labeled internal standard [2H3] sarcosine (25 μM, 40 μl), water (40 μl), and sodium tetraborate solution (0.1 M, 50 μl) prior to derivatization with 5-(dimethylamino) naphthalene-1-sulfonyl chloride (dansyl chloride; 20 mM, 100 μl) at room temperature for 30 min. After evaporation to dryness by vacuum centrifugation, the derivatized samples were dissolved in 200 μl of mobile phase A and transferred to autosampler vials for HPLC-ESI-MS analysis on a Thermo Fisher Q Exactive mass spectrometer used in conjunction with a Thermo Fisher/Dionex Ultimate 3000 HPLC. Peak areas were determined by processing through Quan Browser (Thermo Fisher) and compared to calibration curves that were generated by analysis of authentic standards.

Risk factors and serum sarcosine levels were compared between cases and controls using the chi-square test for categorical outcomes and Wilcoxon test for continuous measures. The AUC was computed for sarcosine and tested using the Wilcoxon rank test for all cases and controls, and in addition restricted to the group of cases and controls with PSA in the 2 to 10 ng/mL range. Logistic regression was used to assess the independent predictive power of sarcosine to PSA, DRE, age, race, history of a prior negative biopsy, and family history of prostate cancer. Among prostate cancer cases, multinomial logistic regression was used to assess whether sarcosine was associated with the trivariate outcome of no cancer, low-grade cancer (Gleason score < 7), and high-grade cancer.

Table 1 SABOR case control demographic and clinical variables

	Control Median (range) or *N* (%) *n* = 251	Prostate cancer Median (range) or *N* (%) *n* = 246	*P* value
Age	64.8 (45.0–83.5)	64.1 (46.0–88.5)	0.80
Race			0.02
White	171 (68.1)	139 (56.5)	
African American	34 (13.5)	38 (15.4)	
Other	46 (18.3)	69 (28.0)	
At least one previous prostate biopsy	43 (17.1)	53 (21.5)	0.26
Abnormal Digital Rectal Exam	7 (2.8)	70 (28.5)	<0.001
Family history of prostate cancer	28 (11.2)	62 (25.2)	<0.001
Prostate-specific antigen (ng/mL)	1.0 (0.1–8.4)	3.4 (0.0–93.8)	<0.001
Sarcosine uM in 20 uL serum (all samples)	16.2 (6.4–53.6)	15.8 (6.2–42.5)	0.40
Sarcosine (only PSA 2–10 ng/mL)	16.3 (8.1–37.6)	15.8 (6.2–42.5)	0.34
Gleason grade			N/A
5		7 (2.8)	
6		158 (64.2)	
7		56 (22.8)	
8		12 (4.9)	
9		8 (3.3)	
Missing		5 (2.0)	

Results

Characteristics of the 251 prostate cancer cases and 246 controls participating in the SABOR screening study are shown in Table 1. Participants diagnosed with prostate cancer were more likely to be of other races than Caucasian, have an abnormal DRE, have a positive family history of prostate cancer, and have a higher PSA value (all $p < 0.05$). Controls had similar ages and history of prior negative biopsy to the cancer cases.

Sarcosine levels were overlapping between the prostate cancer cases (median 15.8 uM, range 6.2 to 42.5 uM) and controls (median 16.2 uM, range 6.4 to 53.6 uM); see Fig. 1 and Table 1. The AUC of sarcosine was not statistically different from random chance either for participants with any PSA value (52.2 %) or those with PSA values in the range of 2 to 10 ng/mL ($n = 53$ controls, 188 cases, AUC 54.3 %). There was no independent predictive power of sarcosine for prediction of prostate cancer, controlling for PSA, DRE, and the other risk factors for prostate cancer (all $p > 0.05$, Table 2). Sarcosine similarly failed to be predictive of high- versus low-grade cancer (all $p > 0.05$).

Discussion

Several studies have postulated that sarcosine is causally linked with the development and progression of prostate

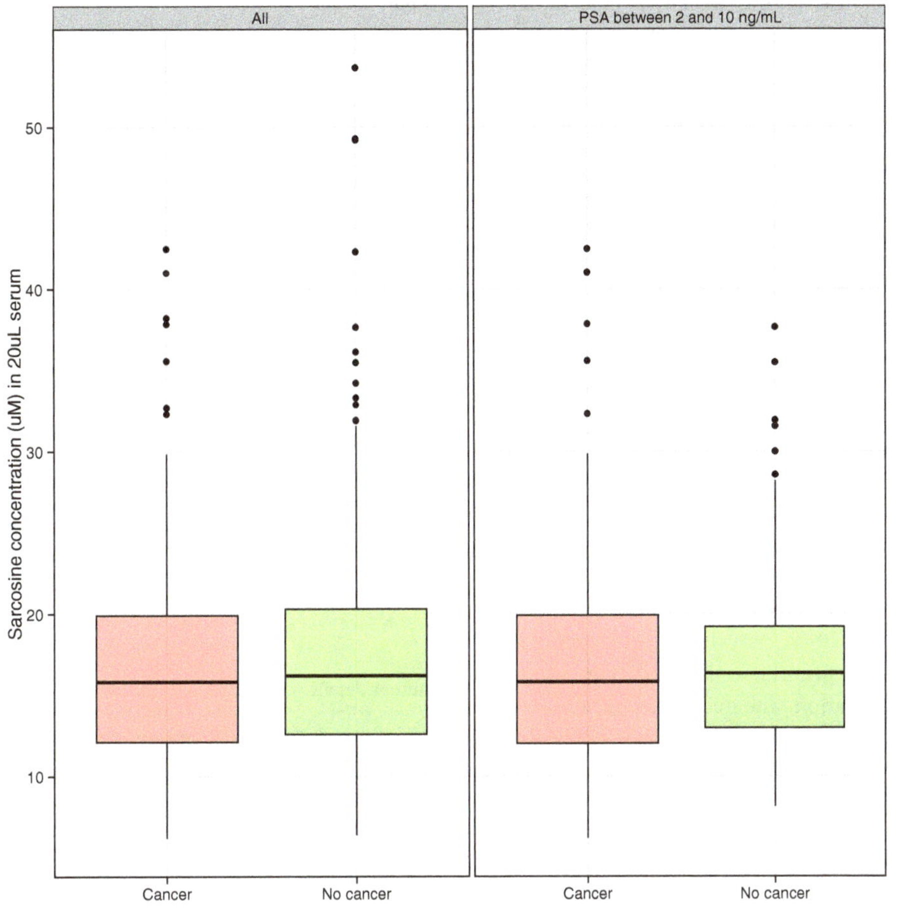

Fig. 1 Boxplots of sarcosine measurements among cancer cases (*red*) and controls (*green*) in the SABOR study for all cases and controls (*left*, 246 cases, 251 controls) and those with PSA in the 2 to 10 ng/mL range (*right*, 188 cases, 53 controls)

Table 2 Multivariable logistic regression model results for prediction of prostate cancer detection based on sarcosine and standard risk factors

	Odds ratio (95 % confidence interval)	*P*-value
Age	1.0 (0.9–1.1)	0.11
Race		
African American	1.3 (0.6–3.0)	0.47
Other	1.2 (0.7–2.3)	0.49
At least one previous prostate biopsy	0.7 (0.3–1.3)	0.26
Abnormal Digital Rectal Exam	30.5 (11.8–92.2)	<0.001
Family history of prostate cancer	3.5 (1.8–6.8)	<0.001
Prostate-specific antigen (ng/mL)[a]	4.4 (3.3–5.9)	<0.001
Sarcosine uM in 20uL serum[a]	1.1 (0.7–1.8)	0.64

[a]Variable was $\log_2$ transformed in the model

cancer. A large Norwegian study ($n = 6000$) concluded that sarcosine should be used as an early detection serum marker, but in contrast to other studies it found a decreased association with risk of prostate cancer rather than an increased one [3]. The reverse association could be due to the fact that baseline sarcosine measurements were used rather than those closer to the time of the biopsy as used in this study (92.7 % within 1 year prior to the biopsy, all the rest within 2.5 years prior). Two other studies, one from the US ($n = 2234$) and one from Italy ($n = 602$), found statistically significant increased associations between sarcosine and prostate cancer risk [4, 6]. The US study did not report an AUC for sarcosine, but rather reported its odds ratio with the outcome of prostate cancer to be 1.30 (95 % confidence interval 1.02 to 1.65). It noted that its inclusion in a clinical model did not improve the AUC. The Italian study investigated the AUC of sarcosine for all possible subsets of PSA, finding its max value of 64 % for use in men with PSA < 4 ng/mL, and its worst performance, which was no different from random chance, for men either with PSA > 10 ng/mL or between 4 and 10 ng/mL. The AUC remained marginally but statistically significantly better than chance for use among men with any value of PSA (AUC 57 %, 95 % CI 53 % to 61 %) as well as among men with PSA in the 2 to 10 ng/mL range (AUC 57 %, 95 % CI 52 % to 62 %).

The discordant findings of the SABOR prospectively-collected cohort with findings of some previous studies may have a number of explanations. First and foremost, previous studies noting an association between serum sarcosine and prostate cancer risk may be simply due to chance. The tendency to false positives is increased because of the multiple comparisons typically evaluated for sarcosine across different ranges of PSA; for example the Italian study reported 5 AUCs [6]. The previous US study did not report an AUC for sarcosine alone, but its inability to budge the AUC based on clinical risk factors in the study indicates the AUC may not have been statistically significantly different from 50 % in accordance with this study [4]. With the initial flurry of interest in this potential biomarker, publication bias may have led to submission and acceptance of only those studies that thereafter *confirmed* this association, meaning that other negative studies were not published. Other biases may also be operational, including the fact that few previous evaluations were conducted on prospectively-assembled cohorts of patients at risk of prostate cancer, or that the sarcosine measurements were taken too far in advance of the biopsy, as was the case for the large Norwegian study [3]. Unfortunately biomarker studies typically fail to report the time interval between biomarker measurement and the biopsy, which is particularly relevant for the prostate cancer cases. SABOR followed a rigorous protocol in which only cases were included where the biomarker was measured within a window of 2.5 years prior to the biopsy.

With its rigorous design, we believe this study eliminates serum sarcosine for further investigation as an early detection marker for prostate cancer. However, sarcosine may have a role in urine. Four studies investigating urine sarcosine for early detection all reported AUCs in the upper 60s and lower 70s, all statistically significantly better than chance in prediction [1, 7–9]. Urinary sarcosine seems to be more predictive of prostate cancer and may be utilized along with PSA and DRE in screening protocols.

Conclusions

Serum sarcosine, while exhibiting promising results for the early detection of prostate cancer in in some prior studies, had no value in this independent analysis of men undergoing screening in San Antonio, Texas. Serum sarcosine should not be pursued further as a marker for the early detection of prostate cancer.

Abbreviations

AUC: Area underneath the receiver-operating characteristic curve; DRE: Digital rectal examination; EDRN: Early Detection Research Network; GNMT: Glycine-N-methyltransferase; HR: Hazard ratio; OR: Odds ratio; PSA: Prostate-specific antigen; SABOR: San Antonio Biomarkers of Risk; US: United States; UTHSCSA: University of Texas Health Science Center at San Antonio.

Competing interests

The authors declare that they have no competing interests.

Authors' contributions

ML and DZ performed the systematic review, while ML wrote the background, conclusions and part of the methods section of the manuscript. DPA designed the case control study, directed the statistical analyses, wrote the statistical methods and part of the results section, and critically revised the manuscript. JH performed all statistical analyses and constructed all graphs. RJL performed the sarcosine analyses and critically revised the draft. IMT designed the study and critically revised the draft. All authors read and approved the final manuscript.

Acknowledgement

The authors of this work are grateful for the participants in the SABOR study, for funding provided by the US National Institutes of Health grants U01 CA86402 and P30 CA0541474, and for publication fees provided by the German Research Foundation (DFG) of the Technische Universität München within the Open Access Publishing Funding Programme.

Author details

[1]Department of Mathematics, Technische Universitaet Muenchen, Boltzmannstr 3, Garching 85748, Germany. [2]Department of Urology, University of Texas Health Science Center at San Antonio, 7703 Floyd Curl Dr, San Antonio, TX 78229, USA. [3]Department of Epidemiology and Biostatistics, University of Texas Health Science Center at San Antonio, 7703 Floyd Curl Dr, San Antonio, TX 78229, USA. [4]Department of Cellular and Structural Biology, University of Texas Health Science Center at San Antonio, 7703 Floyd Curl Dr, San Antonio, TX 78229, USA.

References

1. Sreekumar A, Poisson LM, Rajendiran TM, Khan AP, Cao Q, Yu J, et al. Metabolomic profiles delineate potential role for sarcosine in prostate cancer progression. Nature. 2009;457(7231):910–4.
2. Cernei N, Heger Z, Gumulec J, Zitka O, Masarik M, Babula P, et al. Sarcosine as a potential prostate cancer biomarker–a review. Int J Mol Sci. 2013;14(7):13893–908.
3. de Vogel S, Ulvik A, Meyer K, Ueland PM, Nygard O, Vollset SE, et al. Sarcosine and other metabolites along the choline oxidation pathway in relation to prostate cancer–a large nested case–control study within the JANUS cohort in Norway. Int J Cancer. 2014;134(1):197–206.
4. Koutros S, Meyer TE, Fox SD, Issaq HJ, Veenstra TD, Huang WY, et al. Prospective evaluation of serum sarcosine and risk of prostate cancer in the Prostate, Lung, Colorectal and Ovarian Cancer Screening Trial. Carcinogenesis. 2013;34(10):2281–5.
5. Liang Y, Ankerst DP, Ketchum NS, Ercole B, Shah G, Shaughnessy JD, et al. Prospective evaluation of operating characteristics of prostate cancer detection biomarkers. J Urol. 2011;185(1):104–10.
6. Lucarelli G, Fanelli M, Larocca AM, Germinario CA, Rutigliano M, Vavallo A, et al. Serum sarcosine increases the accuracy of prostate cancer detection in patients with total serum PSA less than 4.0 ng/ml. Prostate. 2012;72(15):1611–21.
7. Jentzmik F, Stephan C, Miller K, Schrader M, Erbersdobler A, Kristiansen G, et al. Sarcosine in urine after digital rectal examination fails as a marker in prostate cancer detection and identification of aggressive tumours. European Urol. 2010;58(1):12–8. discussion 20–21.
8. Wu H, Liu T, Ma C, Xue R, Deng C, Zeng H, et al. GC/MS-based metabolomic approach to validate the role of urinary sarcosine and target biomarkers for human prostate cancer by microwave-assisted derivatization. Anal Bioanal Chem. 2011;401(2):635–46.
9. Cao DL, Ye DW, Zhu Y, Zhang HL, Wang YX, Yao XD. Efforts to resolve the contradictions in early diagnosis of prostate cancer: a comparison of different algorithms of sarcosine in urine. Prostate Cancer Prostatic Dis. 2011;14(2):166–72.

3

Ultra-early versus early salvage androgen deprivation therapy for post-prostatectomy biochemical recurrence in pT2-4N0M0 prostate cancer

Satoru Taguchi, Hiroshi Fukuhara*, Takeshi Azuma, Motofumi Suzuki, Tetsuya Fujimura, Tohru Nakagawa, Akira Ishikawa, Haruki Kume, Yasuhiko Igawa and Yukio Homma

Abstract

Background: The optimal timing of salvage androgen deprivation therapy (ADT) for biochemical recurrence after radical prostatectomy is controversial. We compared the outcomes of ultra-early versus early salvage ADT.

Methods: Among 855 patients undergoing radical prostatectomy at our institution between 2000 and 2012, we identified 121 with adjuvant-treatment-naïve pT2-4N0M0 prostate cancer who received salvage ADT for biochemical recurrence. These patients were divided into an ultra-early salvage ADT group (n = 51), who started salvage ADT before meeting the standardized definition of biochemical recurrence in Japan (two consecutive prostate-specific antigen [PSA] values ≥0.2 ng/ml), and an early salvage ADT group (n = 70) who started salvage ADT when they met the definition. The ultra-early ADT group consisted of those who started salvage ADT with a single PSA value ≥0.2 ng/ml (n = 30) or with two consecutive PSA values >0.1 ng/ml and rising (n = 21). The primary endpoint was biochemical recurrence after salvage ADT, defined as a single PSA value ≥0.2 ng/ml after PSA nadir following salvage ADT. Secondary endpoints were clinical metastasis and cancer-specific survival. A Cox proportional hazards model was used for multivariate analysis. The median follow-up was 65.5 months.

Results: Biochemical recurrence occurred in one patient (2.0%) in the ultra-early group and in 12 (17.1%) in the early salvage ADT group. Multivariate analysis identified ultra-early salvage ADT and preoperative Gleason score ≤7 as independent negative predictors of biochemical recurrence after salvage ADT. Only one patient in the early salvage ADT group developed clinical metastasis to a left supraclavicular lymph node, and no patient died from prostate cancer during follow-up. The major limitations of this study were its retrospective design, selection bias, and the possibility that the ultra-early salvage ADT group may have included patients without biochemical recurrence.

Conclusions: Ultra-early salvage ADT was an independent negative predictor of biochemical recurrence after salvage ADT in post-prostatectomy patients. Further consideration should be given to the use of salvage ADT before meeting the current definition of biochemical recurrence.

Keywords: Androgen deprivation therapy, Biochemical recurrence, Prostate cancer, Radical prostatectomy, Salvage androgen deprivation therapy

* Correspondence: hfukuhara-jua@umin.ac.jp
Department of Urology, Graduate School of Medicine, The University of Tokyo, 7-3-1 Hongo, Bunkyo-ku, Tokyo 113-8655, Japan

Background

Approximately 25–35% of patients develop evidence of biochemical recurrence after radical prostatectomy for clinically localized prostate cancer [1,2]. Although salvage androgen deprivation therapy (ADT) is a popular option for the management of biochemical recurrence, uncertainty remains regarding which patients benefit from early salvage ADT and the ideal time at which to initiate therapy [3]. A retrospective analysis of 1,740 patients who underwent radical prostatectomy between 1990 and 1999 found no difference in systemic progression or cancer-specific survival between men who started salvage ADT at a prostate-specific antigen (PSA) level of ≥0.4 ng/ml compared with those who did not receive salvage ADT [4]. According to a similar analysis of 1,352 patients who underwent radical prostatectomy between 1988 and 2002, early salvage ADT for biochemical recurrence after radical prostatectomy was an independent predictor of delayed clinical metastases in high-risk cases, but not in the overall cohort [5].

However, these studies were mainly conducted before the era of ultrasensitive PSA assays, since when the definition of biochemical recurrence has changed. For example, Mir et al. recently advocated definitions of biochemical recurrence as any PSA ≥0.05 ng/ml in patients with nomogram-predicted 5-year progression-free probabilities of <50% [6].

We therefore compared the outcomes of early and very early administration of salvage ADT in patients treated with radical prostatectomy for localized prostate cancer.

Methods

We retrospectively reviewed 855 patients who underwent radical prostatectomy at our institution between 2000 and 2012 and identified 121 patients with adjuvant-treatment-naïve localized (pT2-4N0M0) prostate cancer who subsequently received continuous salvage ADT because of biochemical recurrence. Patients who underwent radiotherapy prior to or concomitant with hormonal therapy and patients who received any neo-adjuvant therapy were excluded from the study. The included patients were further divided into two groups: an ultra-early salvage ADT group (n = 51), in which patients started salvage ADT before meeting the standardized definition of post-prostatectomy biochemical recurrence in Japan (two consecutive PSA values ≥0.2 ng/ml [7]); and an early salvage ADT group (n = 70), in which patients started salvage ADT when they met the definition. The ultra-early salvage ADT group consisted of those who started salvage ADT with a single PSA value ≥0.2 ng/ml (n = 30) or with two consecutive PSA values >0.1 ng/ml and rising (n = 21). Patient allocation was not randomized. Doctors generally recommended early salvage ADT according to the General Rule for Clinical and Pathological Studies on Prostate Cancer of the Japanese Urological Association [8], but some patients were anxious and chose to have ultra-early salvage ADT. The clinicopathologic backgrounds of the two groups were similar, and the median durations of salvage ADT were 41 months in the ultra-early and 46 months in the early salvage ADT groups, respectively (Table 1). Patients who discontinued salvage ADT were treated as censored at the point of discontinuation. The median follow-up for all patients was 65.5 months (interquartile range [IQR]: 46–90.5 months) after radical prostatectomy, and an average of 33 PSA values were available per patient (i.e. total of 3,957 PSA values). We began using ultrasensitive PSA assays in September 2003.

The primary endpoint was biochemical recurrence after salvage ADT, defined as a confirmed single PSA value ≥0.2 ng/ml after PSA nadir following salvage ADT. Secondary endpoints were clinical metastasis and cancer-specific survival. Univariate analysis was conducted using the log-rank test and multivariate analysis was performed using the Cox proportional hazards model. All statistical analyses were carried out using JMP version 9.0.2 (SAS Institute, Cary, NC, USA). A value of $p < 0.05$ was considered significant.

This study was approved by the Ethics Committee, Graduate School of Medicine and Faculty of Medicine, The University of Tokyo. Written informed consent for participation in this study was obtained from all participants.

As of 2014, the standardized definition of biochemical recurrence after radical prostatectomy in Japan was two consecutive PSA values ≥0.2 ng/ml at intervals of 2–4 weeks, as stated above [7], which is one of six standard definitions that have been used in published studies or are in current clinical use [6].

Results

One of 51 (2.0%) patients in the ultra-early salvage ADT group developed biochemical recurrence, compared with 12 of 70 (17.1%) patients in the early salvage ADT group (Figure 1). Univariate analysis demonstrated that timing of treatment (ultra-early salvage ADT versus early salvage ADT, p = 0.0279), preoperative PSA value (<20 ng/ml versus ≥20 ng/ml, p = 0.0493), and pathologic Gleason score (≤7 versus ≥8, p = 0.0043) were associated with the risk of biochemical recurrence after salvage ADT (Table 2).

Multivariate analysis identified ultra-early salvage ADT (p = 0.0118) and preoperative Gleason score ≤7 (p = 0.0182) as independent negative predictors of biochemical recurrence after salvage ADT (Table 3).

Regarding secondary endpoints, only one patient from the early salvage ADT group developed clinical metastasis to a left supraclavicular lymph node (p = 0.4233, log-

Table 1 Clinicopathologic characteristics of patients treated with ultra-early or early salvage ADT

Variable	Ultra-early salvage ADT (n = 51)	Early salvage ADT (n = 70)	p-value
Median age at prostatectomy, yr (IQR)	65 (61 - 69)	67 (60.75 - 72.25)	0.2992
Age at prostatectomy, no. (%):			0.0804
<70 yr	39 (76.5)	43 (61.4)	
≥70 yr	12 (23.5)	27 (38.6)	
Median preoperative PSA, ng/ml (IQR)	10.65 (7.3 - 15.56)	9.55 (6.3 - 12.07)	0.1903
Preoperative PSA, no (%):			0.6041
<20 ng/ml	46 (90.2)	61 (87.1)	
≥20 ng/ml	5 (9.8)	9 (12.9)	
Pathologic Gleason score, no. (%):			0.3256
≤6	12 (23.5)	23 (32.9)	
7	28 (54.9)	38 (54.3)	
8-10	11 (21.6)	9 (12.9)	
Pathologic tumor stage, no. (%):			0.8619
T2	32 (62.7)	45 (64.3)	
T3/4	19 (37.3)	25 (35.7)	
Extraprostatic extension, no. (%)	17 (33.3)	25 (35.7)	0.7859
Lymphovascular invasion, no. (%)	13 (25.5)	16 (22.9)	0.7376
Positive resection margin, no. (%)	37 (72.5)	43 (61.4)	0.2019
Seminal vesicle invasion, no. (%)	2 (3.9)	2 (2.9)	0.7464
Perineural invasion, no. (%)	35 (68.6)	43 (61.4)	0.4139
Median duration time of salvage ADT, months (IQR)	41 (22 - 66)	46 (27 - 73.25)	0.1326

ADT, androgen deprivation therapy; PSA, prostate-specific antigen; IQR, interquartile range.

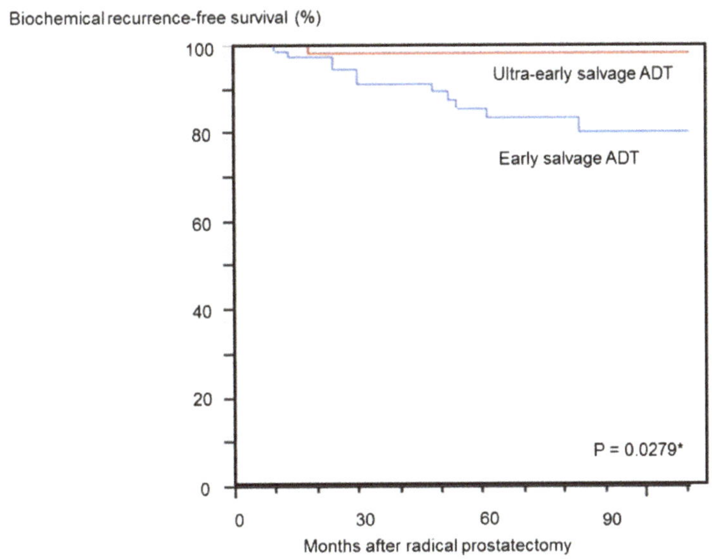

< Number at risk >

Ultra-early salvage ADT	51	41	26	7
Early salvage ADT	70	62	37	21

Figure 1 Kaplan-Meier curve depicting biochemical recurrence-free survival in patients treated with ultra-early versus early salvage ADT.

Table 2 Univariate analysis of the impact of various clinicopathologic factors on the risk of biochemical recurrence after salvage ADT

	No. of patients	p-value
Treatment group		0.0279*
Ultra-early salvage ADT	51	
Early salvage ADT	70	
Age, years		0.0798
<70	82	
≥70	39	
Preoperative PSA, ng/ml		0.0493*
<20	107	
≥20	14	
Pathologic Gleason score		0.0043*
≤7	101	
≥8	20	
Pathologic tumor stage		0.5690
≤2	77	
≥3	44	
Extraprostatic extension		0.7106
0	79	
1	42	
Lymphovascular invasion		0.4606
0	92	
1	29	
Positive resection margin		0.4467
0	41	
1	80	
Seminal vesicle invasion		0.3978
0	117	
1	4	
Perineural invasion		0.5035
0	43	
1	78	

ADT, androgen deprivation therapy; *statistically significant; PSA, prostate-specific antigen.

rank test), and no patient died from prostate cancer during the follow-up period. We were therefore unable to detect any differences in secondary endpoints between the two groups. This might be because the follow-up period was not long enough.

Discussion

ADT is a well-established treatment modality for patients with advanced prostate cancer. However, despite its proven efficacy in improving the quality of life in patients with metastatic disease, there is currently no consensus regarding the optimal timing of ADT after definitive local therapy [9]. Although a small randomized trial has supported the use of adjuvant ADT after radical prostatectomy in the setting of lymph node metastases [10,11], no randomized study has yet evaluated the utility of ADT for failure after radical prostatectomy, especially in patients without lymph node metastases [9].

Table 3 Multivariate Cox proportional hazards regression analysis evaluating the impact of various clinicopathologic factors on the risk of biochemical recurrence after salvage ADT

	HR (95% CI)	p-value
Treatment group		
Ultra-early salvage ADT	Reference	
Early salvage ADT	7.691 (1.466-141.6)	0.0118*
Preoperative PSA, ng/ml		
<20	Reference	
≥20	2.065 (0.529-6.761)	0.2744
Pathologic Gleason score		
≤7	Reference	
≥8	4.739 (1.330-15.73)	0.0182*

ADT, androgen deprivation therapy; *statistically significant; PSA, prostate-specific antigen.

Previous retrospective studies found no effect of salvage ADT on systemic progression-free survival or cancer-specific survival. Siddiqui et al. reviewed 1,740 patients who underwent radical prostatectomy between 1990 and 1999 and compared various PSA thresholds in relation to the timing of salvage ADT administration. They found no advantage in terms of systemic progression-free survival or cancer-specific survival in men who started salvage ADT at a PSA of 0.4, 1.0, or 2.0 ng/ml compared with those who did not receive salvage ADT [4]. A similar analysis by Moul et al. of 1,352 patients who underwent radical prostatectomy between 1988 and 2002 found that early salvage ADT for biochemical recurrence after radical prostatectomy was an independent predictor of delayed clinical metastases in high-risk patients (Gleason score ≥8 or PSA-doubling time ≤12 months), but had no impact on clinical metastases in the overall cohort [5].

However, these studies were mainly conducted before the era of ultrasensitive PSA assays. Ultrasensitive PSA assays allow a more precise measurement of ultrasensitive PSA values, possibly resulting in an optimal definition of biochemical recurrence after radical prostatectomy. For example, Mir et al. recently advocated the use of biochemical recurrence defined as any PSA ≥0.05 ng/ml in patients with nomogram-predicted 5-year progression-free probabilities of <50%, who might thereby benefit from early salvage radiotherapy [6]. While radiotherapy has been established as the most common salvage treatment for recurrence after radical prostatectomy in Europe and the

United States, ADT still plays an important role as salvage treatment in Asia. The Asia Consensus Statement 2013 in the NCCN Clinical Practice Guidelines in Prostate Cancer states that androgen deprivation is a candidate treatment option for post-radical prostatectomy recurrence in Asian patients negative for distant metastasis [12]. Indeed, radical prostatectomy and immediate adjuvant androgen deprivation therapy achieved excellent results, including a 10-year cancer-specific survival rate of 96.3% and 10-year estimated overall survival rate of 85.7% in Japanese patients with pT3N0 prostate cancer after a median follow-up period of 8.2 years [13]. Nevertheless, studies concerning the optimal timing of salvage ADT in the era of ultrasensitive PSA assays are lacking.

In the present study, patients who started salvage ADT before meeting a currently accepted definition of biochemical recurrence were less likely to develop subsequent biochemical recurrence after salvage ADT than those who started salvage ADT when they met the definition. By its very nature, ADT is less likely to contribute to local control than radiotherapy. However, ADT may improve local control when the residual tumor burden is very small, and adjuvant ADT after radical prostatectomy improved the clinical outcome in patients with adverse pathologic findings [10,11]. In a randomized prospective controlled trial, Messing et al. demonstrated that adjuvant ADT benefited patients with nodal metastases who had undergone prostatectomy and lymphadenectomy, compared with those who receive deferred treatment [10,11]. Referring to the results of European Organization for Research and Treatment of Cancer (EORTC) trial 30846, which found no benefit of immediate ADT compared with deferred therapy in men without definitive local treatment of the primary tumor [14], Messing et al. concluded that ADT was probably most effective against very small tumors [10,11,15]. The estimated tumor burden in EORTC 30846 was ≥12.5 cm^3 of cancer tissue, which was the mean local-tumor volume in Messing et al.'s patients [11]. Several experimental systems have provided collateral evidence to support the benefit of early ADT in inhibiting tumorigenesis [16-18].

A similar concept was recently demonstrated in the setting of salvage radiotherapy. Briganti et al. reported that timely administration of early salvage radiotherapy (given at PSA ≤0.5 ng/ml) was comparable to adjuvant radiotherapy for improving biochemical recurrence-free survival in pT3N0 prostate cancer, and suggested that initial observation followed by early salvage radiotherapy delivered at low PSA levels might be a viable option for the majority of surgically-managed patients with pT3N0 prostate cancer [19]. The present study may imply that we should consider using a PSA threshold below the currently accepted definition of biochemical recurrence in order to maximize the benefit from salvage ADT. Together with an excellent result of adjuvant ADT post-prostatectomy against pT3N0 prostate cancer [13], ADT might be more efficacious than other treatments in small tumors. However, ADT is associated with some real risks related to metabolic syndrome.

Our study had several limitations. The ultra-early salvage ADT group may have included patients without evidence of biochemical recurrence, which may have resulted in overestimation of the outcomes of ultra-early salvage ADT. Other limitations were its retrospective design, selection bias, lead-time bias, small sample size, and the inclusion of only Japanese subjects. Randomized prospective studies with longer follow-up periods are thus needed to confirm the benefits of ultra-early salvage ADT.

Conclusions

Ultra-early salvage ADT is an independent negative predictor of biochemical recurrence after salvage ADT in adjuvant-treatment-naïve pT2-4 pN0 M0 radical prostatectomy patients. The currently accepted definition of biochemical recurrence should be challenged in relation to the optimal timing of initiating salvage ADT.

Abbreviations

ADT: Androgen deprivation therapy; PSA: Prostate-specific antigen; IQR: Interquartile range; EORTC: European Organization for Research and Treatment of Cancer.

Competing interests

The authors declare that they have no competing interest.

Authors' contributions

ST made substantial contributions to study conception and design, data analysis and interpretation, and was involved in drafting the manuscript. HF made substantial contributions to study conception and design, data analysis and interpretation, and was involved in revising the manuscript critically for important intellectual content. TA, MS, TF, TN, AI, HK, and YI made substantial contributions to data acquisition. YH supervised the study, helped to draft the manuscript and was involved in revising it critically for important intellectual content. All authors read and approved the final manuscript.

Acknowledgements

We acknowledge the support and assistance provided by all the staff and residents of the Department of Urology, Graduate School of Medicine, The University of Tokyo.

References

1. Hull GW, Rabbani F, Abbas F, Wheeler TM, Kattan MW, Scardino PT: **Cancer control with radical prostatectomy alone in 1,000 consecutive patients.** *J Urol* 2002, **167**:528–534.
2. Roehl KA, Han M, Ramos CG, Antenor JA, Catalona WJ: **Cancer progression and survival rates following anatomical radical retro-pubic prostatectomy in 3,478 consecutive patients: long-term results.** *J Urol* 2004, **172**:910–914.
3. Punnen S, Cooperberg MR, D'Amico AV, Karakiewicz PI, Moul JW, Scher HI, Schlomm T, Freedland SJ: **Management of biochemical recurrence after primary treatment of prostate cancer: a systematic review of the literature.** *Eur Urol* 2013, **64**:905–915.
4. Siddiqui SA, Boorjian SA, Inman B, Bagniewski S, Bergstralh EJ, Blute ML: **Timing of androgen deprivation therapy and its impact on survival after**

radical prostatectomy: a matched cohort study. *J Urol* 2008, **179:**1830–1837.

5. Moul JW, Wu H, Sun L, McLeod DG, Amling C, Donahue T, Kusuda L, Sexton W, O'Reilly K, Hernandez J, Chung A, Soderdahl D: **Early versus delayed hormonal therapy for prostate specific antigen only recurrence of prostate cancer after radical prostatectomy.** *J Urol* 2004, **171:**1141–1147.
6. Mir MC, Li J, Klink JC, Kattan MW, Klein EA, Stephenson AJ: **Optimal definition of biochemical recurrence after radical prostatectomy depends on pathologic risk factors: identifying candidates for early salvage therapy.** *Eur Urol.* In press. http://dx.doi.org/10.1016/j.eururo.2013.08.022 DOI:10.1016/j.eururo.%202013.08.022.
7. Hirao Y: *Clinical Practice Guidelines for Prostate Cancer: The Japanese Urological Association 2012 update.* Tokyo: Kanehara-shuppan Press; 2012 (in Japanese).
8. The Japanese Urological Association, the Japanese Society of Pathology and Japan Radiological Society: *General Rule for Clinical and Pathological Studies on Prostate Cancer, the fourth edition.* Tokyo: Kanehara and Co., Ltd; 2010 (in Japanese).
9. Ryan CJ, Small EJ: **Early versus delayed androgen deprivation for prostate cancer: new fuel for an old debate.** *J Clin Oncol* 2005, **23:**8225–8231.
10. Messing EM, Manola J, Yao J, Kiernan M, Crawford D, Wilding G, Di'SantAgnese PA, Trump D, Eastern Cooperative Oncology Group study EST 3886: **Immediate versus deferred androgen deprivation treatment in patients with node-positive prostate cancer after radical prostatectomy and pelvic lymphadenectomy.** *Lancet Oncol* 2006, **7:**472–479.
11. Messing EM, Manola J, Sarosdy M, Wilding G, Crawford ED, Trump D: **Immediate hormonal therapy compared with observation after radical prostatectomy and pelvic lymphadenectomy in men with node-positive prostate cancer.** *N Engl J Med* 1999, **341:**1781–88.
12. Akaza H, Umbas R: *NCCN Clinical Practice Guidelines in Oncology (NCCN Guidelines®) - Asia Consensus Statement: Prostate Cancer Version 2.2013.* Tokyo: Reno Medical K.K; 2013. http://www.nccn.org/international/PDF/prostate-asia.pdf.
13. Sato YT, Fukuhara H, Suzuki M, Fujimura T, Nakagawa T, Nishimatsu H, Kume H, Morikawa T, Fukayama M, Homma Y: **Long-term results of radical prostatectomy with immediate adjuvant androgen deprivation therapy for pT3N0 prostate cancer.** *BMC Urol* 2014, **14:**13.
14. Schröder FH, Kurth KH, Fossa SD, Hoekstra W, Karthaus PP, De Prijck L, Collette L: **Early versus delayed endocrine treatment of pN1-3 M0 prostate cancer without local treatment of the primary tumor: results of the EORTC 30846—a phase III study.** *J Urol* 2004, **272:**923–927.
15. Messing EM: **A structured debate: immediate vs deferred androgen suppression in prostate cancer—evidence for deferred treatment (editorial).** *J Urol* 2001, **166:**515–16.
16. Isaacs JT: **Relationship between tumor size and curability of prostatic cancer by combined chemo-hormonal therapy in rats.** *Cancer Res* 1989, **49:**6290–6294.
17. Eng MH, Charles LG, Ross BD, Chrisp CE, Pienta KJ, Greenberg NM, Hsu CX, Sanda MG: **Early castration reduces prostatic carcinogenesis in transgenic mice.** *Urology* 1999, **54:**1112–1119.
18. Craft N, Chhor C, Tran C, Belldegrun A, DeKernion J, Witte ON, Said J, Reiter RE, Sawyers CL: **Evidence for clonal outgrowth of androgen-independent prostate cancer cells from androgen-dependent tumors through a two-step process.** *Cancer Res* 1999, **59:**5030–5036.
19. Briganti A, Wiegel T, Joniau S, Cozzarini C, Bianchi M, Sun M, Tombal B, Haustermans K, Budiharto T, Hinkelbein W, Di Muzio N, Karakiewicz PI, Montorsi F, Van Poppel H: **Early salvage radiation therapy does not compromise cancer control in patients with pT3N0 prostate cancer after radical prostatectomy: results of a match-controlled multi-institutional analysis.** *Eur Urol* 2012, **62:**472–487.

4

Reimbursement cuts and changes in urologist use of androgen deprivation therapy for prostate cancer

Vahakn B Shahinian[1*] and Yong-Fang Kuo[2,3,4]

Abstract

Background: We examined the impact of urologist academic affiliation on use of androgen deprivation therapy (ADT) for prostate cancer before and after major reimbursement cuts for ADT in hopes of better understanding the influence of financial incentives on its use. In particular, we hypothesized that if financial incentive was the predominant factor driving use, we should see a narrowing in the previously documented gap of ADT use between non-academic and academic urologists following the reimbursement cuts.

Methods: With the Surveillance, Epidemiology and End-Results (SEER)-Medicare linked database we examined use of ADT for potentially inappropriate indications (primary therapy of localized, lower risk tumors) among patients of 2214 urologists over the period 2000–2002 and 2004–2007, representing eras before and after reimbursement cuts. Multi-level logistic regression models were used to estimate the likelihood of ADT use adjusted for patient, tumor and urologist characteristics (academic affiliation, board certification, years in practice and patient panel size).

Results: Overall, ADT use peaked in 2002 at 46.6% of patients, but dropped dramatically in 2005, with a slow continued decrease through 2007 to 31.1%. A similar pattern was evident within most strata of urologist characteristics, including academic affiliation. In the multilevel model, patients of non-academic urologists had a 30% higher odds of receiving ADT than those of academic urologists in both the eras before and after the reimbursement cuts.

Conclusion: A similar proportionate drop in use of ADT among both academic and non-academic urologists following reimbursement cuts suggests that factors other than financial incentives may have played a role.

Keywords: Androgen deprivation, Prostate cancer, Reimbursement

Background

Androgen deprivation therapy (ADT), either in the form of gonadotropin-releasing hormone (GnRH) agonists or orchiectomy, has long been used for palliation of metastatic prostate cancer [1,2]. Starting in the 1990s, there was an explosive growth in use of ADT with a broadening of its application to earlier stages of disease [3]. Although this was driven in part by clinical trial evidence of benefit in some settings, such as adjuvant ADT together with radiation therapy for high-risk prostate cancer [4], there have been concerns about possible financial motivations for its use. Medicare reimbursement policies made administration of GnRH agonists very profitable (due to large discounts in the acquisition price of the drugs by physicians as compared to reimbursement) [5], and we have previously shown that patients of non-academic urologists (who are more usually paid fee-for-service) were 60% more likely to receive ADT in settings of uncertain benefit than patients of academic urologists (who are more likely salaried) [6]. More recently in 2005, Medicare reimbursement policy changes related to the Medicare Modernization Act in 2003 cut payment for GnRH agonists by over 50%, which was followed by substantial reductions in use of ADT [7]. Although these findings suggested that financial incentives played an important role, other

* Correspondence: vahakn@umich.edu
[1]Department of Internal Medicine, University of Michigan, 1415 Washington Heights, Room 3627, SPH I, Ann Arbor, MI 48109-2029, USA
Full list of author information is available at the end of the article

explanations were also possible. For example, over the same period, there was growing recognition of potentially serious adverse effects related to ADT [8-10]. We therefore examined the impact of urologist characteristics on use of ADT over the period of the reimbursement cuts, with the objective of further clarifying the factors driving the reductions in its use. In particular, we hypothesized that if financial incentive was the sole, or predominant, factor, we should see a narrowing in the gap of ADT use between academic and non-academic urologists following the reimbursement cuts.

Methods

The study protocol was approved by the local institutional review board at the University of Michigan.

Data sources

Surveillance, Epidemiology, and End Results (SEER)-Medicare

The SEER program consists of a group of population-based tumor registries in selected geographic areas of the US [11]. It covered 14% of the US population until 2001, and 26% thereafter. Medicare is a federal program that covers health services for 97% of persons aged 65 years and older. The information in the two programs has been linked. The SEER-Medicare database also contains the Hospital file, which includes information on hospital characteristics such as academic affiliation and is derived from the Provider of Service survey submitted by hospitals to Medicare. The SEER-Medicare database version used for this study contains Medicare claims through 2008 and cancer cases from SEER through 2007.

American Medical Association (AMA) Physician Masterfile

The AMA Physician Masterfile collects information on all physicians in the US, regardless of membership in the AMA [12]. The information is collected from primary sources, such as medical schools, residency training programs, state licensing agencies, and the American Board of Medical Specialties. Physicians are also surveyed every 3 years regarding their current practice.

Study subjects

Men with incident prostate cancer from 2000 through 2002, and from 2004 through 2007, (men diagnosed in the year 2003 were excluded for reasons described below in the Study Variables section) who were at least 66 years old at diagnosis (n = 191,990) were initially selected. To ensure complete information, patients not enrolled in both Medicare Part A and Part B for 12 months before and 6 months following their cancer diagnosis (n = 19160), who died within 6 months of diagnosis (n = 3527), were members of an Health Maintenance Organization (n = 47833), or diagnosed by autopsy or on a death certificate (n = 2388) were excluded. The main interest for this study was the examination of ADT use for potentially inappropriate indications given the large changes in such use noted after the reimbursement cuts [7] and known variations in rates of such use as a function of urologist characteristics [6]. We previously defined this group as men diagnosed with clinically localized (T1 or T2), low to moderate grade (Gleason 2 to 7) tumors, who did not receive treatment with radiation or radical prostatectomy. Use of ADT in that context would be potentially inappropriate given there is no clinical trial evidence supporting its efficacy as primary therapy [13], and even under theoretical considerations, it is difficult to show survival benefit from any intervention in such patients, due to the slow natural progression and competing risk of death from causes other than prostate cancer [14]. This led to the exclusion of an additional n = 91913 patients (in whom ADT use would have been categorized as either discretionary or appropriate), leaving n = 27169 eligible patients for the main analysis.

Physicians providing care to patients within a year of diagnosis were initially identified through encrypted Unique Physician Identifier Numbers (UPINs) on Medicare physician claims, as previously published [15]. Briefly, UPINs were linked to the AMA Physician Masterfile and only physicians with urology as their primary specialty code were selected. Patients who did not see at least one urologist in the year after diagnosis on at least two different days were excluded. If a patient saw 2 or more urologists, they were assigned to the urologist with ≥75% of urologist visits in the year after diagnosis. If no single urologist accounted for ≥75% of the visits, the patient was excluded.

Study variables

Patient demographic and tumor characteristics were derived from the SEER records in the linked database and used to categorize patients by age, ethnicity, SEER region of residence at the time of diagnosis, year of diagnosis, clinical stage (T1 through T4), and grade (low - Gleason 2–4; moderate - Gleason 5–7; poor - Gleason 8–10). Stage was assigned using the SEER Extent of Disease-Clinical Extension classification system prior to 2004 and using the Collaborative Stage Clinical Extension system from 2004 onwards [7]. Cancer grade was categorized only as a range as low (Gleason 2–4), moderate (Gleason 5–7) or high (Gleason 8–10) prior to 2003, but in 2003 only Gleason 7 was switched to the high grade category. From 2004 onwards, individual Gleason scoring has been available, allowing classification into similar groupings as for the data prior to 2003. To ensure comparability across the study period men with incident prostate cancer in 2003 were therefore excluded. The socio-economic characteristics of each patient were based on the percent of adults with less than 12 years of education and median income of the zip code of residence from the 2000 United States Census data. Comorbidity was measured using an adaptation of the Charlson Comorbidity Index for use with Medicare physician claims data, based on the period one year prior to diagnosis of prostate cancer [16,17].

Urologist board certification was available from the AMA based on information from the American Board of Medical Specialties [12]. Patient panel size was defined as the number of patients with incident prostate cancer (regardless of ADT use) assigned to each urologist over the entire study period, and categorized as <14, 14–44, 45–74, and ≥75 patients. The categorization used was similar to an approach we utilized in a previous publication, chosen to ensure a reasonable distribution for the number of patients, with cut-offs roughly corresponding to the 2nd quartile, 3rd quartile and 90th percentile [6]. Hospital academic affiliation was available from the SEER-Medicare Hospital file. Hospitals with a major academic affiliation were those that played an important role in the teaching program of a medical school. Hospitals with a minor academic affiliation had academic involvement limited to hosting of a residency program or occasional medical student rotations [6]. Urologists were categorized as having an academic affiliation if all their inpatient Medicare claims submitted were from a hospital with major or minor academic affiliation. These urologists would be more likely to be salaried, through employment with a medical school, or hospital. All other urologists were categorized as having no academic affiliation. These urologists would be more likely to be in private practice or part of single specialty groups, and therefore derive most of their income from fee-for-service activities. In initial analyses of academic affiliation using three categories (major, minor or none) patterns of ADT use were essentially identical between urologists with major and minor academic affiliation. Therefore, to optimize statistical power the main analyses were presented using a binary classification: major or minor academic affiliation vs. none.

The outcome was receipt of androgen deprivation. Androgen deprivation was defined as the receipt of at least one dose of a GnRH agonist (identified through Medicare claims codes used to designate each dose given of injectable medications [8]) or orchiectomy (defined by the presence of the Current Procedural Terminology codes or International Classification of Diseases, 9th revision [ICD-9] procedure codes in the Medicare claims) in the first six months following diagnosis of cancer.

Statistical analyses

Differences across strata of urologist characteristics in the proportion of patients receiving ADT were tabulated. The effect of urologist characteristics on the outcome of use of androgen deprivation was evaluated using multilevel logistic regression models to account for clustering of patients within urologists. Models entering the urologist, patient and tumor characteristics listed above as independent variables were estimated. Odds ratios (OR) for the use of androgen deprivation for each urologist characteristic were calculated along with 95% confidence intervals (CI). As the main interest was to examine how the effect of urologist characteristics changed related to reimbursement cuts, the model results were stratified into two eras, 2000–2002 (prior to the reimbursement cut) and 2004–2007 (following the reimbursement cut). To specifically assess whether there were significant changes in the effect of urologist characteristics on use of ADT over the course of the two eras, tests of interaction were performed between each urologist characteristic and era, on the outcome of ADT use. In addition, the median urologist rates of androgen deprivation use as a function of academic affiliation were estimated from the models, and plotted by calendar year of diagnosis to show change in use over time. Analyses were performed with SAS version 9.3 (Cary, NC). All tests of statistical significance were two sided, with P values of less than .05 being considered significant.

Results

A total of 2,214 urologists were identified as providing care to patients with incident prostate cancer over the study period. A majority of urologists were board certified (77.9%), had either a major or minor academic affiliation (66.2%), and were male (97.5%). Trends over time in the proportion of patients receiving ADT for inappropriate indications are presented in Table 1, stratified by urologist characteristics. In the overall cohort, such use peaked in 2002 at 46.6% of patients, but dropped dramatically in 2005, with a slow continued decrease through 2007 to 31.1%. A similar pattern was evident within most strata of urologist characteristics. Patients of older urologists, those practicing longer, and those without an academic affiliation tended to have higher rates of ADT use.

Table 2 presents multilevel models showing the odds of ADT use for inappropriate indications as a function of urologist characteristics, stratified by era of use (2000–2002 vs. 2004–2007). The only significant finding was an increase in the odds of ADT use for patients of non-academically affiliated urologists (vs. urologists with either a major or minor academic affiliation), which was similar in both eras. None of the tests for interaction between era and urologist characteristics on the outcome of ADT use were significant.

The Figure 1 shows a plot of median urologist rates of ADT use for inappropriate indications over time for

Table 1 Proportion of patients receiving androgen deprivation therapy for inappropriate indications by year, stratified by urologist characteristics

Urologist characteristics	Categories	Urologist sample		ADT use for inappropriate indications by year						
		N	%	2000	2001	2002	2004	2005	2006	2007
Total		2214	100	44.2	44.3	46.6	44.7	36.2	33.4	31.1
Age (years):	<45	694	31.3	40.9	45.4	48.2	40.4	33.5	30.2	29.6
	45 - 54	630	28.5	44.2	44.1	44.4	46.0	37.8	32.4	30.2
	55 - 64	672	30.4	45.2	42.4	46.1	45.7	35.4	35.0	32.5
	≥65	218	9.8	48.7	49.2	55.1	45.6	38.9	41.7	35.5
Sex:	Female	55	2.5	38.5	44.4	26.9	31.8	33.3	34.4	34.5
	Male	2159	97.5	44.3	44.3	46.7	44.8	36.2	33.4	31.1
Years in practice:	<15	864	40.1	39.7	43.2	46.1	41.7	33.5	30.8	28.4
	15 - 24	548	25.4	43.5	42.6	44.0	46.3	39.9	32.9	33.2
	25 - 34	488	22.6	47.6	44.5	47.9	44.4	33.5	35.4	31.3
	≥35	255	11.8	48.1	47.1	53.0	46.4	40.7	40.7	34.0
Board certification:	Yes	1725	77.9	44.6	44.1	46.0	44.2	36.1	33.5	30.9
	No	489	22.1	42.7	44.9	48.8	46.4	36.8	33.0	31.9
Academic affiliation:	Major or Minor	1338	66.2	41.5	43.2	44.7	41.9	33.3	31.9	28.9
	None	684	33.8	47.6	46.0	49.0	48.2	40.1	35.5	33.6
Patient panel size (no. of patients):	<14	685	30.9	37.7	44.7	42.1	46.1	34.7	35.6	29.2
	14 - 44	603	27.2	39.8	40.6	47.3	43.1	36.7	32.0	30.1
	45 - 74	452	20.4	47.2	48.2	47.2	44.9	37.8	33.4	36.0
	≥75	474	21.4	47.6	43.7	49.3	44.6	35.6	32.9	29.0

patients of urologists with either a major or minor academic affiliation versus urologists without an academic affiliation. Among both groups, there was a drop in use starting in 2004, but the gap between them remained relatively constant throughout the study period.

Discussion

This study shows a drop in use of ADT for inappropriate indications following reimbursement cuts for GnRH agonists in 2004 and 2005, which occurred among patients of both academic and non-academic urologists.

Table 2 Odds of ADT use in multilevel models as a function of urologist characteristics, stratified by era

Urologist characteristics	ADT use by era				
	[a]2000-2002		[a]2004-2007		
	Odds ratio	95% CI	Odds ratio	95% CI	p-value interaction with era
Years in practice (per 5 years)	1.01	(0.97, 1.05)	1.03	(1.00 ,1.07)	0.47
Board certification					
Yes	ref		ref		
No	1.01	(0.82, 1.24)	1.06	(0.89, 1.28)	0.94
Academic affiliation					
Major or minor	ref		ref		
None	1.32	(1.17, 1.56)	1.34	(1.15, 1.56)	0.68
Patient panel size					
<14	ref		ref		0.13
14 - 44	1.02	(0.84, 1.25)	0.93	(0.77, 1.12)	
45 - 74	1.23	(0.99, 1.54)	1.03	(0.84, 1.26)	
≥75	1.10	(0.86, 1.10)	0.89	(0.71, 1.11)	

[a]Based on multilevel model with patient age, comorbidity, ethnicity, SEER region, tumor stage, grade, year of diagnosis, census tract education, and census tract poverty entered as "level 1" variables and urologist characteristics entered as "level 2" variables. Urologist sex was not entered into the models due to low female sample size. Urologist age was not entered into the models due to collinearity with the years in practice variable.

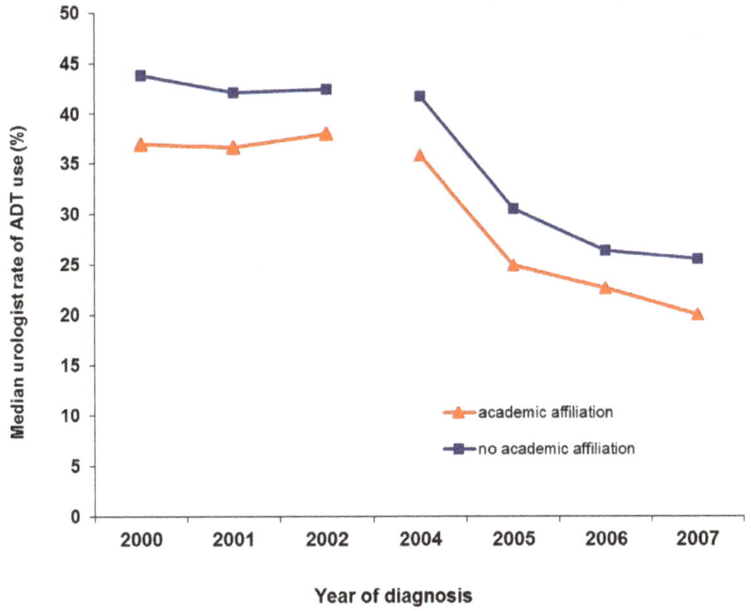

Figure 1 Median urologist rate of androgen deprivation (ADT) for inappropriate indications, based on the multilevel model from Table 2, by calendar year of diagnosis and stratified by urologists with academic (major or minor) versus no academic affiliation.

Notably, although overall rates of use were higher among non-academic urologists, the gap between them and academic urologists remained constant from the period before through the period after the reimbursement cuts.

We initially argued that if the reductions in use of ADT were purely financially motivated, we would expect to see a narrowing in the gap between academic and non-academic urologists as the latter would be most affected in a direct manner by cuts in reimbursement for GnRH agonists. Our findings were not consistent with such a pattern, suggesting that factors other than financial incentives may have also played a role. In support of this, previous work done in other health care contexts in which financial incentives were absent has also demonstrated a decrease in use of ADT over a similar period [18,19]. A Canadian study examining the Ontario province-wide database showed a slow but steady decline in the rate of new ADT initiation starting in the late 1990s and continuing through 2005 [19]. Most of that reduction was for use of ADT as a primary therapy. In a US study utilizing data from the Veterans Health Administration, pharmacy claims for use of GnRH agonists declined 16.8% from 2004 to 2007 [18]. However, the data presented was limited to counts, without examination of rates, or indications for use. The main competing explanation for the recent reductions in use of ADT is the concern for adverse effects. Recognition of the impact of ADT on quality of life, anemia and osteoporosis was evident as early as the 1990s [20-23]. However, it was not until 2005 and later that a series of high impact publications demonstrated potentially life threatening consequences such as fractures, cardiovascular disease and diabetes mellitus, which may have strongly discouraged use of ADT in settings without clear evidence of benefit [8-10]. Ultimately it is likely that a number of factors in combination led to the observed findings in our study, with contributions from both concerns over adverse effects as well as reduced financial incentives.

The persistent gap in use as a function of academic affiliation even after much of the financial incentive was removed may relate to differences in the interactions between urologists and patients. The pressure to provide some sort of treatment in the face of a cancer diagnosis may be a strong factor in the decision to use ADT in place of watchful waiting for patients with localized prostate cancer who are otherwise not good candidates for radiation treatment or radical prostatectomy. Physicians in academic settings may have more time for discussion of risks and benefits, leading patients to choose more conservative courses of action [24]. However, no studies have directly examined whether discussion between patients and urologists about ADT differ between academic versus non-academic urologists.

There are limitations to this study. Only men 66 years and older were included, and use of androgen deprivation in health maintenance organizations could not be examined. Assignment of urologist academic affiliation, based on Medicare claims, may have been imperfect. However, misclassification would tend to bias the results to the null, so that significant associations should still be valid. The statistical power to detect interactions between era and the effect of urologist characteristics on ADT use may have been limited. Nevertheless, inspection of the point estimates reveals no obvious differences in effect between the two eras, making it less likely that an interaction was missed due to insufficient sample size. Finally, due to limitations in the granularity of clinical detail available in a claims-based analysis, not all ADT use deemed inappropriate by our study definition is necessarily unreasonable. However, our main intention was to examine differences in ADT use between academic and non-academic urologists, which we felt (and had previously demonstrated) would be most prominent in settings where evidence of efficacy was most lacking.

Conclusion

In conclusion, although the study findings do not rule out a role of financial incentive in the observed patterns of ADT use, they suggest that the explanation is likely to be more complex.

Abbreviations

ADT: Androgen Deprivation Therapy; AMA: American Medical Association; GnRH: Gonadotropin-releasing hormone; SEER: Surveillance Epidemiology and End Results; UPIN: Unique Physician Identifier Number.

Competing interests

VBS is a paid consultant to Amgen, Inc.

Authors' contributions

Both authors (VBS and YK) made substantial contributions to the conception, design, analysis and interpretation of the data; VBS drafted the first draft of the manuscript and YK provided critical revision; both authors give final approval for the manuscript and agree to be accountable for all aspects of the work herein.

Acknowledgments

Funding: This work was supported by an American Cancer Society Research Scholar Grant (118244-RSGI-10-076-01-CPHPS to VBS). The sponsor had no role in the design or conduct of the study, nor in the interpretation of data, or in the preparation of the manuscript.
This study used the linked SEER-Medicare database. The interpretation and reporting of these data are the sole responsibility of the authors. The authors acknowledge the efforts of the Applied Research Program, NCI; the Office of Research, Development and Information, CMS; Information Management Services (IMS), Inc.; and the Surveillance, Epidemiology, and End Results (SEER) Program tumor registries in the creation of the SEER-Medicare database.

Author details

[1]Department of Internal Medicine, University of Michigan, 1415 Washington Heights, Room 3627, SPH I, Ann Arbor, MI 48109-2029, USA. [2]Department of Internal Medicine, University of Texas Medical Branch, Galveston, TX, USA. [3]Sealy Center on Aging, University of Texas Medical Branch, Galveston, TX, USA. [4]Department of Preventive Medicine and Community Health, University of Texas Medical Branch, Galveston, TX, USA.

References

1. Crawford ED, Eisenberger MA, McLeod DG, Spaulding JT, Benson R, Dorr FA, et al. A controlled trial of leuprolide with and without flutamide in prostatic carcinoma. N Engl J Med. 1989;321(7):419–24.
2. Huggins C, Hodges CV. Studies on prostatic cancer: I. The effect of castration, of estrogen and of androgen injection on serum phosphatases in metastatic carcinoma of the prostate. 1941. J Urol. 2002;168(1):9–12.
3. Shahinian VB, Kuo YF, Freeman JL, Orihuela E, Goodwin JS. Increasing use of gonadotropin-releasing hormone agonists for the treatment of localized prostate carcinoma. Cancer. 2005;103(8):1615–24.
4. Bolla M, Collette L, Blank L, Warde P, Dubois JB, Mirimanoff RO, et al. Long-term results with immediate androgen suppression and external irradiation in patients with locally advanced prostate cancer (an EORTC study): a phase III randomised trial. Lancet. 2002;360(9327):103–6.
5. Painter MR. Reimbursement issues with hormonal therapies for prostate cancer. Rev Urol. 2005;7 Suppl 5:S44–7.
6. Shahinian VB, Kuo YF, Freeman JL, Orihuela E, Goodwin JS. Characteristics of urologists predict the use of androgen deprivation therapy for prostate cancer. J Clin Oncol. 2007;25(34):5359–65.
7. Shahinian VB, Kuo YF, Gilbert SM. Reimbursement policy and androgen-deprivation therapy for prostate cancer. N Engl J Med. 2010;363(19):1822–32.
8. Shahinian VB, Kuo YF, Freeman JL, Goodwin JS. Risk of fracture after androgen deprivation for prostate cancer. N Engl J Med. 2005;352(2):154–64.
9. Smith MR, Lee WC, Brandman J, Wang Q, Botteman M, Pashos CL. Gonadotropin-releasing hormone agonists and fracture risk: a claims-based cohort study of men with nonmetastatic prostate cancer. J Clin Oncol. 2005;23(31):7897–903.
10. Keating NL, O'Malley AJ, Smith MR. Diabetes and cardiovascular disease during androgen deprivation therapy for prostate cancer. J Clin Oncol. 2006;24(27):4448–56.
11. Warren J, Klabunde C, Schrag D, Bach PB, Riley GF. Overview of the SEER-medicare data: content, research applications, and generalizability to the United States elderly population. Med Care. 2002;40(suppl IV):3–18.
12. Baldwin L-M, Adamache E, Klabunde CN, Kenward K, Dahlman C, Warren J, et al. Linking physician characteristics and medicare claims data: issues in data availability, quality and measurement. Med Care. 2002;40(suppl IV):82–95.
13. Chodak GW, Keane T, Klotz L. Critical evaluation of hormonal therapy for carcinoma of the prostate. Urology. 2002;60(2):201–8.
14. Welch HG, Albertsen PC, Nease RF, Bubolz TA, Wasson JH. Estimating treatment benefits for the elderly: the effect of competing risks. Ann Intern Med. 1996;124(6):577–84.
15. Shahinian VB, Kuo YF, Freeman JL, Goodwin JS. Determinants of androgen deprivation therapy use for prostate cancer: role of the urologist. J Natl Cancer Inst. 2006;98(12):839–45.
16. Charlson ME, Pompei P, Ales KL, MacKenzie CR. A new method of classifying prognostic comorbidity in longitudinal studies: development and validation. J Chronic Dis. 1987;40(5):373–83.
17. Klabunde CN, Potosky AL, Legler JM, Warren JL. Development of a comorbidity index using physician claims data. J Clin Epidemiol. 2000;53:1258–67.
18. Chang SL, Liao JC, Shinghal R. Decreasing use of luteinizing hormone-releasing hormone agonists in the United States is independent of reimbursement changes: a medicare and veterans health administration claims analysis. J Urol. 2009;182(1):255–60. discussion 261.
19. Krahn M, Bremner KE, Tomlinson G, Luo J, Ritvo P, Naglie G, et al. Androgen deprivation therapy in prostate cancer: are rising concerns leading to falling use? BJU Int. 2011;108(10):1588–96.
20. Strum SB, McDermed JE, Scholz MC, Johnson H, Tisman G. Anaemia associated with androgen deprivation in patients with prostate cancer receiving combined hormone blockade. Br J Urol. 1997;79(6):933–41.
21. McDermed J, Strum S, Scholz M. The androgen deprivation syndrome (ADS): the incidence and severity in prostate cancer (PC) patients (PTS) receiving hormone blockade (HB). Proc Am Soc Clin Oncol. 1998;17:315a.
22. Maillefert JF, Sibilia J, Michel F, Saussine C, Javier RM, Tavernier C. Bone mineral density in men treated with synthetic gonadotropin-releasing hormone agonists for prostatic carcinoma. J Urol. 1999;161(4):1219–22.
23. Herr HW, O'Sullivan M. Quality of life of asymptomatic men with nonmetastatic prostate cancer on androgen deprivation therapy. J Urol. 2000;163(6):1743–6.
24. Voss JD, Schectman JM. Prostate cancer screening practices and beliefs. J Gen Intern Med. 2001;16(12):831–7.

5

Terminal dribbling in male patients with lower urinary tract symptoms: relationship with International Prostate Symptom Score and with intravesical prostatic protrusion

Jae Heon Kim[1], Ji Sung Shim[2,3], Hoon Choi[2,3], Du Geon Moon[3], Jeong Gu Lee[3], Je Jong Kim[3], Jae Hyun Bae[2,3] and Jae Young Park[2,3*]

Abstract

Background: Terminal dribbling is one of the lower urinary tract symptoms (LUTS) that has not been widely studied. The aim of this study was to investigate the associations between terminal dribbling (TD) and other parameters such as International Prostate Symptom Score (IPSS) and intravesical prostatic protrusion (IPP).

Methods: Medical records of male patients with LUTS aged 40 years and older were prospectively collected. Data regarding TD defined by the International Continence Society standardization subcommittee, IPSS, prostate-specific antigen, total prostate volume, and IPP on transrectal ultrasonography were obtained. TD was confirmed by the subsequent uroflowmetry (uroflowmetry-confirmed TD). Logistic regression analysis was performed to identify the parameters affecting TD and uroflowmetry-confirmed TD.

Results: Among the 578 men, 226 patients (39.1 %) complained of TD and 157 patients (27.2 %) had objective findings of TD on uroflowmetry. In the logistic regression analysis, IPSS voiding subscore were correlated with TD (Odds ratio 1.06). In addition, IPP was the only significant risk factor for uroflowmetry-confirmed TD (Odds ratio 2.83). Each question of IPSS is not correlated with TD or uroflowmetry-confirmed TD.

Conclusions: While the symptom of TD is well correlated with IPSS voiding subscore, objective evidence of TD on uroflowmetry had strong correlation with IPP. TD should be investigated further to reveal its clinical impact and guide a proper management.

Background

Terminal dribbling (TD) is known to be common in men with or without benign prostate hyperplasia (BPH), and has been shown to have a negative impact on quality of life [1–3]. TD has been included in the symptom score suggested by Boyarsky et al. and the International Continence Society (ICS) male questionnaire [4, 5]. In 1996, the study done by Abrams et al. pointed out that objective evidence of TD is significantly related with bladder outlet obstruction [6].

* Correspondence: jaeyoungpark@korea.ac.kr
[2]Department of Urology, Korea University Ansan Hospital, Ansan, Republic of Korea
[3]Department of Urology, Korea University College of Medicine, Seoul, Republic of Korea
Full list of author information is available at the end of the article

TD is newly defined by the ICS standardization subcommittee in 2002 [7]. However, no study has been carried out according to this definition up to now even though it is the most common symptom among lower urinary tract symptom (LUTS) in BPH patients or community people [4]. In the present study, we sought to investigate the prevalence of TD among LUTS patients and its relationship with intravesical prostatic protrusion (IPP) and with International Prostate Symptom Score (IPSS).

Methods

Study population

The study comprised 635 consecutive male LUTS patients aged 40 years and older attending as new patients at the outpatient clinic between January 2008 and July 2013. This study was conducted in accordance with the ethical standards laid down in the 1964 Declaration of Helsinki and its later amendments; appropriate ethical review boards (Korea University Medical Center Ansan Hospital IRB No. AS 14156) approved this retrospective study. The patients with LUTS mean that the patients who have storage symptoms, voiding symptoms or post micturition symptoms as described in the previous study [7]. Fifty seven of these men were excluded from our study due to biopsy proven prostate cancer, other malignancies, previous medication for LUTS, past history of surgery for BPH or other pelvic diseases, neurologic abnormalities, or missing data. IPSS, prostate-specific antigen (PSA), prostate volume, prostate transitional zone volume and IPP on transrectal ultrasonography (TRUS), and the answer to the TD item on the ICS male questionnaire were recorded for each subject.

Terminal dribbling definition and confirmation

TD was defined in the ICS guidelines as "when an individual describes a prolonged final part of micturition when the flow has slowed to a trickle/dribble" [7]. The questionnaire item regarding TD was stated as follows: "Do you have a prolonged final part of micturition when the flow has slowed to a trickle/dribble?" Answer choices for this question included yes and no. Uroflowmetry-confirmed TD means that TD confirmed by the uroflowmetry when the typical finding of slowly decreasing flow with trickling/dribbling at the end of the void was observed.

Features measured using transrectal ultrasonography

The prostate was measured in three dimensions on TRUS, and its volume and transitional volume were estimated using a modification of the prolate ellipsoid formula and expressed in cm3 (0.523 [length (cm) × width (cm) × height (cm)]) [8]. IPP was measured as the vertical distance from the tip of the protruding prostate to the base of the urinary bladder in the sagittal plane, and it was graded as mild (less than 5 mm), moderate (from 5 to less than 10 mm), severe (10 mm or more) [9, 21]. Urology residents performed this procedure under the supervision of attendings. We divided patients into two groups based on the presence of IPP when performing logistic regression analysis.

Acquisition of IPSS questionnaires

The severity of LUTS was measured using the IPSS, which is based on the American Urological Association symptom index with one additional question on quality of life (QoL). After the patients were asked to complete the IPSS questionnaire, voiding subscore (sum of scores in 1st, 3rd, 5th, and 6th question of IPSS) and storage subscore (sum of scores in 2nd, 4th, and 7th question of IPSS) were calculated [10]. The Korean version of the IPSS was also validated in terms of relevance and reliability, and is now used as a diagnostic tool for LUTS [11].

Statistical analysis

Continuous variables were expressed as either the mean ± standard deviation, or median [inter-quartile range]. Categorical variables were reported as the number of occurrences and frequency. Student t-test and the Pearson $\chi 2$ test were used for statistical comparisons of continuous and categorical variables, respectively. Simple and multiple logistic regressions with a backward variable selection procedure were performed to identify the parameters affecting TD. Simple logistic regressions were performed to reveal the association between TD and IPSS. Data were analyzed using PASW Statistics version 18.0 (SPSS, Inc. Chicago, IL, USA). We regarded a p value <0.05 as statistically significant.

Results

Characteristics of enrolled patents

The mean age of subjects was 62.4 years, the median prostate volume was 31.0 cm^3, and the median transitional volume was 12.0 cm^3 (Table 1). Among 578 men with LUTS, 226 men (39.1 %) complained of TD. Among these 226 men who complained of TD, TD was confirmed in 157 men (uroflowmetry-confirmed TD group) by subsequent uroflowmetry. Typical findings such as slowly decreasing flow with trickling/dribbling at the end of the void were observed in these patients (Fig. 1). When the patients were classified with age, 23 men (10.1 %) in their 40's complained of TD, 65 men (28.6 %) in their 50's complained of TD, 81 men (35.7 %) in their 60's, and 58 men (25.6 %) in their 70's, respectively. There were no significant differences between TD and non-TD groups with respect to age, PSA, prostate volume or prostate transitional zone volume. However, IPSS total score, IPSS voiding subscale score, IPSS storge subscale score, and IPSS QoL score in TD group were significantly higher than those in non-TD group. Among 578 men with LUTS, IPP was observed in 248 patients (42.9 %). The number of patients with IPP was not significantly different in TD group than that in non-TD group (p value 0.402). When classified by uroflowmetry-confirmed TD, the number of patients with IPP was significantly higher in uroflowmetry-confirmed TD group (95 out of 157) than that in patients who did not show the typical finding of TD in uroflowmetry test (153 out of 421) (Odds ratio 2.67).

The risk factors for terminal dribbling in the logistic regression analysis

In the logistic regression analysis with a backward variable selection procedure, voiding subscore was the only

Table 1 Baseline characteristics of enrolled patients

Variables	All cases ($n = 578$)	Terminal dribbling ($n = 226$)	Non-Terminal dribbling ($n = 352$)	p value
Age (years), mean ± SD	62.4 ± 10.8	62.2 ± 10.3	62.6 ± 11.03	0.775
PSA (ng/ml), median [IQR]	2.22 [0.75-5.46]	1.70 [0.73-4.81]	2.65 [0.76-5.87]	0.098
Prostate volume (cm^3), median [IQR]	31.0 [23.0-44.0]	29.0 [22.0-43.0]	32.0 [23.0-45.0]	0.261
Prostate transitional zone volume (cm^3), median [IQR]	12.0 [7.0-20.0]	10.0 [6.0-18.0]	13.0 [7.25-22.0]	0.116
IPSS total score, Mean ± SD	14.1 ± 8.67	15.7 ± 8.33	13.1 ± 8.72	<0.001
Voiding subscale score, mean ± SD	8.13 ± 5.76	9.23 ± 5.44	7.43 ± 5.85	<0.001
Storage subscale score, mean ± SD	5.99 ± 3.70	6.49 ± 3.67	5.66 ± 3.66	0.008
IPSS QoL score, Mean ± SD	3.64 ± 1.15	3.83 ± 1.07	3.51 ± 1.20	0.002
IPP (%)	248 (42.9 %)	100 (44.2 %)	148 (40.2 %)	0.402
Mild (%)	362 (15.3 %)	12 (12.0 %)	26 (17.6 %)	
Moderate (%)	149 (60.1 %)	64 (64.0 %)	85 (57.4 %)	
Severe (%)	65 (24.6 %)	24 (24.0 %)	37 (25.0 %)	

IPSS = International Prostate Symptom Score; QoL = Quality of Life; IPP = intravesical prostatic protrusion

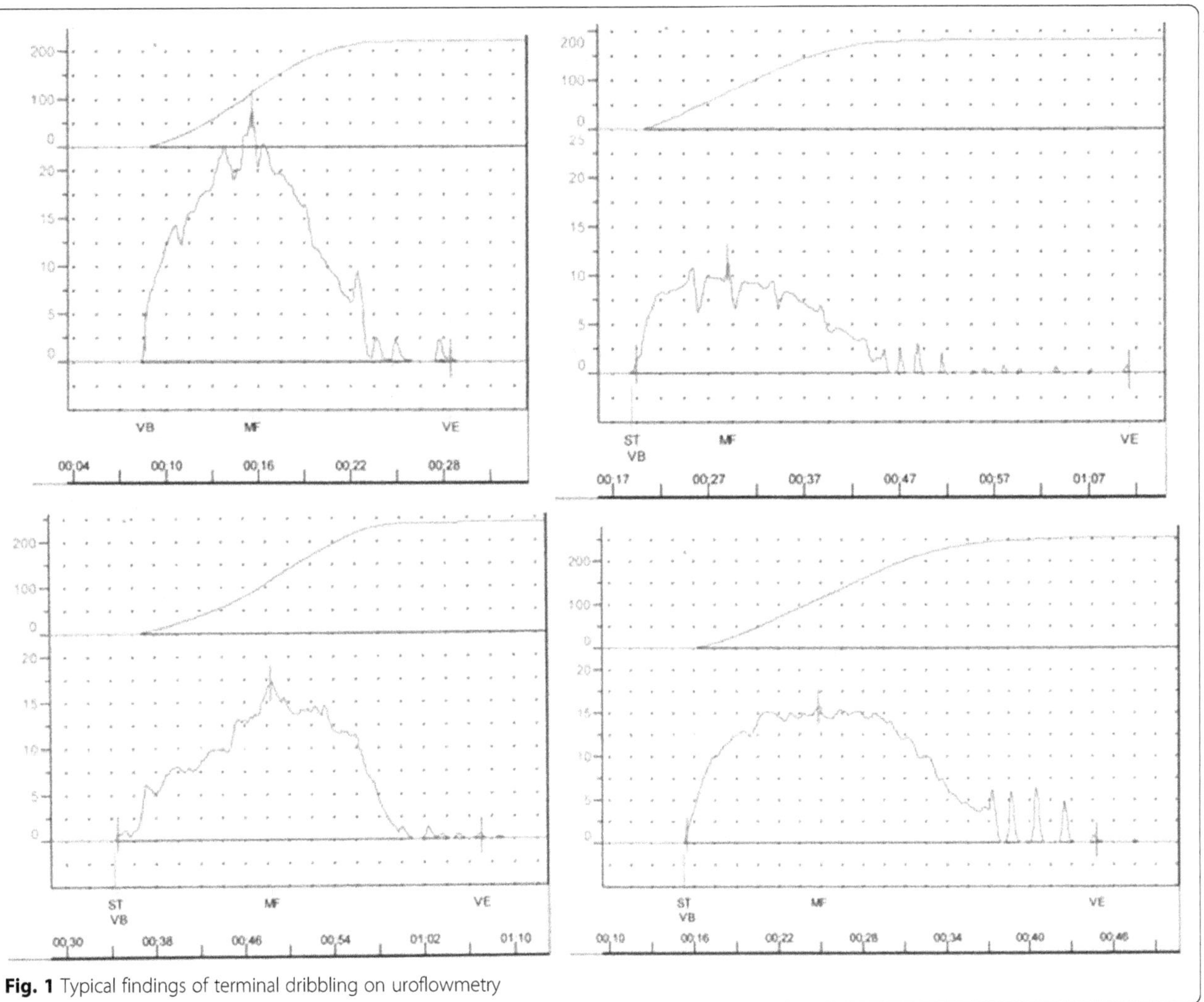

Fig. 1 Typical findings of terminal dribbling on uroflowmetry

significant risk factor for TD in the enrolled patients (Odds ratio 1.06, Table 2). In addition, when the multiple logistic regression analysis was performed to reveal the significant factor for uroflowmetry-confirmed TD, IPP was the only significant risk factor (Odds ratio 2.83, Table 3). Each question of IPSS is not correlated with TD or uroflowmetry-confirmed TD in the logistic regression analysis.

Discussion

One of the difficulties encountered in earlier studies regarding TD was the lack of a clear definition ensuring that patients could discriminate it from post-void dribbling. The current concept of TD was first addressed on the ICS male questionnaire and has been defined by ICS recommendations in 2002 [4, 7]. Before this definition, the studies performed in 1990s used various definitions of TD [12–16]. Moreover, several reports have regarded TD as an initial or mild form of post-void dribbling [13–15]. Post-void dribbling was recently determined to be one of post-micturition symptoms that is distinct from TD. The pathogenesis of post-micturition dribbling involves weakness of the bulbocavernosus muscle, which results in failure to evacuate urine that has pooled and trapped in the bulbar area of the urethra after voiding [17]. Additionally, the ICS previously removed the term "terminal dribbling" because of its similarity with post-void dribbling, which could be the main reason why there have been few studies on this issue [18]. To achieve the consistency, we conducted face-to-face interview by a single investigator using standardized definition of TD. Clinical studies on this topic should describe the demographic characteristics of the subjects, the prevalence of TD, the questionnaire used, and the definition of TD. Table 4 summarizing the previous studies related with TD indicates that the prevalence of TD is much greater in the LUTS patients than in the community people.

Table 2 The logistic regression analysis identifying the factors affecting terminal dribbling

Variable	Logistic Regression		
	OR	95 % Confidence interval	p value
Age	1.00	0.98 – 1.02	0.707
PSA	0.98	0.94 – 1.02	0.262
Prostate volume (cm^3)	1.00	0.99 – 1.01	0.626
Prostate transitional zone volume (cm^3)	0.98	0.96 – 1.00	0.089
IPP	1.41	0.96 – 2.09	0.083
IPSS total	1.00	0.93 – 1.07	0.901
Voiding subscore	1.06	1.02 – 1.09	0.001
Storage subscore	0.96	0.88 – 1.05	0.384
IPSS QoL	1.15	0.94 – 1.41	0.170

OR = odds ratio; PSA = prostate-specific antigen; IPP = intravesical prostatic protrusion; IPSS = International Prostate Symptom Score; QoL = Quality of Life
*Backward variable selection procedure was applied

Table 3 The logistic regression analysis identifying the factors affecting uroflowmetry-confirmed terminal dribbling

Variable	Logistic Regression		
	OR	95 % Confidence interval	p value
Age	0.99	0.97 – 1.01	0.530
PSA	0.97	0.92 – 1.02	0.273
Prostate volume (cm^3)	1.00	0.99 – 1.01	0.752
Prostate transitional zone volume (cm^3)	1.00	0.99 – 1.02	0.713
IPP	2.83	1.91 – 4.21	<0.001
IPSS total	0.96	0.89 – 1.04	0.363
Voiding subscore	1.03	0.93 – 1.15	0.561
Storage subscore	1.01	0.96 – 1.07	0.600
IPSS QoL	1.23	0.98 – 1.55	0.070

OR = odds ratio; PSA = prostate-specific antigen; IPP = intravesical prostatic protrusion; IPSS = International Prostate Symptom Score; QoL = Quality of Life
*Backward variable selection procedure was applied

Although few studies have been perform to investigate TD, high rates have been observed in patients with LUTS in both Western and Asian populations [2, 4, 19]. The ICS–'BPH' study reported 91–96 % of symptom prevalence of TD in BPH patients and 73–79 % in community people by ICS male questionnaire [4]. Korean study using translated version of ICS male questionnaire also showed that 86 % of male patients with LUTS had the symptom of TD, which was the second most common symptom even though TD has not been regarded as a bothersome symptom [2]. In addition, the reported prevalence of TD in elderly men was less than that of middle aged men [4]. This may imply that TD is an early obstructive symptom and that the patients with TD get used to this symptom as time passes by. Interestingly, our results were consistent with the previous study that the prevalence of TD in male LUTS patients was higher in their 60's compared with in their 50's and 70's. TD does not seem to be the sign of the early stages of LUTS because IPSS total score and IPSS QoL score in TD group were significantly higher than those in non-TD group.

Since there have been few studies investigating TD, its associations with LUTS and several clinical parameters have not been well characterized so far. In this study, TD had an association with voiding subscore in IPSS but no associations with serum PSA level, prostate volume, and prostate transitional zone volume. Traditionally, TD has been regarded as one of the voiding symptoms [4, 6, 13]. In addition, IPP has been reported to be associated with voiding symptoms [9, 20, 21]. In the present study, IPSS voiding subscore had a strong correlation with TD and

Table 4 Summary of previous studies on terminal dribbling

Source	Study sample	Prevalence	Questionnaires used	Definition of terminal dribbling	Remark
Boyarsky *et al.* (1977) [4]	Not a clinical study	Not determined	A pilot questionnaire with 10 items	No specific definition of terminal dribbling.	Suggested a guideline with a 10 item questionnaire including terminal dribbling.
Garraway *et al.* (1991)[20]	Community sample	45 %	A pilot questionnaire by Fowler[16]	Patients were asked to rate the frequency of dribbling after urination. (Confusion with post-void dribbling)	Uroflowmetry and transrectal ultrasonography were done. Undetermined impact of terminal dribbling
Meyhoff *et al.* (1993)[12]	LUTS patients	Not determined	DAN-PSS-1	"Do you experience dribbling after voiding, when you feel you have finished urination?" (Confusion with post-void dribbling)	Post-void dribbling was aggravated after transurethral prostatectomy.
Chute *et al.* (1993) [13]	Community sample	36–44 %	A pilot questionnaire by Epstein[18]	"Dribbling after urinating." (Confusion with post-void dribbling)	Uroflowmetry and transrectal ultrasonography were done. Terminal dribbling was noted to be bothersome.
Reynard *et al.* (1996)[6]	LUTS patients	44 % in questionnaire, 27 % in uroflowmetry	Not determined	"Does your urinary stream end with a dribble?" Gradient of a line drawn between the maximum flow rate and the end of flow was <0.25 and if, in the terminal 15 s of uninterrupted flow, the flow rate did not exceed 5 ml/s at any point.	Pressure-flow study was done. Terminal dribbling on questionnaire was not related to BOO defined by pressure-flow study.
Hughes *et al.* (2000)[1]	Community sample	35 %	ICS male questionnaire	"Do you have any trickle/dribble at the final part of micturition?"	Terminal dribbling was the single- most bothersome symptom.
Scarpa *et al.* (2001)[2]	LUTS patients	88 %	ICS male questionnaire	"Do you have any trickle/dribble at the final part of micturition?"	Terminal dribbling was the both most common and bothersome symptom
Jin *et al.* (2003)[3]	LUTS patients	85.6 %	ICS male questionnaire	"Do you have any trickle/dribble at the final part of micturition?"	Translated questionnaire in Korean. Pressure-flow study was done. IPP was not checked.
Yano *et al.* (2004)[16]	LUTS patients	Not determined	Saitama Prostate Symptom Score	"Do you experience dribbling after voiding, when you feel you have finished urination?"	Validation study with IPSS. Pressure-flow study was done. Undetermined impact of terminal dribbling.
Shiri *et al.* (2005)[14]	Community sample	52 %	DAN-PSS-1[20]	"Do you consider your urinary stream as dribbling?"	Relationship between LUTS and ED. Terminal dribbling was related to ED.

LUTS = lower urinary tract symptoms; ICS = International Continence Society; BOO = bladder outlet obstruction; IPSS = International Prostate Symptom Score; IPP = intraprostatic protrusion; DAN-PSS-1 = Danish Prostate Symptom Score; ED = erectile dysfunction

IPP emerged as a significant risk factor for uroflowmetry-confirmed TD.

Earlier reports have tended to put an emphasis on objective tools such as uroflowmetry. However, 48 % of the patients who reported TD did not show any objective evidence of TD on uroflowmetry [6]. In our study, about 30 % of the patients did not show the typical finding of TD on uroflowmetry. One of the reasons of this result is probably that TD does not happen all the time in some patients. Another reason to be considered is the large amount of urine volume that the patients try to void when they are taking the uroflowmetry test.

This study has several limitations. First, pressure flow studies were not performed, and as a result we could not confirm bladder outlet obstruction of each patient. However, the recent guideline recommends that pressure flow studies should be considered before invasive treatment in men with a Qmax greater than 10 ml per second and are not necessarily needed in the patients whose maximum flow rate is less than 10 ml per second [22]. Second, we did not use the entire ICS male questionnaire because it contains a large number of questions. Notably, however, the initial developers of the questionnaire have recommended the short form ICSmaleSF questionnaire omitting duplicate or redundant items [19].

Conclusions

Among men with LUTS attending outpatient clinic, about 40 % of them complained of TD. IPSS voiding subscore had a strong correlation with TD and IPP was the only significant risk factor for uroflowmetry-confirmed TD. On the other hand, the parameters such as age, PSA, prostate volume and prostate transitional zone volume did not show any significant association with it. TD is not correlated with each question of IPSS, which means that TD is the specific symptom among several LUTS. Further studies on TD will reveal the clinical impact of this underestimated symptom on LUTS patients, and make it possible to guide a proper management.

Abbreviations

TD: Terminal dribbling; BPH: Benign prostate hyperplasia; ICS: International continence society; LUTS: Lower urinary tract symptom; IPSS: International prostate symptom score; PSA: Prostate-specific antigen; TRUS: Transrectal ultrasonography; QoL: Quality of life.

Competing interests

The authors declare that they have no competing interests.

Authors' contributions

JHK and JYP contributed to conception, study design, analysis and interpretation of data. JHK and JYP were also involved in drafting and revising the manuscript. JSS, HC, JYP, JHB contributed to acquisition of data. JHB, DGM, JGL, and JJK conceived and supervised the study, helped to draft the manuscript and was involved in revising it critically for important intellectual content. All authors read and approved the final manuscript.

Acknowledgements

This work was supported by the National Research Foundation of Korea (NRF) grant funded by the Korea government (MSIP) (No. 2011-0020128) and Soonchunhyang University Research Fund.

Author details

[1]Department of Urology, Soonchunhyang University Hospital, Soonchunhyang University College of Medicine, Seoul, Republic of Korea. [2]Department of Urology, Korea University Ansan Hospital, Ansan, Republic of Korea. [3]Department of Urology, Korea University College of Medicine, Seoul, Republic of Korea.

References

1. Scarpa RM. Lower urinary tract symptoms: what are the implications for the patients? Eur Urol. 2001;40 Suppl 4:12–20.
2. Jin MH, Ko YS, Lee JG, Park HS, Park WH, Chung HC, et al. The Correlation of an ICS-male Questionnaire for Lower Urinary Tract Symptoms and Bladder Outlet Obstruction Parameters in Korea. Korean J Urol. 2003;44(1):64–76.
3. Hughes AM, Sladden MJ, Hirst GH, Ward JE. Community study of uncomplicated lower urinary tract symptoms among male Italien immigrants in Sydney, Australia. Eur Urol. 2000;37(2):191–8.
4. Donovan JL, Abrams P, Peters TJ, Kay HE, Reynard J, Chapple C, et al. The ICS-'BPH' Study: the psychometric validity and reliability of the ICSmale questionnaire. Br J Urol. 1996;77(4):554–62.
5. Boyarsky S, Jones G, Paulson DF, Prout Jr GR. A new look at bladder neck obstruction by the food and drug administration regulators: guide lines for investigation of benign prostatic hypertrophy. Trans Am Assoc Genitourin Surg. 1976;68:29–32.
6. Reynard JM, Lim C, Peters TJ, Abrams P. The significance of terminal dribbling in men with lower urinary tract symptoms. Br J Urol. 1996;77(5):705–10.
7. Abrams P, Cardozo L, Fall M, Griffiths D, Rosier P, Ulmsten U, et al. The standardisation of terminology of lower urinary tract function: report from the Standardisation Sub-committee of the International Continence Society. Neurourol Urodyn. 2002;21(2):167–78.
8. Park JY, Yoon S, Park MS, Cho DY, Park HS, du Moon G, et al. Initial biopsy outcome prediction in Korean patients-comparison of a noble web-based Korean prostate cancer risk calculator versus prostate-specific antigen testing. J Korean Med Sci. 2011;26(1):85–91.
9. Keqin Z, Zhishun X, Jing Z, Haixin W, Dongqing Z, Benkang S. Clinical significance of intravesical prostatic protrusion in patients with benign prostatic enlargement. Urology. 2007;70(6):1096–9.
10. Oelke M, Bachmann A, Descazeaud A, Emberton M, Gravas S, Michel MC, et al. EAU guidelines on the treatment and follow-up of non-neurogenic male lower urinary tract symptoms including benign prostatic obstruction. Eur Urol. 2013;64(1):118–40.
11. Choi HR, Chung WS, Shim BS, Kwon SW, Hong SJ, Chung BH, et al. Translation Validity and Reliability of I-PSS Korean Version. Korean J Urol. 1996;37(6):659–65.
12. Chute CG, Panser LA, Girman CJ, Oesterling JE, Guess HA, Jacobsen SJ, et al. The prevalence of prostatism: a population-based survey of urinary symptoms. J Urol. 1993;150(1):85–9.
13. Meyhoff HH, Hald T, Nordling J, Andersen JT, Bilde T, Walter S. A new patient weighted symptom score system (DAN-PSS-1). Clinical assessment of indications and outcomes of transurethral prostatectomy for uncomplicated benign prostatic hyperplasia. Scand J Urol Nephrol. 1993;27(4):493–9.
14. Shiri R, Hakkinen JT, Hakama M, Huhtala H, Auvinen A, Tammela TL, et al. Effect of lower urinary tract symptoms on the incidence of erectile dysfunction. J Urol. 2005;174(1):205–9. discussion 209.
15. Sladden MJ, Hughes AM, Hirst GH, Ward JE. A community study of lower urinary tract symptoms in older men in Sydney, Australia. Aust N Z J Surg. 2000;70(5):322–8.
16. Yano M, Kitahara S, Yasuda K, Yamanishi T, Nakai H, Yanagisawa R, et al. A pilot study evaluating a new questionnaire for prostatic symptom scoring, the SPSS, and its sensitivity as constructed to objective measures of outflow obstruction. Int J Urol. 2004;11(5):288–94.

17. Maserejian NN, Kupelian V, McVary KT, Doshi M, Link CL, McKinlay JB. Prevalence of post-micturition symptoms in association with lower urinary tract symptoms and health-related quality of life in men and women. BJU Int. 2011;108(9):1452–8.
18. Robinson J. Post-micturition dribble in men: causes and treatment. Nurs Stand. 2008;22(30):43–6.
19. Donovan JL, Peters TJ, Abrams P, Brookes ST, De AA Rosette JJ, Schafer W. Scoring the short form ICSmaleSF questionnaire. International Continence Society. J Urol. 2000;164(6):1948–55.
20. Aganovic D, Hasanbegovic M, Prcic A, Kulovac B, Hadziosmanovic O. Which is a better indicator of bladder outlet obstruction in patients with benign prostatic enlargement–intravesical protrusion of prostate or bladder wall thickness? Med Arh. 2012;66(5):324–8.
21. Wee JH, Choi YS, Bae WJ, Kim SJ, Cho HJ, Hong SH, et al. Influence of intravesical prostatic protrusion on preoperative lower urinary tract symptoms and outcomes after 120 w high performance system laser treatment in men with benign prostatic hyperplasia. Korean J Urol. 2012;53(7):472–7.
22. Abrams P, Chapple C, Khoury S, Roehrborn C, de la Rosette J, International Consultation on New Developments in Prostate C, et al. Evaluation and treatment of lower urinary tract symptoms in older men. J Urol. 2013;189(1 Suppl):S93–S101.

6

Prostate cancer outcomes in France: treatments, adverse effects and two-year mortality

Philippe Tuppin[1*], Solène Samson[1], Anne Fagot-Campagna[1], Bertrand Lukacs[2], François Alla[1], and the CNAMTS scientific board members[1], Fred Paccaud[1], Jean-Christophe Thalabard[1], Eric Vicaut[1], Michel Vidaud[1] and Bertrand Millat[1]

Abstract

Background: This very large population-based study investigated outcomes after a diagnosis of prostate cancer (PCa) in terms of mortality rates, treatments and adverse effects.

Methods: Among the 11 million men aged 40 years and over covered by the general national health insurance scheme, those with newly managed PCa in 2009 were followed for two years based on data from the national health insurance information system (SNIIRAM). Patients were identified using hospitalisation diagnoses and specific refunds related to PCa and PCa treatments. Adverse effects of PCa treatments were identified by using hospital diagnoses, specific procedures and drug refunds.

Results: The age-standardised two-year all-cause mortality rate among the 43,460 men included in the study was 8.4%, twice that of all men aged 40 years and over. Among the 36,734 two-year survivors, 38% had undergone prostatectomy, 36% had been treated by hormone therapy, 29% by radiotherapy, 3% by brachytherapy and 20% were not treated. The frequency of treatment-related adverse effects varied according to age and type of treatment. Among men between 50 and 69 years of age treated by prostatectomy alone, 61% were treated for erectile dysfunction and 24% were treated for urinary disorders. The frequency of treatment for these disorders decreased during the second year compared to the first year (erectile dysfunction: 41% vs 53%, urinary disorders: 9% vs 20%). The frequencies of these treatments among men treated by external beam radiotherapy alone were 7% and 14%, respectively. Among men between 50 and 69 years with treated PCa, 46% received treatments for erectile dysfunction and 22% for urinary disorders. For controls without PCa but treated surgically for benign prostatic hyperplasia, these frequencies were 1.5% and 6.0%, respectively.

Conclusions: We report high survival rates two years after a diagnosis of PCa, but a high frequency of PCa treatment-related adverse effects. These frequencies remain underestimated, as they are based on treatments for erectile dysfunction and urinary disorders and do not reflect all functional outcomes. These results should help urologists and general practitioners to inform their patients about outcomes at the time of screening and diagnosis, and especially about potential treatment-related adverse effects.

Keywords: Prostate cancer, Treatments, Adverse effects, Prostatectomy, Radiotherapy, Complications, Population-based study

Background

The availability of serum prostate-specific antigen (PSA) testing has led to a dramatic increase in the incidence of localised prostate cancer (PCa), corresponding to well or moderately differentiated tumours with a low risk of progression [1-4]. The discordant results of randomised studies concerning the impact of PSA testing on mortality and the adverse effects of treatments contribute to the debate on overdiagnosis and overtreatment of PCa [4-13].

Adverse effects on sexual and urinary functions are due to specific pathophysiological mechanisms related to each of the main treatment modalities, e.g., radical prostatectomy, brachytherapy, external beam radiotherapy and hormone therapy. Patient quality of life is usually estimated by assessment tools filled in by the patient or completed

* Correspondence: philippe.tuppin@cnamts.fr
[1]National general health insurance scheme (Caisse Nationale d'Assurance Maladie des Travailleurs Salariés, CNAMTS), Paris, France
Full list of author information is available at the end of the article

during telephone interviews, based on samples of less than 2000 individuals [7-13]. The frequency of symptoms is generally high, but depends on the definition used for urinary and erectile problems, as well as on practices, measurement tools and monitoring periods. Quality of life assessment rarely includes comparisons with a control group without PCa.

The purpose of this observational study based on a large population of French men aged 40 and over with newly managed PCa in 2009 was to estimate the two-year all-cause mortality according to the various treatments for PCa, and the frequency of PCa treatments and their adverse effects, when they required health care resources, for survivors compared to two control groups.

Methods

Population and data source

All data were obtained from the French National Health Insurance Information System (SNIIRAM) [14]. Access to data and data analysis are granted by decree only for a period of three years plus the current year and authorisation from the French Data protection Authority (*Commission nationale de l'informatique et des libertés, CNIL*) must also be obtained. This database comprehensively records all hospitalisations, prescriptions, health care services and procedures reimbursed together with their dates. Drugs are identified using their ATC (Anatomical Therapeutic Classification) code, while medical and surgical procedures are identified by a specific classification. The SNIIRAM does not contain any medical information concerning results related to prescriptions or examinations. It nevertheless includes information on the presence of long-term chronic diseases (LTCD), such as PCa, eligible for 100% reimbursement of health care expenditure, after approval by a national health insurance consultant physician. LTCD status is granted at the time of diagnosis of the disease and is renewable for five years. These chronic diseases and hospital diagnoses are coded according to the International Classification of Diseases (ICD 10). The SNIIRAM also includes a permanent sample (EGB: échantillon généraliste des bénéficiares) of individuals selected at random from 1/97th of all beneficiaries of the French general health insurance schemes, i.e. approximately 600,000 individuals.

The study population was composed of men aged 40 years and over, covered by the general health insurance scheme, with newly managed PCa in 2009. In 2009, 73% of French men aged 40 and over (11 million people) were covered by the general health insurance scheme. The rest of the French population was covered by other specific health insurance schemes. One of the reasons for limiting the study to individuals covered by the general scheme was the availability of survival status and date of death from the National Institute for Statistics and Economic Studies for the study period.

Definitions and data analysis

Men with PCa were identified by the presence of at least one of the following criteria in 2009: a hospital stay with a PCa code as primary diagnosis, PCa *in situ* or prostate tumour with an unpredictable course; LTCD for PCa; hospitalisation for radical prostatectomy, subcapsular orchidectomy or specific brachytherapy; hospitalisation for chemotherapy or radiotherapy with a PCa-related diagnosis; at least one reimbursement for GnRH analogues, antiandrogens or oestrogens and estramustine. To select only newly diagnosed cases in 2009, men with any of the above criteria in 2008 were excluded.

PCa treatments and their combinations were identified during the two-year follow-up after the first treatment criterion identified in 2009. Two groups of patients without treatment over the next two years were formed: one group with a hospitalisation corresponding to a primary diagnosis of PCa (with or without LTCD for PCa in 2009) and the other group with only LTCD status for PCa granted in 2009. These patients were considered to be on watchful waiting for PCa. For the study of treatment combinations, subcapsular orchidectomy, which is rarely performed, was grouped together with hormone therapy.

Complications were defined on the basis of at least one hospitalisation with a main diagnosis corresponding to the specific codes of complications or the presence of a surgical procedure to treat these complications. Urinary disorders were identified by reimbursements of external devices to treat incontinence (urine collectors and penile sheaths). Reimbursements of specific drugs were also considered (ATC G04BD: oxybutynin, flavoxate, trospium and solifenacin). Erectile dysfunction was identified by reimbursements for penile prostheses or intracavernous injections of vasoactive agents (sildenafil was not reimbursed). Drug treatments were defined on the basis of at least one reimbursement for specific drugs for patients still alive at one year and at two years.

The two-year mortality rate for patients with treated PCa was compared to that of all male health insurance beneficiaries aged 40 years and over. A standardised mortality ratio (SMR) was calculated for each age group and the overall SMR was age-standardised using data for men aged 40 years and over in the general scheme. Frequencies of treatments and complications were studied among men of the general scheme who were still alive with a follow-up of two years. Among men between the ages of 50 and 69, complication rates according to the type of medical treatment were compared to those of two control groups without PCa, selected from the EGB according to the presence of a surgical or endoscopic procedure performed for BPH between 2008 and 2011. The 50–69 years age-group was selected because radical prostatectomy, associated with a higher complication rate than other treatments, is more frequent at these ages and also has a greater impact on erectile dysfunction and quality of life and is therefore more frequently treated. The frequencies for each of these groups were age-standardised for all males aged 50–69. Chi-square tests were used to compare frequencies between groups. Statistical analyses were performed using SAS Enterprise Guide 4.3 software (SAS Institute Inc., Cary, NC, USA).

Results

Survival

Newly diagnosed PCa in 2009 was found in 43,460 men with a mean age of 70.2 years. The crude one-year and two-year all-cause mortality rates were 7% and 13%, respectively, and the age-standardised rates were 4.6% and 8.4%, respectively (Table 1). The age-standardised mortality rate was slightly higher before the age of 50 (7%) and was 47% for men aged 85 years and over. The patients of this population had a significant excess two-year all-cause mortality rate compared to all men aged 40 and over (SMR = 2). The SMR was higher for the youngest age groups. In this group of 43,460 patients, 1,169 subjects still alive at two years were excluded because they were no longer covered by the general health insurance scheme or had been admitted to an institution that managed medicinal products directly with no reimbursements reported in the SNIIRAM database.

Age-standardised two-year mortality rates varied according to age and type of PCa treatment (Table 2). Lowest two-year mortality rates were observed for patients treated by radical prostatectomy (4%) and hormone therapy (9%) and highest two-year mortality rates were observed for patients treated by external beam radiotherapy (14% overall, and 30% for those treated by external beam radiotherapy alone) and chemotherapy (38%). The two-year mortality rate for men not treated for PCa was 15% for men hospitalised for PCa and 8% for men with only LTCD status.

Prostate cancer treatment

In the population of 36,734 men with PCa still alive after two years, 38% had been treated by radical prostatectomy, 35% by hormone therapy, 29% by external beam radiotherapy, 2.5% by brachytherapy, 0.3% by subcapsular orchidectomy and 1.6% by chemotherapy (2). Twenty per cent of patients had not received any active treatment, but had been hospitalised with a specific code for PCa (15%) or had been granted LTCD status (5%).

The frequency of prostatectomy decreased from 67% in men between the ages of 50 and 54 to 6% among men between the ages of 75 and 79. The frequency of hormone therapy, stable at around 20% between the ages of 50 and 64, increased to 65% for men aged 80 and over. The frequency of external beam radiotherapy reached a peak of 41% in men between the ages of 75 and 79. The most common treatment combination was hormone therapy and external beam radiotherapy (13%). Prostatectomy was often performed alone (31%), especially among the youngest patients (more than half), and was combined with radiotherapy and hormone therapy in only 2% of men treated for PCa.

Table 1 One-year and two-year mortality rates among men with newly managed prostate cancer in 2009 by age and comparison with all male general scheme beneficiaries aged 40 and over, according to age after two years

	40-49	50-54	55-59	60-64	65-69	70-74	75-79	80-84	85 and over	All ages
Patients with cancer										
N	**478**	**1,567**	**4,079**	**7,371**	**7,435**	**7,876**	**6,663**	**4,351**	**3,640**	**43,460**
%	1.1	3.6	9.4	17.0	17.1	18.1	15.3	10.0	8.4	100.0
One-year follow-up										
Patients still alive*	443	1,481	3,857	7,026	7,070	7,368	6,022	3,568	2,526	39,361
Deceased										
N	15	40	101	186	242	392	532	727	1,047	3,282
%	3.3	2.6	2.6	2.6	3.3	5.1	8.1	16.9	29.3	4.6**
Two-year follow-up										
Patients still alive*	414	1,433	3,727	6,782	6,792	7,033	5,554	3,106	1,893	36,734
Deceased										
N	31	71	192	369	456	665	948	1,159	1,656	5,547
%	7.0	4.7	4.9	5.2	6.3	8.6	14.6	27.2	46.7	8.4**
SMR§	11.4	3.7	2.6	2.1	1.9	1.8	1.9	2.1	1.9	2.0**

*Excluding deaths, regime changes and patients lost to follow-up.
**Age-standardised.
§$p < 0.001$ for all SMR.

Table 2 Age-standardised two-year mortality rates among men with newly managed prostate cancer (PCa) in 2009 according to treatment, and frequency of treatments and their combinations among men still alive at two-years according to age

	Death rate	Frequency of treatment									
	Age-standardised	40-49	50-54	55-59	60-64	65-69	70-74	75-79	80-84	≥85	Total
N	43,460	414	1,433	3,727	6,782	6,792	7,033	5,554	3,106	1,893	36,734
Treatments (at least one)	%	%	%	%	%	%	%	%	%	%	%
Total prostatectomy	4.3	46.9	66.9	65.8	60.6	54.2	32.4	6.0	0.2	0.3	38.1
- laparoscopy	3.5	20.3	37.7	36.6	33.2	30.9	19.7	3.8	0.1	0.2	21.6
- laparotomy	5.1	26.6	29.2	29.2	27.4	23.3	12.7	2.1	0.1	0.1	16.5
Hormone therapy	9.4	40.3	21.4	20.3	20.5	25.4	34.9	53.3	65.4	66.8	35.5
Subcapsular orchidectomy	12.7	1.2	0.3	0.2	0.1	0.1	0.2	0.4	1.2	1.3	0.3
Chemotherapy	38.5	4.3	2.5	1.6	1.6	1.4	1.5	1.7	1.8	1.1	1.6
Brachytherapy	0.8	2.4	3.0	4.2	4.0	2.8	2.7	1.2	0.1	0.0	2.5
External beam radiotherapy	14.0	18.4	21.1	24.8	26.0	28.8	39.7	40.6	12.2	3.5	28.6
No treatment*:	13.6	12.1	13.9	14.7	16.9	17.8	20.7	24.6	30.2	31.2	20.4
- Hospitalisation with PCa diagnosis	15.0	10.4	11.0	11.5	12.8	13.6	15.3	17.9	22.9	25.5	15.5
- Isolated LTCD for PCa	8.1	1.7	2.9	3.2	4.2	4.2	5.3	6.7	7.2	5.7	4.9
Treatment combinations	%	%	%	%	%	%	%	%	%	%	%
Prostatectomy, all types											
Alone	4.4	37.4	53.5	52.3	49.4	43.7	25.4	4.8	0.2	0.1	30.6
Combined with:											
- Hormone therapy	1.2	1.9	3.6	3.4	2.8	3.0	2.1	0.6	0.0	0.1	2.1
- External beam radiotherapy	4.2	4.1	5.7	5.6	5.0	4.1	2.8	0.4	0.0	0.0	3.1
- External beam radiotherapy + Hormone therapy	0.4	2.9	4.0	4.1	3.2	3.2	1.9	0.3	0.0	0.0	2.2
Hormone therapy											
Alone	9.5	28.3	6.8	4.0	3.8	5.6	9.8	26.4	55.9	64.0	16.6
Combined with:											
- External beam radiotherapy	8.9	4.3	4.9	6.7	8.7	11.6	19.1	23.9	8.5	2.5	12.8
External beam radiotherapy alone	30.0	2.2	2.5	3.4	4.7	6.7	12.9	14.3	3.0	0.7	7.5

LTCD: long term chronic disease status.
*Absence of the above treatments during the two-year follow-up.

Adverse effects of PCa treatments

In the population of 36,734 men with PCa still alive after two years, regardless of the PCa treatment, 54% presented no health care consumption corresponding to adverse effects of PCa treatments (Table 3).

The frequency of reimbursement for at least one intracavernous injection for erectile dysfunction was 21% for all ages and ranged between 33% and 47% for men under the age of 65. A penile prosthesis was used by 0.2% of men under 55 years of age. The frequency of reimbursement for drugs used to treat urinary disorders was 15% for all ages, and varied slightly according to age (from 9% to 17%), while external devices were reimbursed in 4.8% of cases and 1% of cases were treated by surgery. The frequency of surgical procedures for acute urinary retention was 11% for all ages, but was higher among older men. Surgical treatment of complications was more common during the first year of follow-up.

The frequency of treatment for adverse effects varied according to the type of PCa treatment (Table 4). Among patients between the ages of 50 and 69, intracavernous injection for erectile dysfunction was more common for patients treated by prostatectomy alone (61%) compared to patients treated by radiotherapy alone (7%). Similar results were observed for urinary disorders, with reimbursement of drugs in 18% versus 12% of patients and reimbursement of external devices in 8% and 2% of patients, respectively. Patients treated by prostatectomy alone more frequently received reimbursements for drugs used to treat erectile dysfunction than those treated by prostatectomy combined with external beam radiotherapy or hormone therapy.

Table 3 Frequency of treatments* for various complications, according to age, among men with newly managed prostate cancer in 2009, still alive after two years

Complications	40-49 414 %	50-54 1,433 %	55-59 3,727 %	60-64 6,782 %	65-69 6,792 %	70-74 7,033 %	75-79 5,554 %	80-84 3,106 %	≥85 1,893 %	All ages 36,734 %
Erectile dysfunction	34.1	46.9	43.9	37.1	27.6	11.8	2.1	0.5	0.1	21.2
Intracavernous injection	33.8	46.7	43.8	37.0	27.5	11.7	2.0	0.4	0.1	21.1
Penile prosthesis	0.2	0.2	0.2	0.1	0.1	0.1	0.0	0.0	0.0	0.1
Urinary disorders	14.0	20.4	20.5	19.4	21.8	19.5	17.1	14.6	14.4	18.9
Drug treatment	10.6	15.6	16.4	14.7	17.1	15.9	14.5	11.6	9.3	15.0
External devices	3.9	6.1	5.6	5.8	6.2	4.8	2.6	2.8	4.2	4.8
Surgical procedure	1.0	1.0	1.3	1.4	1.6	1.2	0.4	0.1	0.0	1.0
Clot removal										
Surgical procedure	1.2	1.4	1.0	1.3	1.0	1.3	1.4	1.9	2.3	1.4
Urethral stricture										
Surgical procedure	1.4	1.5	1.4	1.5	2.0	2.4	2.0	2.0	2.6	1.9
Bladder neck stenosis										
Surgical procedure	1.4	2.2	1.7	1.8	1.9	2.0	1.8	1.3	1.2	1.8
Radiation-induced inflammation										
Hospitalisation	0.0	0.6	0.5	0.6	0.9	1.4	2.0	0.5	0.1	1.0
Acute urinary retention										
Surgical procedure	5.1	3.8	5.4	7.5	8.6	12.6	17.2	20.6	19.4	11.5
Urethral or rectal fistula										
Hospitalisation	0.7	0.4	0.2	0.2	0.3	0.1	0.1	0.0	0.0	0.2
None	55.1	40.5	40.5	45.2	49.4	60.0	65.4	66.4	64.3	54.1
Drug treatment										
Antidepressants	14.5	15.6	12.4	9.2	9.4	9.3	11.6	15.9	18.8	11.3
Anxiolytics	19.3	19.0	17.2	15.0	15.4	17.0	18.2	21.7	23.9	17.4

*Hospitalisation: primary diagnosis, surgical treatment: presence of a specific surgical procedure code, external devices and medication: reimbursement codes.

Among patients with untreated PCa, 10% had received medication for erectile dysfunction, 12% had received medication for urinary disorders, and 19% had received medication for acute urinary retention. For the subgroup of patients not hospitalised for PCa, these frequencies were 20%, 12% and 5%, respectively. In contrast, the frequencies of the various treatments for erectile dysfunction and urinary disorders in the two control groups without PCa were very low, even in men who had undergone BPH surgery. The highest treatment frequencies observed in these men concerned medication for urinary disorders (4.8%), acute urinary retention (3.6%) and, to a lesser degree, erectile dysfunction (1.5%).

The frequency of treatment for erectile dysfunction decreased during the second year compared to the first year among patients treated by radical prostatectomy and patients with untreated PCa, while the frequency of treatment for erectile dysfunction increased between the first and second year among men treated by external beam radiotherapy alone. The frequency of drug treatment for urinary disorders decreased during the second year for men treated by prostatectomy and men with untreated PCa. However, men with untreated PCa had a high frequency of treatment for acute urinary retention.

Discussion

This study reports outcomes for men diagnosed with PCa based on health care consumption data concerning a very large population followed for two years. We report a low 8% mortality rate which is nevertheless twofold higher than that of the general male population and a higher frequency of radical treatments in men under the age of 70. Very high frequencies of erectile dysfunction and urinary disorders requiring treatment were observed among men between the ages of 50 and 69 treated by radical prostatectomy, compared to controls and men with untreated PCa.

This study demonstrated a crude one-year survival rate of 95% with variations related to age, which is

Table 4 Frequencies of the various complications according to type of treatment* among men aged between 50 and 69 with newly managed prostate cancer (PCa) in 2009 and still alive after two years, and comparison with two control groups without PCa, with or without surgical treatment for benign prostatic hyperplasia (BPH)

	Prostatectomy		External beam radiotherapy	Hormone therapy	Treated PCa	Untreated PCa***	Control groups without PCA	
	Alone	With another treatment**	Alone	Alone	All		Without BPH surgery	With BPH surgery
N	**9,035**	**2,159**	**941**	**882**	**15,623**	**3,107**	**43,099**	**1,026**
Mean age (years)	**61.8**	**61.8**	**63.6**	**62.4**	**62.1**	**62.5**	**57.8**	**60.5**
Complications	%	%	%		%	%	%	%
Erectile dysfunction								
Two years	61.4	47.9°	7.2°	6.8°	45.8	9.6°	0.3°	1.5°
Drug treatment	61.3	47.9	7.2	6.8	45.7	9.5	0.3	1.5
Penile prosthesis	0.2	0.2	0.04	0.0	0.2	0.1	0.00	0.00
First year	**53.2**	**38.1°**	**2.6°**	**4.7°**	**38.7**	**8.1°**	**0.2°**	**1.0°**
Drug treatment	53.1	38.1	2.6	4.7	38.6	8.0	0.2	1.0
Penile prosthesis	0.1	0.0	0.0	0.0	0.0	0.0	0.0	0.0
Second year	**41.5**	**31.8°**	**6.3°**	**4.4°**	**30.8**	**6.4°**	**0.2°**	**1.1°**
Drug treatment	41.3	31.8	6.3	4.4	30.7	6.3	0.2	1.1
Penile prosthesis	0.2	0.2	0.0	0.0	0.1	0.0	0.0	0.0
Urinary disorders								
Two years	**23.7**	**27.9°**	**14.4°**	**8.7°**	**21.6**	**12.3°**	**0.4°**	**5.6°**
Drug treatment	18.0	21.6	12.3	7.4	17.0	9.4	0.3	4.8
External devices	7.7	9.3	2.4	1.8	6.3	3.8	0.1	0.8
Surgical procedure	2.1	1.2	0.00	0.1	1.4	0.6	0.00	0.00
First year	**20.1**	**22.8**	**10.9°**	**4.7°**	**17.5**	**10.4°**	**0.2°**	**3.7°**
Drug treatment	14.7	16.0	8.9	4.0	13.1	7.5	0.2	3.2
External devices	7.2	8.9	2.2	1.1	5.8	3.3	0.1	0.5
Surgical procedure	0.5	0.2	0.0	0.1	0.3	0.5	0.0	0.0
Second year	9.0	11.5°	7.6	6.0°	9.0	5.5°	0.2°	3.5°
Drug treatment	7.2	10.3	5.7	4.8	7.6	4.2	0.2	3.0
External devices	1.4	1.5	1.9	1.2	1.3	1.6	0.1	0.4
Surgical procedure	1.7	1.0	0.0	0.1	1.1	0.2	0.0	0.0
Clot removal								
Surgical procedure	1.2	1.2	1.0	1.3	1.2	1.2	0.00°	0.3°
Urethral stricture								
Surgical procedure	1.6	1.9	1.5	1.1	1.4	2.2	0.0°	1.3
Bladder neck stenosis								
Surgical procedure	2.0	2.2	0.3°	1.0°	1.9	1.7	0.00°	0.9°
Radiation-induced inflammation								
Hospitalisation	0.0	1.1°	3.2°	0.1	0.7	0.3°	0.00°	0.00°
Acute urinary retention								
Surgical procedure	1.4	1.3	12.2	9.9°	3.5	19.3°	0.00°	3.6
Urethral-rectal fistula								
Hospitalisation	0.5	0.4	0.00	0.1°	0.3	0.0°	0.00°	0.00°
None	28.1	35.8°	69.3°	76.9°	40.1	63.5°	99.3°	89.0°

Table 4 Frequencies of the various complications according to type of treatment* among men aged between 50 and 69 with newly managed prostate cancer (PCa) in 2009 and still alive after two years, and comparison with two control groups without PCa, with or without surgical treatment for benign prostatic hyperplasia (BPH) *(Continued)*

Drug treatment								
Antidepressants	11.3	11.4	12.2	15.9	12.0	12.2	7.1°	11.7
Anxiolytics	15.3	18.1	21.1°	19.8	17.1	15.0°	10.4°	16.5

*Hospitalisation: primary diagnosis, surgical treatment: presence of a specific surgical procedure code, external devices and medication: reimbursement codes.
**Patients without treatment during the two years but with a primary diagnosis of PCa during hospitalisation or long-term chronic disease status for PCa.
***External beam radiotherapy and/or hormone therapy.
Frequencies are age-standardised for men aged between 50 and 69 covered by the general scheme.
°$p < 0.05$ for comparisons of frequencies between prostatectomy alone and prostatectomy combined with another treatment, external beam radiotherapy, for comparisons between untreated PCa and treated PCa, for comparisons between treated PCa and each control group.

similar to estimates from French cancer registries (92% one-year overall survival, and a specific survival rate of 96%) [15]. Causes of death other than PCa were reported for 80% of deceased patients in the United States and 65% of deceased patients in Sweden [16]. Patients with PCa, especially with metastatic disease, presented a higher risk of death by suicide or cardiovascular disease than the general population [17]. These data highlight the high survival rate and the fact that mortality is due to causes other than PCa. Although no information was available concerning specific mortality rates, the two-year mortality rate in this population was twofold higher than that of men covered by the general health insurance scheme. More specifically, the highest SMR was observed for the 40–49 year age-group, which was less frequently treated by prostatectomy and more frequently treated by chemotherapy and hormone therapy, which could suggest more advanced disease, although no information on disease stage was available in our database.

In this study, the estimated frequencies of the various treatments for PCa were 38% for prostatectomy, 35% for hormone therapy, 29% for external beam radiotherapy and 20% of patients did not receive any treatment during the two-year follow-up. This group can be considered to correspond to watchful waiting, but some of these patients may have received treatment for PCa before 2008 and were wrongly considered to have newly diagnosed PCa. However, it is much more likely that the watchful waiting group was underestimated, as newly diagnosed patients who were not hospitalised and who did not require treatment or LTCD status were not included in this database. A French registry study conducted in 2001 on 1,840 men of all ages with stage T1 or T2 PCa reported slightly lower frequencies for prostatectomy (31%) and hormone therapy (22%) and nearly the same rate for radiotherapy (26%) and watchful waiting (19%) [18]. The proportion of patients managed by watchful waiting has most likely increased since 2001. The more recent Swedish registry provides different figures. Among the 31,903 patients of all ages with localised PCa between 1996 and 2006, 41% had undergone prostatectomy (66% between 55 and 59 years of age, as for all stages in this study), 20% had received external beam radiotherapy (24% for those between 65 and 69) and 30%, a very high proportion, were on watchful waiting [19]. The Australian state of New South Wales registry showed that, in a group of 1,636 patients under the age of 70 with localised PCa between 2000 and 2002, 60% had been treated by prostatectomy, 28% by external beam radiotherapy, 14% by hormone therapy and 12% by watchful waiting [8]. For the same age-group, at all stages, our study found similar frequencies for prostatectomy (60%) and external beam radiotherapy (26%) but higher frequencies for hormone therapy (23%) and watchful waiting (16%). The choice of treatment probably varies from one series to another depending on the tumour grades included, the study period, patient characteristics and comorbidity. However, it is very likely that the choice of treatment also depends on PCa screening frequency and medical practices. For example, brachytherapy is less commonly used in France [20].

This study demonstrated a very high rate of PCa treatment-related adverse effects. Over a 2-year period, treatments for urinary and erectile disorders were reported in 19% and 21% of all men with newly diagnosed Pca, respectively. These rates were even higher among men aged 50–54 years (20% and 47%) and men of all ages who had undergone prostatectomy (24% and 61%). In contrast with studies on urinary disorders and erectile dysfunction based on the presence of symptoms or quality of life assessment, using various definitions and instruments, in the present study, these disorders were estimated on the basis of health care consumption. These estimates depend on the patient's perception of the disorder, the efficacy of treatment of the disorder and the physician's or surgeon's impression.

These adverse effect rates, although underestimated, can nevertheless be considered to accurately reflect the impact of PCa treatments on quality of life. Specific health care consumption was very rare in the control group without PCa and who had not undergone BPH surgery. As expected, treatment rates for acute urinary retention and urinary disorders were higher among controls that had undergone BPH surgery. Higher rates of treatment for acute urinary retention were observed for men with untreated PCa compared to men with treated PCa, which may be linked to tumour progression [13]. As also reported in quality of life studies, lower rates of adverse effects were observed after external beam radiotherapy than after prostatectomy [7–13]. In our study, surgery for incontinence during the two years following prostatectomy was performed in 2.1% of patients versus 2.6% in a Canadian study based on 25,436 patients of all ages with a five-year follow-up [21,22]. Patients treated by prostatectomy in combination with another treatment such as hormone therapy also had a lower rate of treatment for erectile disorders, which could be explained by the lack of available treatment for sexual dysfunction induced by hormone therapy.

Urinary disorders and erectile dysfunction are much less common after external beam radiotherapy: 7% of patients experienced erectile dysfunction and 15% experienced urinary disorders. A recent American study based on 1,201 patients of all ages with stage T1 or T2 PCa between 2003 and 2006, analysing first-line treatments, reported urinary disorders in 30% of patients after two months and 7% of patients after two years [10]. The present study showed lower rates of adverse effects of treatment after the first year following PCa treatment, in line with the results of quality of life studies that reported improvement of symptoms after the first year of treatment, with an impact on quality of life, but without return to baseline conditions [7,8,10,11].

This study presents a number of limitations. Certain groups of the French population (25%) were not included due to their occupation, such as civil servants, liberal professions and farmers, which may influence epidemiological characteristics (exposure) or health care consumption, and who are covered by other health insurance schemes. The data of this study were derived from administrative databases comprising the classical limitations concerning the modalities of data collection and coding. However, these databases are useful for economic purposes for hospitals and ambulatory services, which could be an argument in favour of the quality and exhaustiveness of data on the medicinal products and health care provided. The availability of data for a period of three years plus the current year constitutes a limit to the duration of follow-up of prospective studies, especially concerning medium-term or long-term adverse effects, such as those of hormone therapy. Some products, such as sildenafil or vacuum pumps, are not reimbursed. The database does not include any information on PCa stage, type of tumour or the severity of the disorders, in contrast with qualitative studies, and only allows analysis of treatments prescribed and reimbursed. PCa considered to be newly managed could also correspond to recurrences requiring further treatment, but a one- to two-year treatment-free period prior to inclusion was required. These patients were also required to have LTCD status for PCa granted before 2009. As already emphasized, outcomes based on health care consumption data may not reflect all complications experienced nor their severity, but this aspect must be considered case by case for each database [23,24]. The strengths of our observational study are that it was based on a very large, comprehensive population of men covered by the French national health insurance scheme and comprised comparisons with control groups. Given the differences in health care systems between Western countries, the results of this study cannot be directly extrapolated in other settings. In France, PCa incidence was estimated to be 71,000 cases for 2011 using data from regional cancer registries. Recently, a new estimation provided a lower incidence of 53,465 cases for 2009. National extrapolation of the 43,460 cases of PCa in 2009 identified by this study would give an incidence of 59,500 cases, close to the 2009 estimation.

Conclusions

In this population of men with treated or diagnosed PCa, we report, as expected, a high two-year survival rate and describe the frequencies of various PCa treatments. More importantly, we report a high frequency of men treated for adverse effects induced by PCa treatments, especially prostatectomy. These results can be used as a basis to provide patients with information about outcomes at the time of screening and diagnosis, and to choose treatments according to national guidelines and PCa clinical characteristics.

Abbreviations

PSA: Prostate-specific antigen; PCa: Prostate cancer; SNIIRAM: National health insurance information system (SNIIRAM); LTCD: Long-term chronic diseases; INSEE: National institute for statistics and economic studies; ICD10: International classification of diseases 10 revision; ATC: Anatomical therapeutic classification.

Competing interests

All authors declare that they have no competing financial interests. There was no specific funding for this study, which was conducted by the employees of the French national health insurance general scheme.

Authors' contributions

PT participated in the conception and design, data interpretation, manuscript drafting, SS participated in design, data analysis and interpretation. AFC, BL and FA participated in design and data interpretation. FP, JCT, EV, MV and BM participated in design, interpretation, manuscript validation and supervision. All authors have read and approved the final manuscript.

Acknowledgements

The authors would like to thank all participants in the study and colleagues from the statistical information department.

Author details

[1]National general health insurance scheme (Caisse Nationale d'Assurance Maladie des Travailleurs Salariés, CNAMTS), Paris, France. [2]Department of Urology, Tenon Hospital, Assistance Publique- Hôpitaux de Paris, 4 Rue de la Chine, 75020 Paris, France.

References

1. Lucia MS, Bokhoven AV: **Temporal changes in the pathologic assessment of prostate cancer.** *J Natl Cancer Inst Monogr* 2012, **45:**157–161.
2. Albertsen PC, Hanley JA, Fine J: **20-year outcomes following conservative management of clinically localized prostate cancer.** *JAMA* 2005, **293:**2095–2101.
3. Lu-Yao GL, Albertsen PC, Moore DF, Shih W, Lin Y, DiPaola RS, Barry MJ, Zietman A, O'Leary M, Walker-Corkery E, Yao SL: **Outcomes of localized prostate cancer following conservative management.** *JAMA* 2009, **302:**1202–1209.
4. Sandhu GS, Andriole GL: **Overdiagnosis of prostate cancer.** *J Natl Cancer Inst Monogr* 2012, **45:**146–151.
5. Schroder FH, Hugosson J, Roobol MJ, Schröder FH, Hugosson J, Roobol MJ, Tammela TL, Ciatto S, Nelen V, Kwiatkowski M, Lujan M, Lilja H, Zappa M, Denis LJ, Recker F, Berenguer A, Määttänen L, Bangma CH, Aus G, Villers A, Rebillard X, van der Kwast T, Blijenberg BG, Moss SM, de Koning HJ, Auvinen A, ERSPC Investigators: **Screening and prostate-cancer mortality in a randomised European study.** *N Engl J Med* 2009, **360:**1320–1328.
6. Andriole GL, Crawford ED, Grubb RL 3rd, Buys SS, Chia D, Church TR, Fouad MN, Isaacs C, Kvale PA, Reding DJ, Weissfeld JL, Yokochi LA, O'Brien B, Ragard LR, Clapp JD, Rathmell JM, Riley TL, Hsing AW, Izmirlian G, Pinsky PF, Kramer BS, Miller AB, Gohagan JK, Prorok PC, PLCO Project Team: **Prostate Cancer Screening in the Randomized Prostate, Lung, Colorectal, and Ovarian Cancer Screening Trial: Mortality Results after 13 Years of Follow-up.** *J Natl Cancer Inst* 2012, **104:**125–132.
7. Resnick MJ, Koyama T, Fan KH, Albertsen PC, Goodman M, Hamilton AS, Hoffman RM, Potosky AL, Stanford JL, Stroup AM, Van Horn RL, Penson DF: **Long-term functional outcomes after treatment for localized prostate cancer.** *N Engl J Med* 2013, **368:**436–445.
8. Smith DP, King MT, Egger S, Berry MP, Stricker PD, Cozzi P, Ward J, O'Connell DL, Armstrong BK: **Quality of life three years after diagnosis of localised prostate cancer: population based cohort study.** *BMJ* 2009, **339:**b4817.
9. Gore JL, Kwan L, Lee SP, Reiter RE, Litwin MS: **Survivorship beyond convalescence: 48-month quality-of-life outcomes after treatment for localized prostate cancer.** *J Natl Cancer Inst* 2009, **101:**888–892.
10. Sandler HM, Northouse L, Hembroff L, Lin X, Greenfield TK, Litwin MS, Saigal CS, Mahadevan A, Klein E, Kibel A, Pisters LL, Kuban D, Kaplan I, Wood D, Ciezki J, Shah N, Wei JT: **Quality of life and satisfaction with outcome among prostate-cancer survivors.** *N Engl J Med* 2008, **358:**1250–1261.
11. Potosky AL, Davis WW, Hoffman RM, Stanford JL, Stephenson RA, Penson DF, Harlan LC: **Five-year outcomes after prostatectomy or radiotherapy for prostate cancer: the prostate cancer outcomes study.** *J Natl Cancer Inst* 2004, **96:**1358–1367.
12. Johansson E, Steineck G, Holmberg L, Johansson JE, Nyberg T, Ruutu M, Bill-Axelson A, SPCG-4 Investigators: **Long-term quality-of-life outcomes after radical prostatectomy or watchful waiting: the Scandinavian Prostate Cancer Group-4 randomised trial.** *Lancet Oncol* 2011, **12:**891–899.
13. Kasperzyk JL, Shappley WV 3rd, Kenfield SA, Mucci LA, Kurth T, Ma J, Stampfer MJ, Sanda MG: **Watchful waiting and quality of life among prostate cancer survivors in the Physicians' Health Study.** *J Urol* 2011, **186:**1862–1867.
14. Tuppin P, de Roquefeuil L, Weill A, Ricordeau P, Merlière Y: **French national health insurance information system and the permanent beneficiaries sample.** *Rev Epidemiol Sante Publique* 2010, **58:**286–290.
15. Grosclaude P, Remontet L, Bélot A, Danzon A, Rasamimanana C, Bossard N: *Survie des personnes atteintes de cancer en France, 1989–2007 - Etude à partir des registres des cancers du réseau Francim.* Saint-Maurice: Institut de Veille Sanitaire; 2013. 412 p.
16. Epstein MM, Edgren G, Rider JR, Mucci LA, Adami HO: **Temporal trends in cause of death among Swedish and US men with prostate cancer.** *J Natl Cancer Inst* 2012, **104:**1335–1342.
17. Fang F, Keating NL, Mucci LA, Adami HO, Stampfer MJ, Valdimarsdóttir U, Fall K, Adami HO, Stampfer MJ, Valdimarsdóttir U, Fall K: **Immediate risk of suicide and cardiovascular death after a prostate cancer diagnosis: cohort study in the United States.** *J Natl Cancer Inst* 2010, **102:**307–314.
18. Delpierre C, Lamy S, Kelly-Irving M, Velten M, Tretarre B, Woronoff AS, Buemi A, Lapôtre-Ledoux B, Bara S, Guizard AV, Colonna M, Grosclaude P: **Life expectancy estimates as a key factor in over-treatment: the case of prostate cancer.** *Cancer Epidemiol* 2013, **37:**462–468.
19. Ladjevardi S, Sandblom G, Berglund A, Varenhorst E: **Tumour grade, treatment, and relative survival in a population-based cohort of men with potentially curable prostate cancer.** *Eur Urol* 2010, **57:**631–638.
20. Bauvin E, Soulié M, Ménégoz F, Macé-Lesec'h J, Buémi A, Velten M, Villers A, Grosclaude P: **Medical and non-medical determinants of prostate cancer management: a population-based study.** *Eur J Cancer* 2003, **39:**2364–2371.
21. Nam RK, Herschorn S, Loblaw DA, Liu Y, Klotz LH, Carr LK, Kodama RT, Stanimirovic A, Venkateswaran V, Saskin R, Law CH, Urbach DR, Narod SA: **Population based study of long-term rates of surgery for urinary incontinence after radical prostatectomy for prostate cancer.** *J Urol* 2012, **188:**502–506.
22. Kim PH, Pinheiro LC, Atoria CL, Eastham JA, Sandhu JS, Elkin EB: **Trends in the use of incontinence procedures after radical prostatectomy: a population based analysis.** *J Urol* 2013, **189:**602–608.
23. Tollefson MK, Gettman MT, Karnes RJ, Frank I: **Administrative data sets are inaccurate for assessing functional outcomes after radical prostatectomy.** *J Urol* 2011, **185:**1686–1690.
24. Cathcart P, Connolly S, Walton T, Costello AJ, Murphy DG: **Re: Administrative data sets are inaccurate for assessing functional outcomes after radical prostatectomy: M. K. Tollefson, M. T. Gettman, R. J. Karnes and I. Frank J Urol 2011; 185: 1686–1690.** *J Urol* 2011, **186:**2133–2134.

Cancer of the penis associated with HIV: a report of three cases presenting at the CHU cocody, ivory coast

P. G. Konan*, C. C. Vodi, A. H. Dekou, A. Fofana, E. E. Gowé and K. Manzan

Abstract

Background: We describe three cases of advanced penile cancer associated with HIV infection.

Case presentation: Advanced penile cancer associated with VIH infection were discovered in three patients aged respectively 47, 56 and 40. The prognosis was extremely poor. Two patients died without receiving any treatment and one patient was lost to follow-up after refusing all treatment proposed.

Conclusion: There appears to be a link between HIV infection and penile cancer with concomitant HIV infection worsening the prognosis of the disease.

Keywords: Cancer, Penis, HIV, AIDS

Introduction

Cancer of the penis is extremely rare. In Europe and the USA, the incidence of this form of cancer is estimated as 1.0 per 100,000 men [1]. The incidence varies between different countries worldwide with a higher incidence in Hispanic individuals, in Brazil and in Uganda [2]. Circumcision in the perinatal period or before puberty has a preventative role, but not circumcision carried out in adulthood. Early circumcision decreases the risk 3–5-fold [3], probably by improving local hygiene. Cancer of the penis is usually a disease of older men and its incidence increases with age. The peak in frequency occurs between 60 and 70 years of age [1, 2, 4]. In 95 % of cases penile tumours are squamous cell carcinomas [5]. Penile cancer may present as a flat or ulcerated exophytic papillary lesion, with the latter having a worse prognosis. The most common locations are the glans (48 % of cases) and the foreskin (25 % of cases). Penile cancer patients with advanced disease have a poor prognosis. Grades 2 and 3 disease, T3 stage and positive lymph nodes are adverse prognostic factors for cancer-specific survival in penile squamous cell carcinoma [6, 7]. In a study of eight patients with metastatic penile cancer, the longest and shortest survival times (from diagnosis of the primary cancer to death) were 16 years and 9 months, respectively [8]. Other, rarer histological forms of penile cancer such as melanoma and sarcoma may also occur [9].

There is a higher risk of penile cancer in patients with AIDS although it is not possible to conclude formally about a causal link with immunosuppression [10]. An increasing number of cases of penile cancer associated with HIV are being reported in the literature [1, 10, 11]. The aim of this report is to describe three cases of penile cancer associated with HIV that presented at the Urology Department of the CHU Cocody and to review the literature.

Case reports

Patient 1

A 47-year-old teacher was admitted to the CHU Cocody on the 10th February 2010 with a tumour of the glans evolving over a period of 2 years. He had been circumcised when he was 17-years-old, was married and was the father of 10 children. He has also participated in unprotected extra-marital sexual intercourse. One of his partners had died a year earlier without admission to a health centre; the cause of her death was unknown. He was a drinker and a smoker. His smoking habit was 20 packets-year.

* Correspondence: kpaulgerard@yahoo.com
Service d'Urologie, CHU de Cocody, Abidjan, Ivory Coast, Africa

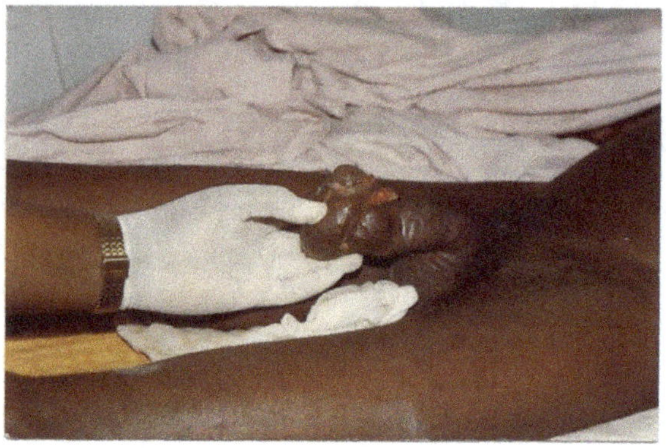
Fig. 1 Cancer of the penis (patient 1), view 1

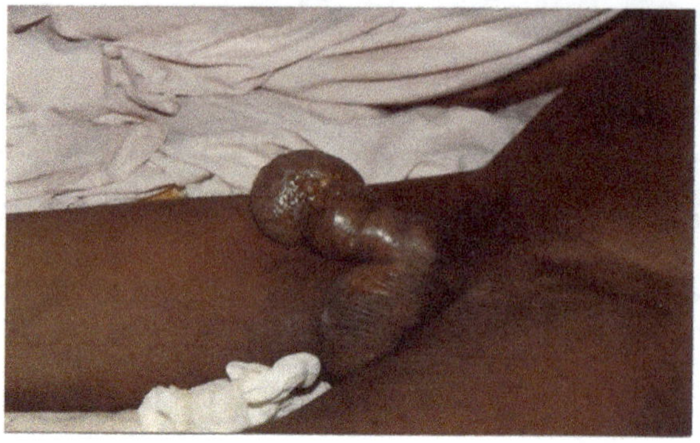
Fig. 3 Cancer of the penis (patient 1), view 3

On physical examination, his general state was good. A hard, painless tumour was noted on his penis infiltrating the glans and approximately 3 cm of the cavernous body (Figs. 1, 2, 3). There was no superficial inguinal lymphadenopathy. Micturition was normal (Fig. 1). A diagnostic incisional biopsy of the tumour with histological examination revealed a mature and invasive differentiated squamous cell carcinoma of the penis. No metastases were discovered. The tumour was TNM stage T4N0M0. No partial or complete penectomy was performed. Serology was positive for HIV-1. The patient was lost to follow-up after the announcement of his examination results and he did not receive any treatment.

Patient 2

A 56-year-old retired soldier was admitted to the urology emergency department of the CHU Cocody on the 12th November 2010 due to a change in his general state, spontaneous amputation of the glans, left suppurative inguinal adenitis and acute urinary retention. His first wife had died 4 years earlier from cervical cancer and he had remarried. He was the father of seven children. His previous history was unremarkable. He was a non-smoker. On physical examination he was in poor general state and spontaneous amputation of the glans was noted, with an irregular crateriform wound on the penis shaft and ureteral obstruction (Figs 4, 5, 6). Polycyclic, painful and ulcerated adenitis was noted in the left inguinal area. A globus vesicalis was found. He was febrile with a temperature of 39 °C. The wound was swabbed, a sample of urine was taken and a sub-pubic cystocatheter was inserted. The patient's condition improved with antibiotics and hydroelectrolyte rehydration. A diagnostic incisional biopsy of the lesion with histological examination revealed a mature and invasive differentiated squamous cell carcinoma of the penis. No metastases were discovered. The tumour was TNM stage T4N + M0. No partial or complete penectomy was performed. The patient was seropositive for HIV-1. He died 10 days after admission. The cause of death was unknown but was attributed to fulminant progression of the penile cancer associated with HIV/AIDS.

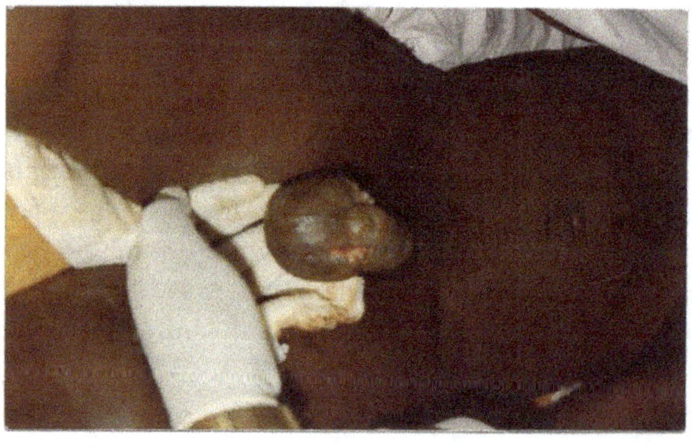
Fig. 2 Cancer of the penis (patient 1), view 2

Patient 3

A 40-year-old statistical engineer was admitted to the urology emergency department with paraphimosis on the 6th June 2011. He was not married and had no children. He had multiple partners and participated in

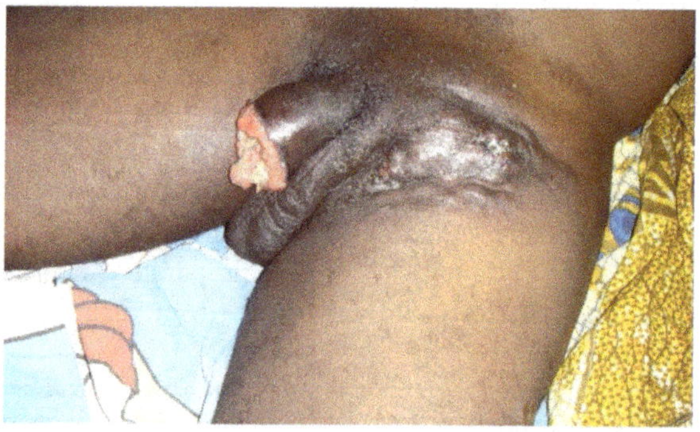
Fig. 4 Ulcerative carcinoma with spontaneous amputation of the glans and widespread inguinal adenopathy at the point of ulceration (patient 2)

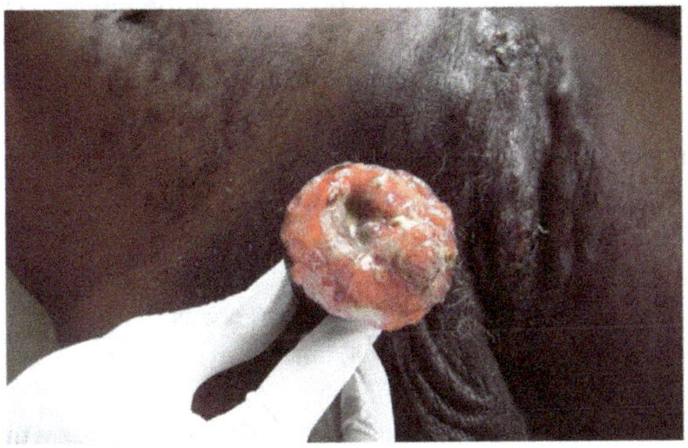

Fig. 5 Cancer of the penis (patient 2)

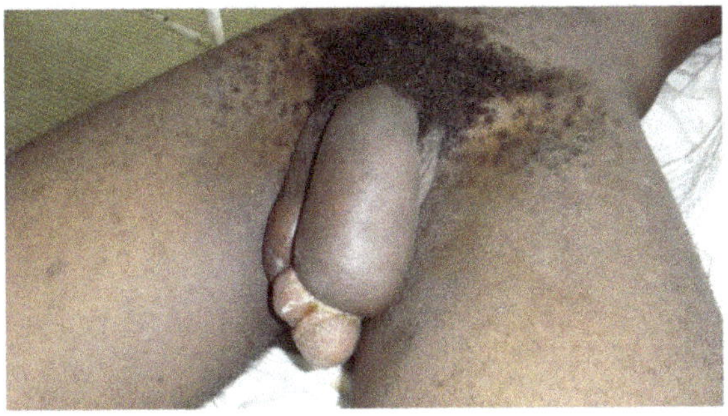

Fig. 7 Paraphimosis seen in patient 3 on admission, view 1

unprotected sexual intercourse. He was not diabetic or hypertensive and did not smoke or drink alcohol. On examination, strangulation of the glans by the foreskin was noted (Figs 7 and 8). On penile palpation, pain in the glans and induration of the penis were noted. His general state was good and he was apyrexial. He had no palpable inguinal lymphadenopathy. After an emergency circumcision, a biopsy was taken of the induration of the penis (Figs 9 and 10) and histological examination revealed a squamous cell carcinoma. He was seropositive for HIV-1. No metastases were discovered. The tumour was TNM stage T3N0M0. He died 15 days later without receiving any specific treatment. The cause of death was unknown but was attributed to fulminant progression of the penile cancer associated with HIV/AIDS.

Discussion

Cancer of the penis is extremely rare. In Europe it represents 0.4-0.6 % of cancers of men and its incidence is decreasing. In Finland, the incidence decreased from 1.4 per 100,000 between 1971 and 1975 to 1.0 per 100,000 between 1991 and 1995. In contrast, in some countries in Africa and Asia, the incidence of this disease is very high and represents 10–20 % of cancers of men [2]. In other regions of Africa, where few cases have been published or most data are old and scattered, the incidence of penile cancer appears to be low. Kebe et al. estimated the incidence of penile cancer as 2.66 % of cancers of men in the Ivory Coast in 1987 [12]. In Senegal, in 1997, the prevalence reported by Guèye et al. was less than 1 % [13]. Finally, in the Congo, only three cases have been reported, two by Bouya et al. [3] in 2000 and one case by Odzébé et al. [14] in 2010.

Cancer of the penis in the Western world is usually a disease of older men and the peak incidence of infiltrating lesions is found around 80 years of age [2, 15, 16]. In Africa, it occurs in younger subjects, aged <50 years. This was the case in our patients and in the reports of other African authors [1, 3, 14]. The mean age of our patients was 47.7 years. Although our cases are devastating examples of presentations of penile cancer, it has been reported that penile cancer can progress explosively in the setting of AIDS [11, 17].

The two most common locations of penile cancer are the glans (48 % of cases) and the foreskin (25 % of cases). The prognosis of squamous cell carcinoma depends on the depth of infiltration, its histological grade and the existence of blood, lymphatic or peripheral nervous system metastases [4, 6–8]. The main risk factors (Odds ratio >10) are maceration and a lack of local

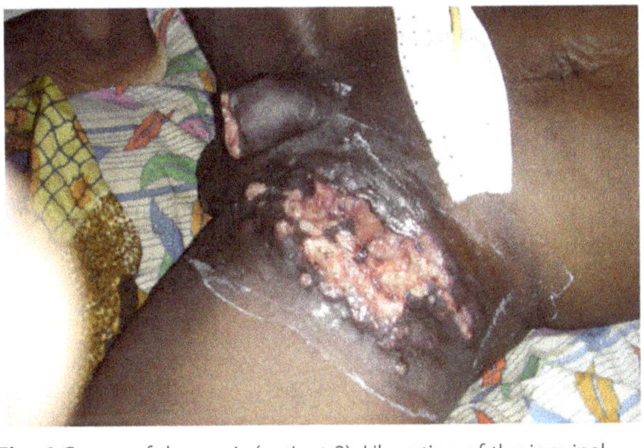

Fig. 6 Cancer of the penis (patient 2). Ulceration of the inguinal lymph nodes; urine drained by cystostomy

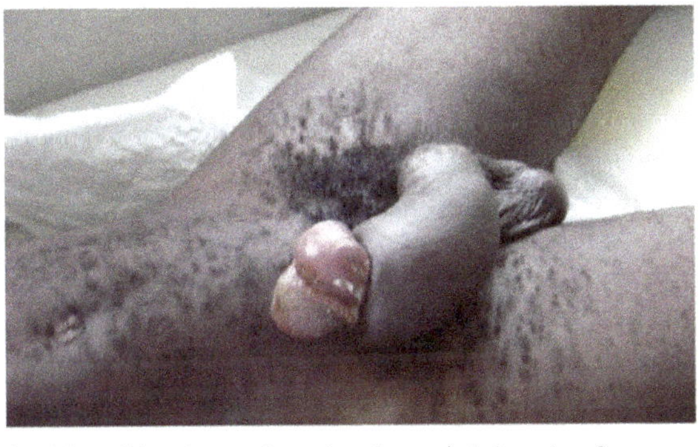

Fig. 8 Paraphimosis seen in patient 3 on admission, view 2

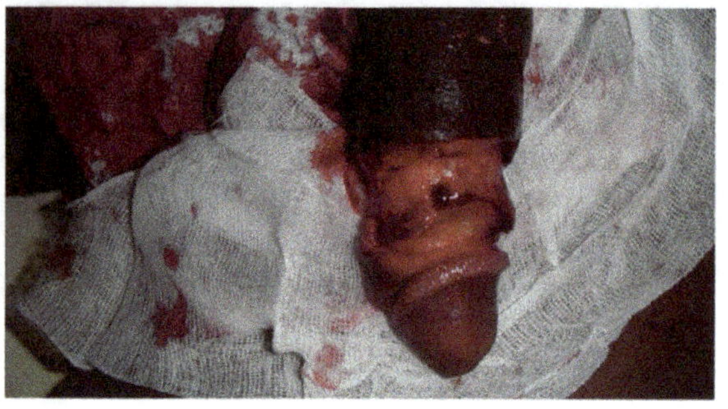

Fig. 9 Penile tumour in patient 3 seen after circumcision and biopsy for histological examination

hygiene as a result of phimosis [4]. This was the case with our third patient whose cancer was discovered during paraphimosis. Other risk factors including chronic inflammation (balanoposthitis, sclera-antrophic lichen), photochemotherapy with psoralen and ultraviolet A, sexual habits (multiple partners, early first sexual relationship) and a previous history of condylomas are associated with a 3–5-fold increase in risk of penile cancer [4]. All of these sexual risk factors were found in our patients.

Squamous cell carcinoma (95 %) occurs in two main forms with a different evolution and prognosis: exophytic papillary lesions which have a late and rare lymph node spread and ulcero-infiltrating lesions which are rapidly associated with lymph node invasion and have a poorer prognosis [18, 19]. Two other forms of cancer merit particular mention: basaloid squamous cell carcinoma affects younger men, is more aggressive and is often linked to human papilloma virus (HPV) and verrucous carcinoma, which is a locally malignant lesion only.

Prior infection with HPV (particularly HPV-16) has been recognised as a risk factor for penile cancer [19–21] and for lesions with a higher histological grade [20–22]. For some authors, infection with HIV is also considered as a risk factor for penile cancer [1]. Smoking is also a risk factor for penile cancer although two of our patients had never smoked. HIV is an aggravating factor for penile cancer and accelerates the progression of the disease. This was the case for two of our patients. The last patient died before the results of the biopsy. The second patient was lost to follow-up at a terminal stage of the disease with acute evolution of the lymph nodes towards ulceration and a rapidly fatal outcome.

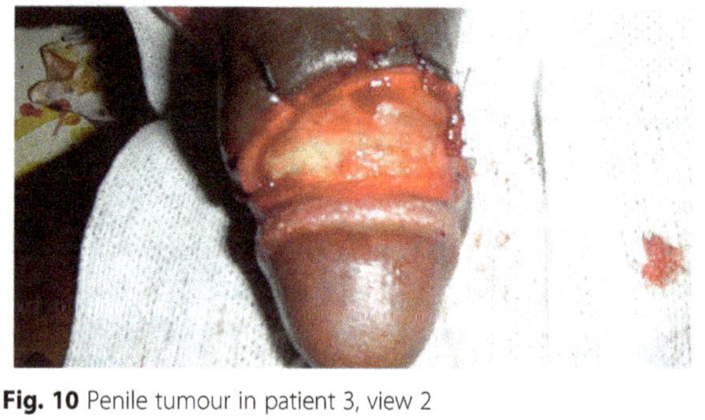

Fig. 10 Penile tumour in patient 3, view 2

The pathogenesis of malignant tumours linked to HIV infection is poorly understood but their association with specific viruses such as Epstein-Barr virus (EBV), human herpes virus type 8 (HHV8) and some HPVs has been clearly demonstrated. HIV could also play a direct role in tumourigenesis [5]. During the HIV epidemic it quickly became apparent that the risk of developing a malignant tumour is higher in subjects infected with HIV than in the general population [5]. Kaposi's sarcoma, early malignant non-Hodgkin's lymphoma (MNHL) of the central nervous system, systemic MNHL and invasive cancer of the cervix are events that classify AIDS in the CDC classification [5].

In industrialised countries, patients infected with HIV have a 2-fold higher risk of presenting with a malignant tumour (other than Kaposi's sarcoma or MNHL) than the general population of the same age and sex [5]. The risk of lung cancer is 2-fold higher in HIV infected individuals, probably due to higher tobacco consumption in this population [5]. A study carried out in the USA distinguished, among the cancers occurring in HIV-infected subjects, those linked with immunosuppression and those occurring at higher rates in this population due to other factors [5]. In addition to lung cancer, penile cancer, because of frequent HPV infection, and malignant tumours of soft tissue, due to probable errors in the differential diagnosis with Kaposi's sarcoma, were more frequent in the HIV-infected population without any relation to the degree of immunosuppression. In contrast, cancer of the lip and testicular seminoma appear to be linked to immunosuppression. Finally, skin cancers (other than melanoma) are more frequent during HIV infection [5]. However, the incidence of other cancers that are common in the general population, such as breast, prostate or colon cancer, is not increased in patients with immunosuppression. Furthermore, as can be observed in patients who have undergone organ transplantation, the improvement in immune status obtained by decreasing the intensity of immunosuppressive treatment may sometimes allow complete regression of the tumour lesions. Defining the current impact of HIV infection on invasive bowel cancer and anal cancer has important implications on an individual and collective level, as screening programmes for anal and genital tumours currently exist.

With the improvements in survival brought about by current and new antiretroviral treatments, it is probable that the risk of developing or dying from cancer during HIV infection will increase in the future [5]. The impact of antiretroviral treatments varies according to the type of tumour. After immune restoration, patients are no longer at risk of developing Kaposi's sarcoma. Conversely, patients with a previous history of severe immunosuppression remain at risk of developing MNHL. Unfortunately, adapted management of our patients was not possible due to the late discovery of their disease.

In conclusion, there appears to be a link between HIV and penile cancer with concomitant HIV infection worsening the prognosis of the disease. There is a benefit in systematically screening HIV-positive patients for penile cancer in order to discover tumours in the early stages which can be treated conservatively. Conversely, the discovery of cancer of the penis should systematically lead to screening for HIV.

Consent

Informed consent was obtained from patient for the publication of this report and any accompanying images.

Competing Interests

The authors declare that they have no competing interests.

Author contributions

All authors read and approved the final manuscript.

References

1. Bah OR, Guirassy S, Diallo AB, et al. Le carcinome épidermoïde de la verge: a propos de deux observations au CHU de Conakry. Afr J Urol. 2007;13:291–5.
2. Bastide C, Lesourd A. Épidémiologie des tumeurs malignes du pénis. Prog Urol. 2005;15:797–8.
3. Bouya PA, Lomina D. Deux observations congolaises de tumeur de la verge. Carcinol Prat Afrique. 2000;3:42–3.
4. Rigaud J, Avancès C, Camparo P, et les membres du CCAFU, et al. Recommandations en onco-urologie 2010: tumeurs malignes du pénis. Prog Urol. 2010;20 Suppl 4:S279–S89.
5. Comité de Cancérologie de l'Association Française d'Urologie. Recommandations 2004 en onco-urologie. Prog Urol. 2004;41:869–1041.
6. Burt LM, Shrieve DC, Tward JD. Stage presentation, care patterns, and treatment outcomes for squamous cell carcinoma of the penis. Int J Radiat Oncol Biol Phys. 2014;88:94–100.
7. Moses KA, Winer A, Sfakianos JP, et al. Contemporary management of penile cancer: greater than 15 year MSKCC experience. Can J Urol. 2014;21:7201–6.
8. Zhang K, Da J, Yao HJ, et al. Metastatic tumors of the penis: a report of 8 cases and review of the literature. Medicine (Baltimore). 2015;94, e132.
9. Mottet N, Avances C, Bastide C, et al. Tumeurs du pénis. Prog Urol. 2007;17:1049–61.
10. Launay O, Guillevin L. Épidémiologie des tumeurs malignes associées à l'infection par le VIH. Bull Cancer. 2003;90:387–92.
11. Théodore C, Androulakis N, Spatz A, et al. An explosive course of squamous cell penile cancer in an AIDS patient. Ann Oncol. 2002;13:475–9.
12. Kebe M, Leguyader A, Allangba K, et al. Le cancer de la verge en Côte d'Ivoire: aspects épidémiologiques et cliniques et prophylactiques à propos de 99 cas observés en 20 ans. Chirurgie. 1987;113:437–43.
13. Guèye SM, Diagne BA, Ba M, et al. Le cancer de la verge. Aspects épidémiologiques et problèmes thérapeutiques au Sénégal. J Urol. 1992;98:159–61.
14. Odzébé AWS, Bouya PA, Nkoua Mbon JB, et al. Le cancer de la verge: à propos d'un cas et revue de la littérature. Andrologie. 2010;20:273–5.
15. Frisch M, Biggar RJ, Engels EA, et al. Association of cancer with AIDS-related immunosuppression in adults for the AIDS-cancer match registry study group. JAMA. 2001;285:1736–45.
16. Marconnet L, Bouchot O, Culine S, et les membres du CCAFU-OGE, et al. Prise en charge ganglionnaire dans le carcinome épidermoïde du pénis : revue de la littérature par le comité de cancérologie de l'Association française d'urologie-groupe organes génitaux externes (CCAFU-OGE). Prog Urol. 2010;20:332–42.
17. Aboulafia DM, Gibbons R. Penile cancer and human papilloma virus (HPV) in a human immunodeficiency virus (HIV)-infected patient. Cancer Invest. 2001;19:266–72.
18. Lesourd A. Anatomo-pathologie des tumeurs malignes du pénis. Prog Urol. 2005;15:801–4.
19. Bissuel F, Sarrouy J, Stegmann-Planchard S, et al. Importance du dépistage systématique des cancers péniens liés au papillomavirus humain chez les patients infectés par le VIH. Med Mal Infect. 2011;41:76–8.
20. Cubilla AL, Lloveras B, Alejo M, et al. The basaloid cell is the best tissue marker for human papillomavirus in invasive penile squamous cell carcinoma: a study of 202 cases from Paraguay. Am J Surg Pathol. 2010;34:104–14.
21. Bezerra SM, Chaux A, Ball MW, et al. Human papillomavirus infection and immunohistochemical p16(INK4a) expression as predictors of outcome in penile squamous cell carcinomas. Hum Pathol. 2015;46:532–40.
22. Nascimento PS, Ornellas AA, Campos MM, et al. Déséquilibre de Bax, Bcl-2, et infection par HPV dans les tumeurs du pénis et les tissus adjacents. Prog Urol. 2004;14:353–9.

8

Site-dependent and interindividual variations in Denonvilliers' fascia: a histological study using donated elderly male cadavers

Kuniyasu Muraoka[1], Nobuyuki Hinata[2], Shuichi Morizane[1], Masashi Honda[1], Takehiro Sejima[1], Gen Murakami[3], Ashutosh K Tewari[4] and Atsushi Takenaka[1*]

Abstract

Background: Site-dependent and interindividual histological differences in Denonvilliers' fascia (DF) are not well understood. This study aimed to examine site-dependent and interindividual differences in DF and to determine whether changes in the current approach to radical prostatectomy are warranted in light of these histological findings.

Methods: Twenty-five donated male cadavers (age range, 72–95 years) were examined. These cadavers had been donated to Sapporo Medical University for research and education on human anatomy. Their use for research was approved by the university ethics committee. Horizontal sections (15 cadavers) or sagittal sections (10 cadavers) were prepared at intervals of 2–5 mm for hematoxylin and eosin staining. Elastic–Masson staining and immunohistochemical staining were also performed, using mouse monoclonal anti-human alpha-smooth muscle actin to stain connective tissues and mouse monoclonal anti-human S100 protein to stain nerves.

Results: We observed that DF consisted of disorderly, loose connective tissue and structures resembling "leaves", which were interlacing and adjacent to each other, actually representing elastic or smooth muscle fibers. Variations in DF were observed in the following: 1) configuration of multiple leaves, including clear, unclear, or fragmented behind the body and tips of the seminal vesicles, depending on the site; 2) connection with the lateral pelvic fascia at the posterolateral angle of the prostate posterior to the neurovascular bundles, being clear, unclear, or absent; 3) all or most leaves of DF fused with the prostatic capsule near the base of the seminal vesicles, and periprostatic nerves were embedded in the leaves at the fusion site; and 4) some DF leaves fused with the prostatic capsule anteriorly and/or the fascia propria of the rectum posteriorly.

Conclusions: Site-dependent and interindividual variations in DF were observed in donated elderly male cadavers. All or most DF leaves are fused with the prostatic capsule near the base of the seminal vesicles and some DF leaves are fused with the fascia propria of the rectum posterior. Based on our results, surgeons should be aware of variations and search for them to create a suitable dissection plane to avoid iatrogenic positive margins and rectal injury.

Keywords: Denonvilliers' fascia, Fascia propria of the rectum, Neurovascular bundle, Prostatic capsule, Prostate, Robot-assisted radical prostatectomy

* Correspondence: atake@med.tottori-u.ac.jp
[1]Division of Urology, Department of Surgery, Tottori University Faculty of Medicine, Yonago 683-8504, Japan
Full list of author information is available at the end of the article

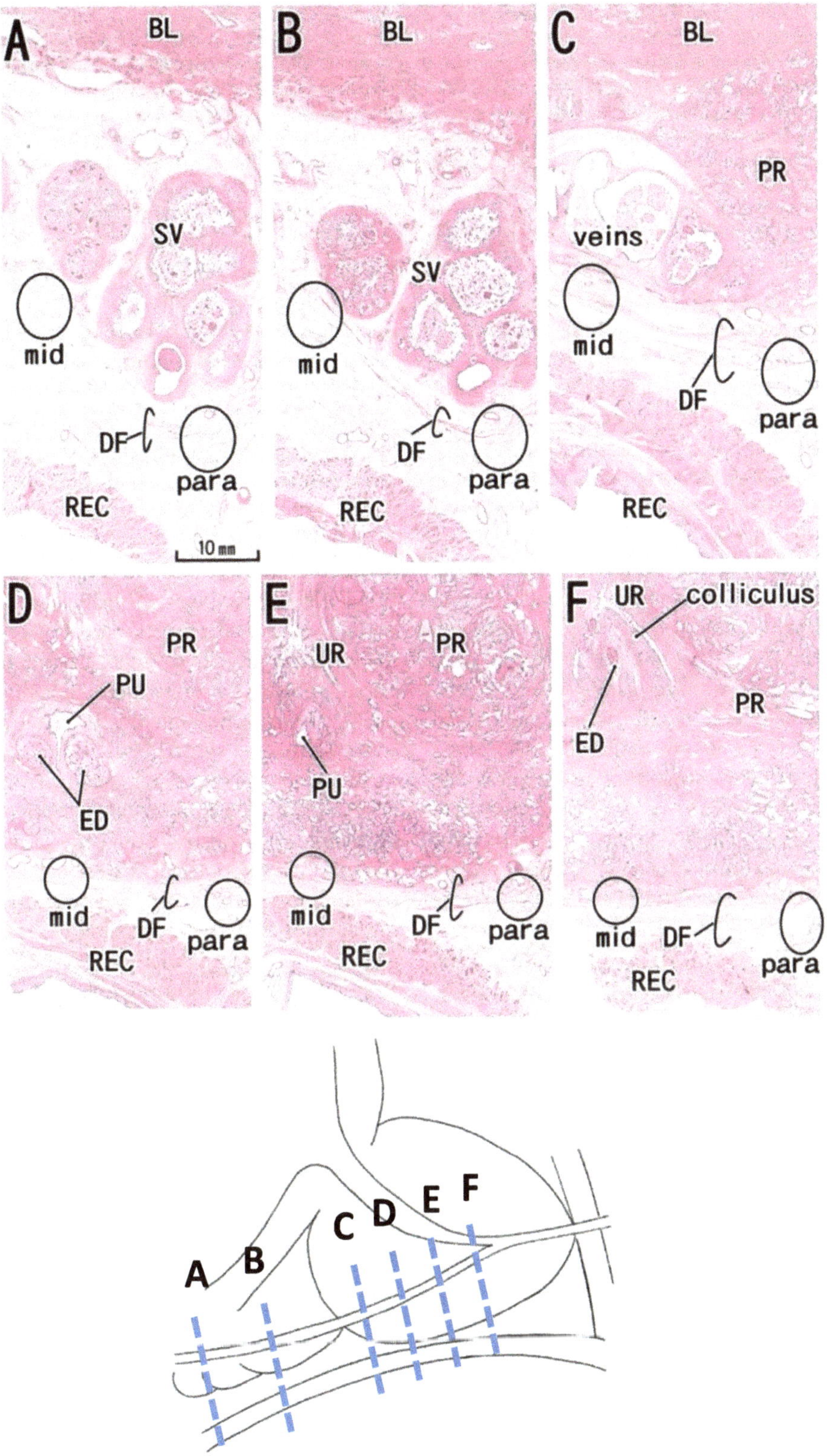

Figure 1 (See legend on next page.)

(See figure on previous page.)

Figure 1 Site-dependent difference in Denonvilliers' fascia in horizontal sections from a 90-year-old man. Panel **A (F)** displays the most superior (inferior) level in the figure. Intervals between panels are 3 mm **(A–B)**, 13 mm **(B–C)**, 11 mm **(C–D, D–E)**, and 6 mm **(E–F)**. Denonvilliers' fascia (DF) shows a multiple-leaf configuration at all levels and sites. In the midsagittal areas (circle with "mid"), the fascia is unclear or fragmented in panels **A**, **B**, and **D**, while in the parasagittal areas (circle with "para"), DF is most evident in panels **B**, **C**, and **E**. The fascia thus appears more clearly identifiable in the lateral sites than in medial sites. The site more lateral to this figure is shown in Figure **2C** (near panel **B**) and Figure **2D** (near panel **E**). All panels were prepared at the same magnification (scale bar is in panel **A**). BL; bladder; ED: ejaculatory duct; PR: prostate; PU: prostatic utricle; REC: rectum; SV: seminal vesicle; UR: urethra.

Background

Since Charles-Pierre Denonvilliers first discovered the firm, membranous structure between the rectum and prostate or bladder in 1836, now called "Denonvilliers' fascia" (DF), the origin of DF has remained controversial. The most widely accepted theory is that DF represents fusion of the embryonic peritoneum of the retrovesical cul-de-sac [1,2]. Disorderly, loose connective tissue is present between the cul-de-sac and the rectourethralis muscle (RUM), with a tight, thick membrane that includes smooth muscle fibers between the cul-de-sac and the posterior aspect of the prostate near the base of the seminal vesicle [3]. DF is often fused with the prostatic capsule at the center of the posterior prostatic surface [4-6]. DF is not well adhered to the prostatic capsule toward the posterolateral aspect of the prostate. The space between DF and this capsule is filled by areolar tissue and the neurovascular bundle (NVB) [5-7]. Costello et al. [8] demonstrated plexus- or mesh-like nerves extending along the posterior aspect of the prostate after removal of DF using cadaveric dissection. Laterally, DF becomes continuous with the "pararectal fascia" posteriorly and the "lateral pelvic fascia" (LPF) anteriorly.

DF has been used as a surgical landmark during intrapelvic surgery for many years, and is one of the major areas of interest for urological surgeons for cancer control and functional preservation. Since the operative procedure for robot-assisted radical prostatectomy (RARP) was established by Menon et al. [9], it has widely expanded is use. RARP provides a precise, highly magnified view and less venous oozing, leading to a better anatomical understanding of fine membranous structures.

To the best of our knowledge, site-dependent and interindividual histological differences in DF have not previously been investigated. Therefore, this study aimed to examine site-dependent and interindividual differences in DF among 25 donated male cadavers and to determine whether changes in the current approach to radical prostatectomy are warranted in light of these histological findings. In the present study, DF was defined as a structure between the rectum and prostate, bladder, or seminal vesicles.

Methods

Twenty-five donated male cadavers (mean age at death, 85 years; range, 72–95 years) were examined. None of the patients had undergone abdominal surgery based on the medical records and macroscopic observations after opening the abdominopelvic cavity. These cadavers had been donated to Sapporo Medical University for research and education on human anatomy. Their use for research was approved by Sapporo Medical University ethics committee and all the participants provided written informed consent in their lifetime. Each donated cadaver had been fixed by arterial perfusion of 10% v/v formalin solution and stored in 50% v/v ethanol solution for more than 3 months. From each cadaver, one large tissue block including the bladder neck, seminal vesicles, membranous urethra, prostate, and rectal anterior wall, as well as connective tissue around these viscera, was obtained. After trimming the tissue block, routine procedures for paraffin-embedded histological examination were performed. Horizontal sections (15 cadavers) or sagittal sections (10 cadavers) were prepared at 2- to 5-mm intervals for hematoxylin and eosin staining (HE) and immunohistochemistry. When the prostate was large, the superior and inferior halves were included in two separate paraffin blocks. From each cadaver, 20–80 HE-stained and unstained sections were prepared.

Based on observations of HE-stained sections, some sections were used for immunohistochemistry and elastic–Masson staining (a variation of Masson–Goldner staining) [10,11]. The primary antibodies that were used to identify connective tissues and nerves were mouse monoclonal anti-human alpha-smooth muscle actin (1:100, Dako M0851; Dako, Glostrup, Denmark) and mouse monoclonal anti-human S100 protein (1:200 dilution, Dako Z0311; Dako), respectively. The smooth muscle antibody yields positive results not only for any smooth muscle, but also for vascular endothelium [12].

The study was performed in accordance with the provisions of the Declaration of Helsinki 1995 (as revised in Edinburgh 2000).

Results

Basic structure of DF

DF was composed of collagen, elastic, and smooth muscle fibers in all cases. There were structures resembling "leaves", actually representing elastic or smooth muscle fibers, in DF. DF consisted of a configuration of multiple leaves, mainly anteriorly, and a disorderly loose

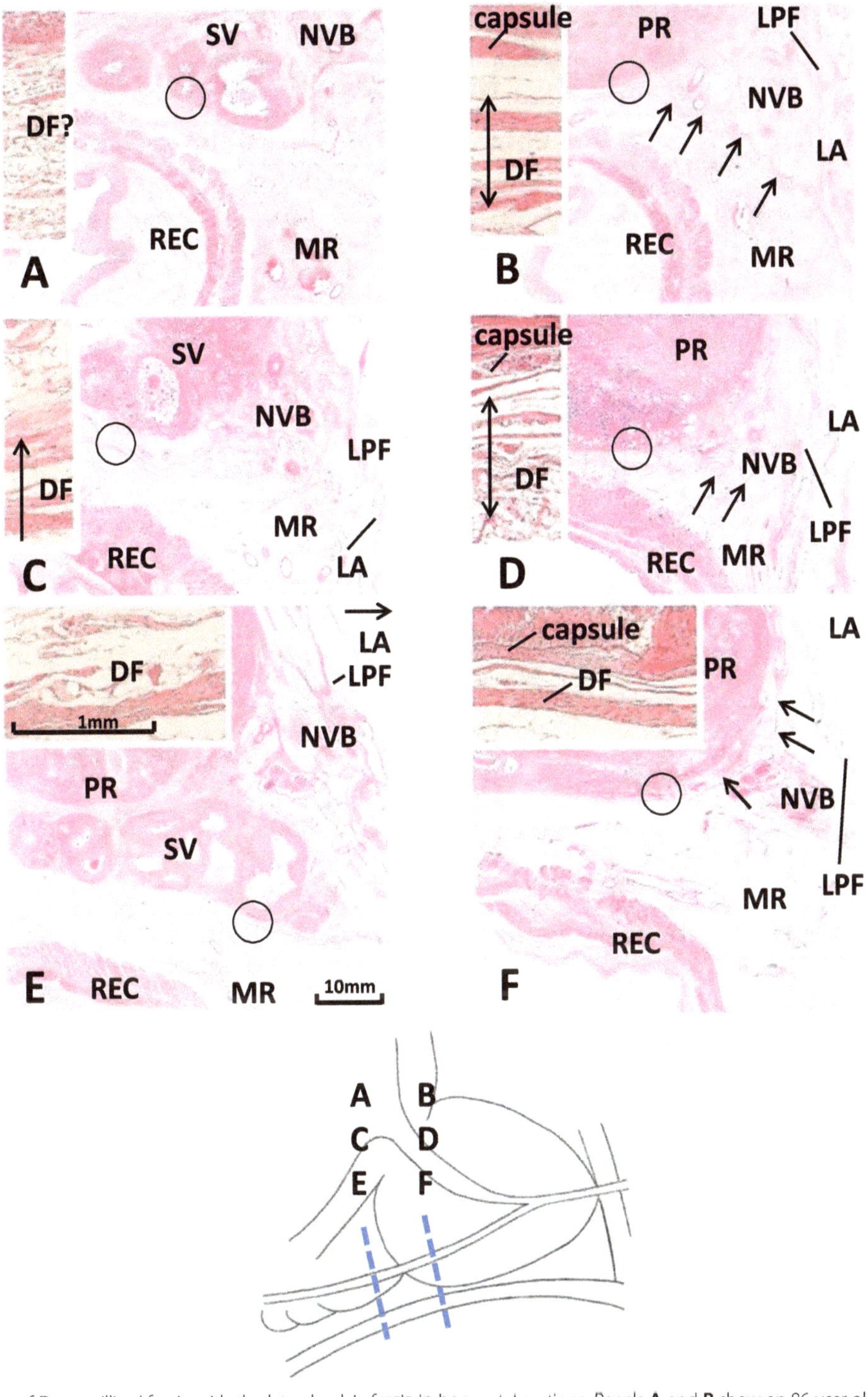

Figure 2 Connection of Denonvilliers' fascia with the lateral pelvic fascia in horizontal sections. Panels **A** and **B** show an 86-year-old man. Panels **C** and **D** show a 90-year-old man. Panels **E** and **F** show an 83-year-old man. The right- and left-hand side columns display Denonvilliers' fascia (DF) behind the base of the seminal vesicle (SV) and prostate (PR), respectively. The insert of each panel shows a higher magnification view of a circle in the panel. In panel **B**, DF (arrows) extends laterally in the posterior side of the neurovascular bundle (NVB) to connect with the lateral pelvic fascia (LPF). In panel **D**, the fascia can be seen (arrows), but the connection is not clear. In panel **F**, the fascia does not extend laterally, but extends anteriorly (arrows) instead along the prostatic capsule. All panels (or all inserts) were prepared at the same magnification (scale bars are in panel **E** and its insert). In the six inserts, DF shows a multiple-leaf configuration in the first and second specimens (86- and 90-year-old men), while the fascia is composed of a thick leaf and other thin leaves in the third specimen (83-year-old man). The multiple-leaf configuration is unclear in the insert of panel **A**. LA: levator ani muscle; LPF: lateral pelvic fascia; MR: mesorectum; REC: rectum.

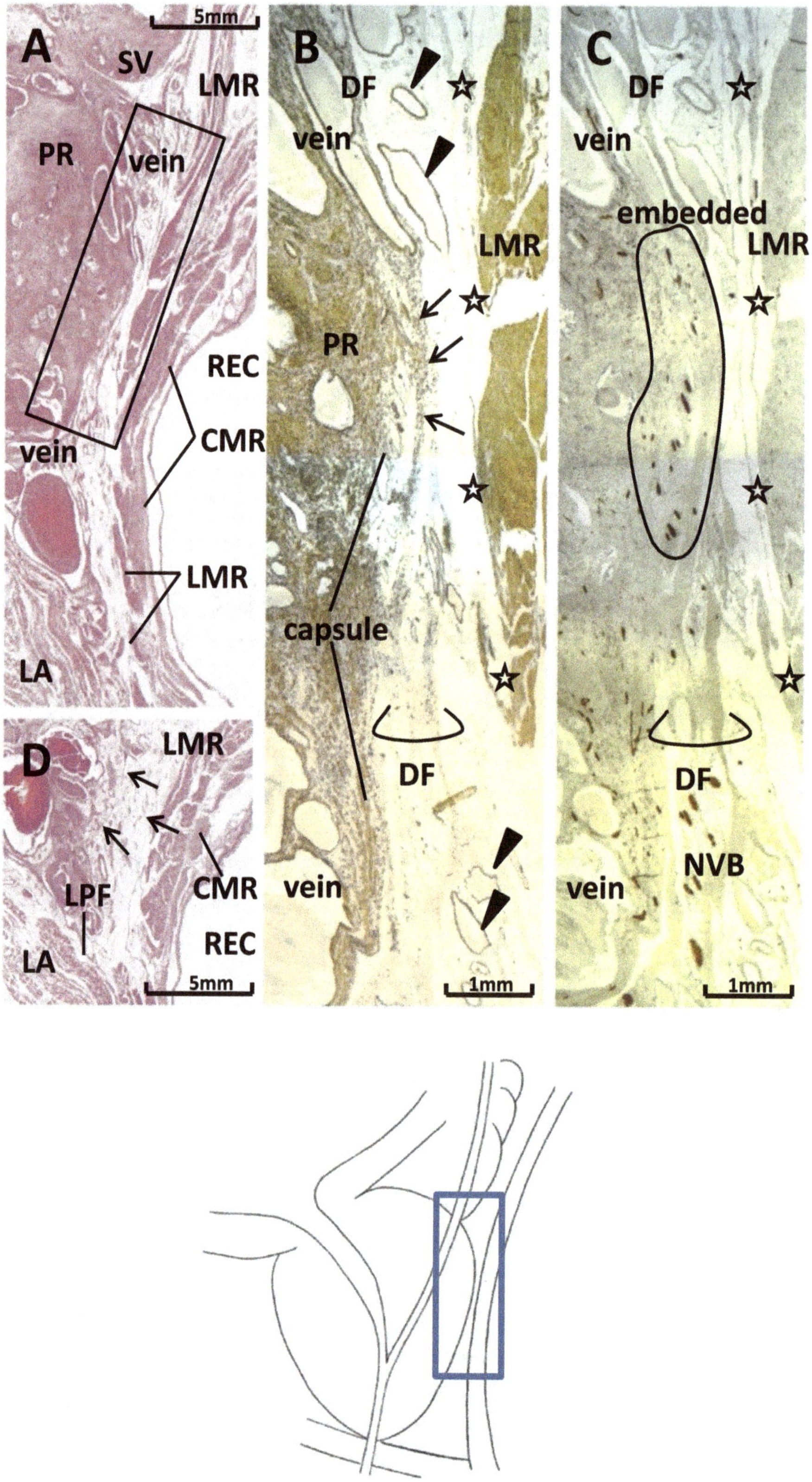

Figure 3 (See legend on next page.)

(See figure on previous page.)
Figure 3 Fascial complex between Denonvilliers' fascia and the prostatic capsule in sagittal sections. Sections from a 75-year-old man are shown. Panel **A** (HE staining) displays topographical anatomy around Denonvilliers' fascia (DF) at the 2- to 3-o'clock position of the rectum. The levator ani muscle (LA) approaches the rectum (REC). Panel **B** (Panel **C**), corresponding to a square in panel **A**, shows immunohistochemistry for smooth muscles (for all nerves). DF, containing smooth muscles, comprises 3–4 leaves (lower part of panel **B**), but the leaves are bundled to fuse with the prostatic capsule (capsule) in the upper part of the panel (arrows). At the fusion area (panel **C**), periprostatic nerves are embedded in the fascial complex between DF and the prostatic capsule (encircled). Stars indicate a candidate for the fascia propria of the rectum. The DAKO antibody that was applied for smooth muscles also strongly stains vascular endothelium (arrowheads). In panel **D**, 4 mm lateral to the area shown in panel **A**, fascial leaves (arrows) become thinner and fewer in number. CMR and LMR: circular and longitudinal muscle layers of the rectum; LP: lateral pelvic fascia; NVB: neurovascular bundle at the posterolateral corner of the prostate; PR: prostate; SV: seminal vesicle.

connective tissue, mainly posteriorly. Furthermore, although the multiple-leaf configuration appeared to be a firm membranous structure, it was actually recognized as a fascicle of multiple leaves with interlacing branches.

Findings of DF from the seminal vesicle to the middle of the prostate in horizontal sections

In contrast to sagittal sections, horizontal sections showed the presence of multiple leaves of DF, and two to eight leaves were consistently observed (Figures 1 and 2). Because of the multiple leaves, we found it difficult to determine whether the leaves were "thick or thin". However, when we compared these sections with those from a specimen from a 90-year-old man, DF leaves tended to be more clearly observed behind the middle of the seminal vesicles (Figure 1B) and near the base of the seminal vesicles (Figure 1C). In contrast, in sites behind the superior half of the seminal vesicles, DF leaves tended to be unclear or fragmented (Figure 1A) in the midsagittal areas.

When individual variations in DF were investigated, clear variation was observed in DF morphology behind the seminal vesicles and at the posterolateral angle of the prostate. With regard to the multiple-leaf configuration of DF behind the base of the seminal vesicles, some were clear (Figure 2C, E), and some were unclear (Figure 2A). DF leaves extended to the posterior side of the NVB to connect with the LPF in seven cadavers (Figure 2B), but the connection was unclear (Figure 2D) or absent (Figure 2F) in eight cadavers. In the seven cadavers in which a lateral fascial connection was evident on the posterolateral side of the prostate, DF usually became unclear on the posterolateral side of the seminal vesicles. In the eight cadavers with an unclear or absent connection, DF extended anteriorly to pass through or disperse in the NVB, and some leaves joined the capsule covering the lateral aspect of the prostate. The mesorectal loose tissue thus appeared to be continuous with the NVB (Figure 2F). Among multiple leaves, a single leaf was sometimes thick at a limited area or level (Figure 2E, F), although quantitative evaluation was difficult because of the use of semiserial sections for observations.

Findings of DF from the middle of the prostate to the apex in sagittal sections

Even when a monolayer configuration appeared in one or several sections, this was restricted to a small area, and DF actually comprised multiple leaves and loose connective tissue (Figures 3 and 4). Notably, when the fascial space between the prostate and rectum was narrower than 3 mm without interposition of the mesorectal loose tissues at or near the midsagittal line, all or most DF leaves were bundled to fuse with the prostatic capsule (Figure 3A, B). The fusion site was equivalent near the base of the seminal vesicles.

Periprostatic nerves ran between multiple leaves, and all or most periprostatic nerves appeared embedded in the fascial complex between DF leaves and the prostatic capsule (i.e., at the fusion site) (Figure 3C). These embedded nerves were not observed in all areas behind the prostate, but were mostly restricted within a region associated with DF midline adherence to the capsule of 10 mm wide × 5 mm high at maximum.

Elastic fibers were rich throughout the entire capsule, the fascia propria of the rectum, and DF (Figure 4A, insert). In the multiple leaves of DF, some leaves were fused with the prostatic capsule (Figures 3B and 4B) and/or the fascia propria of the rectum (Figure 4B). The latter connection was particularly evident in sagittal sections, because the fascia propria of the rectum became evident along the external longitudinal smooth muscles of the rectum.

Leaves of DF were dispersed around the venous plexus on the superior side of the RUM (Figures 3A and 4A), while parts of the longitudinal muscle layer of the rectum were dispersed into the latter smooth muscle mass. At least three specimens showed parts of the DF ending at the RUM (figure not shown). Inferiorly, DF reached a level behind the rhabdosphincter area, but the venous plexus consistently interposed between the striated muscle and the inferior end of DF (Figure 4A). The connection of DF with the LPF was difficult to observe in sagittal sections because of the venous plexus interposed in the lateral site, including the levator ani muscle (Figure 3).

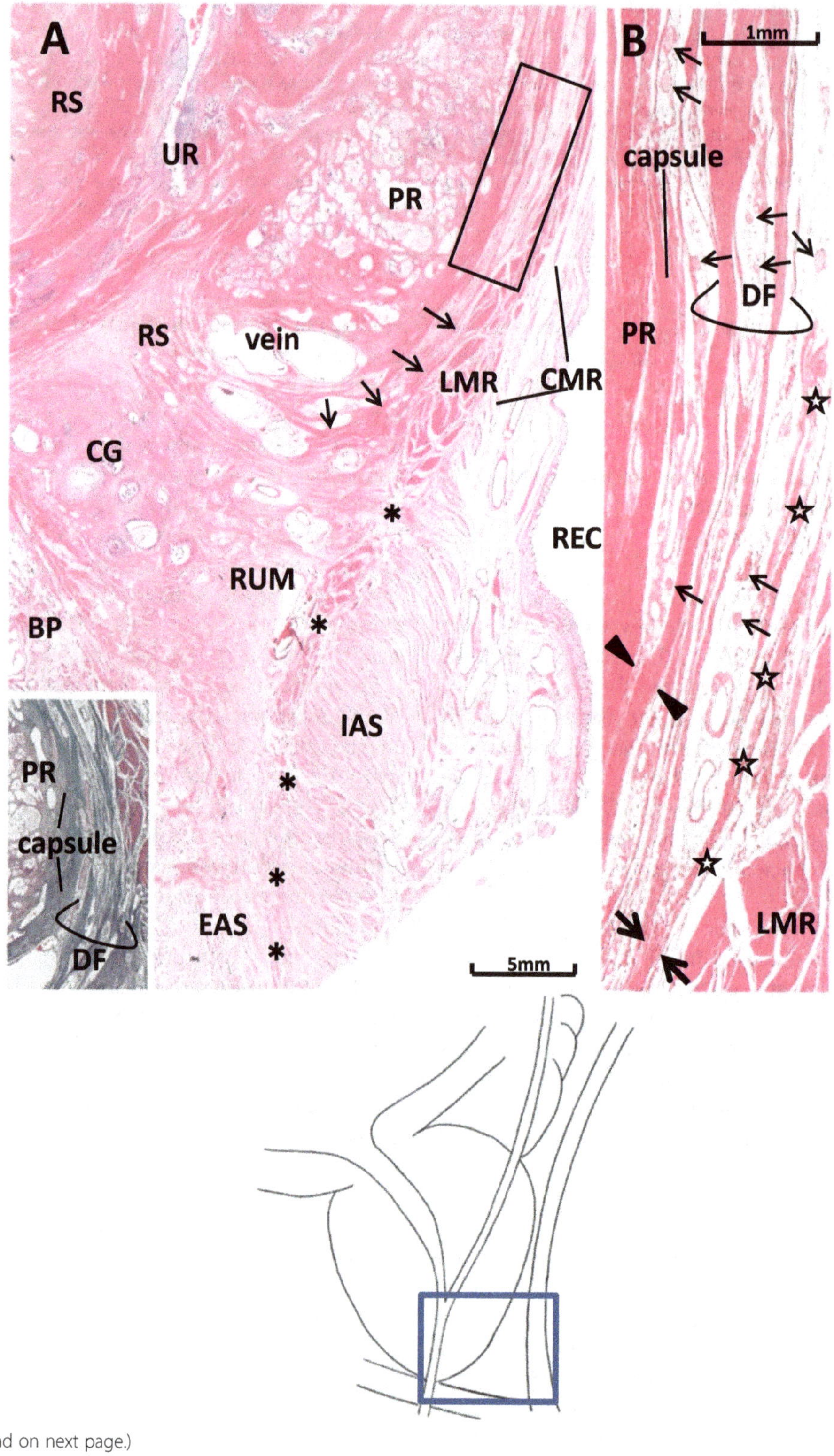

Figure 4 (See legend on next page.)

(See figure on previous page.)

Figure 4 Multiple-leaf configuration of Denonvilliers' fascia in a midsagittal section from a 79-year-old man. Panel **A** displays topographical anatomy around Denonvilliers' fascia (DF). The longitudinal muscle layer of the rectum (LMR) extends inferiorly to continue to the conjoint muscle coat or longitudinal anal muscle (asterisks). The leaves of DF (arrow) are dispersed in a venous plexus (veins) without ending at the rectourethralis muscle (RUM) in this specimen. The insert in the panel **A** (elastic–Masson staining; a section near panel **A**) shows rich content of elastic fibers (black color) in the prostatic capsule, DF, and fascia propria of the rectum. Panel **B**, corresponding to the rectangle in panel **A**, shows the multiple-leaf configuration of DF. Periprostatic nerves (thin arrows) are scattered between the fascial leaves. A thick leaf of the fascia is fused with the prostatic capsule (capsule) at the site indicated by arrowheads, while the other leaf merges with the fascia propria of the rectum (stars) at a site indicated by thick arrows. BP: bulbus penis; CG: Cowper's gland, CMR: circular muscle layer of the rectum; EAS: external anal sphincter; IAS: internal anal sphincter; PR: prostate; REC: rectum; RS: rhabdosphincter area; UR: urethra.

Discussion

The present study showed that the configuration of the firm membranous structure of DF consistently involved multiple leaves. Even when a monolayer configuration appeared, this was restricted to a small area and actually comprised a thick leaf and other thin leaves. As Bertrand et al. [13] suggested, DF variations appeared to depend on differences in mechanical stress from either or both the prostate and rectum. Site-dependent and interindividual variations in DF were also observed, including the following: 1) variations in configuration behind the seminal vesicles; 2) variations in the connection with the LPF at the posterolateral angle of the prostate; 3) fusion of all or most DF leaves with the prostatic capsule near the base of the seminal vesicles; and 4) fusion of some DF leaves with the prostatic capsule anteriorly and/or the fascia propria of the rectum posteriorly.

Between the seminal vesicles and rectum, some DF leaves were clearly evident, while others were unclear or fragmented. During RARP, after bladder neck transection and dissection of the seminal vesicles and vas deferens, the connective tissue is present in the dorsum of the seminal vesicles and vas deferens. When the seminal vesicles, vas deferens, and prostate are pulled ventrally, DF is recognized as a membranous structure between the prostate and the rectum by its tension, irrespective of whether the leaves of the DF are clear or unclear histologically (Figure 5A).

Clear variation in DF morphology was also observed in the connection with the LPF at the posterolateral angle of the prostate on the posterior side of the NVB, as either clear, unclear, or absent. When leaves connecting the DF and LPF were unclear or absent, the mesorectal loose tissue appeared continuous with the NVB. Periprostatic nerves were not restricted at the posterolateral corner of the prostate, but their distribution extended medio-posteriorly in the DF [7,14]. These findings might be useful for understanding that the NVB is not restricted and that colorectal surgeons should pay careful attention to the anterior dissection plane of the rectum during total mesorectal excision.

Our study showed that all or most DF leaves were fused with the prostatic capsule near the base of the seminal vesicles. Notably, when the fascial space between the prostate and rectum was narrower without interposed mesorectal loose tissues at or near the midsagittal line, all or most DF leaves were fused with the prostatic capsule. Therefore, the dissection plane between the prostatic capsule and DF does not exist at the fusion site, because of the fascial complex between DF leaves and the prostatic capsule. Subsequently, periprostatic nerves were embedded in the combined capsule in a small area. Villers et al. [5] reported that muscular bundles and collagenous fibers of DF behind the vas deferens blend with central zone stroma and the ejaculatory duct sheath at the junction of the base of the prostate with the seminal vesicles and vas deferens. Kiyoshima et al. [6] reported that, in 79 surgically obtained specimens, DF was fused with the prostatic capsule at the center of the prostatic posterior aspect in 97% of cases. Hisasue et al. [15] reported the distribution of neuronal nitric oxide synthase positive nerve fibers, which are candidates for parasympathetic pro-erectile nerves [16]. They found that the distribution of these nerve fibers at 5- to 6-o'clock positions on the base of the prostate was 13.4% in the same hemisphere slice around the prostate in 23 specimens from non-nerve-sparing radical prostatectomy. However, what these nerves that are embedded in the fusion site innervate remains unclear. During RARP, DF is recognized as a membranous structure between the prostate and rectum by tension when pulling the seminal vesicles, vas deferens, and prostate ventrally. Simultaneously, the fusion site with DF and the prostatic capsule near the seminal vesicle-prostate junction are visible. DF between the seminal vesicles and rectum should first be cut at the midline to avoid entering the prostatic capsule. After this incision, a mesh-like structure behind the posterior aspect of the prostate corresponds with loose connective tissue and multiple leaves, and a flexible approach to the apex is easily found [17,18]. In cases of intra- or interfascial dissection, the dissection plane should be as close to the prostate as possible to avoid iatrogenic positive margins. Therefore, double cutting of DF while avoiding the fusion site is necessary to perform nerve-sparing procedures [19]. In cases of extrafascial dissection,

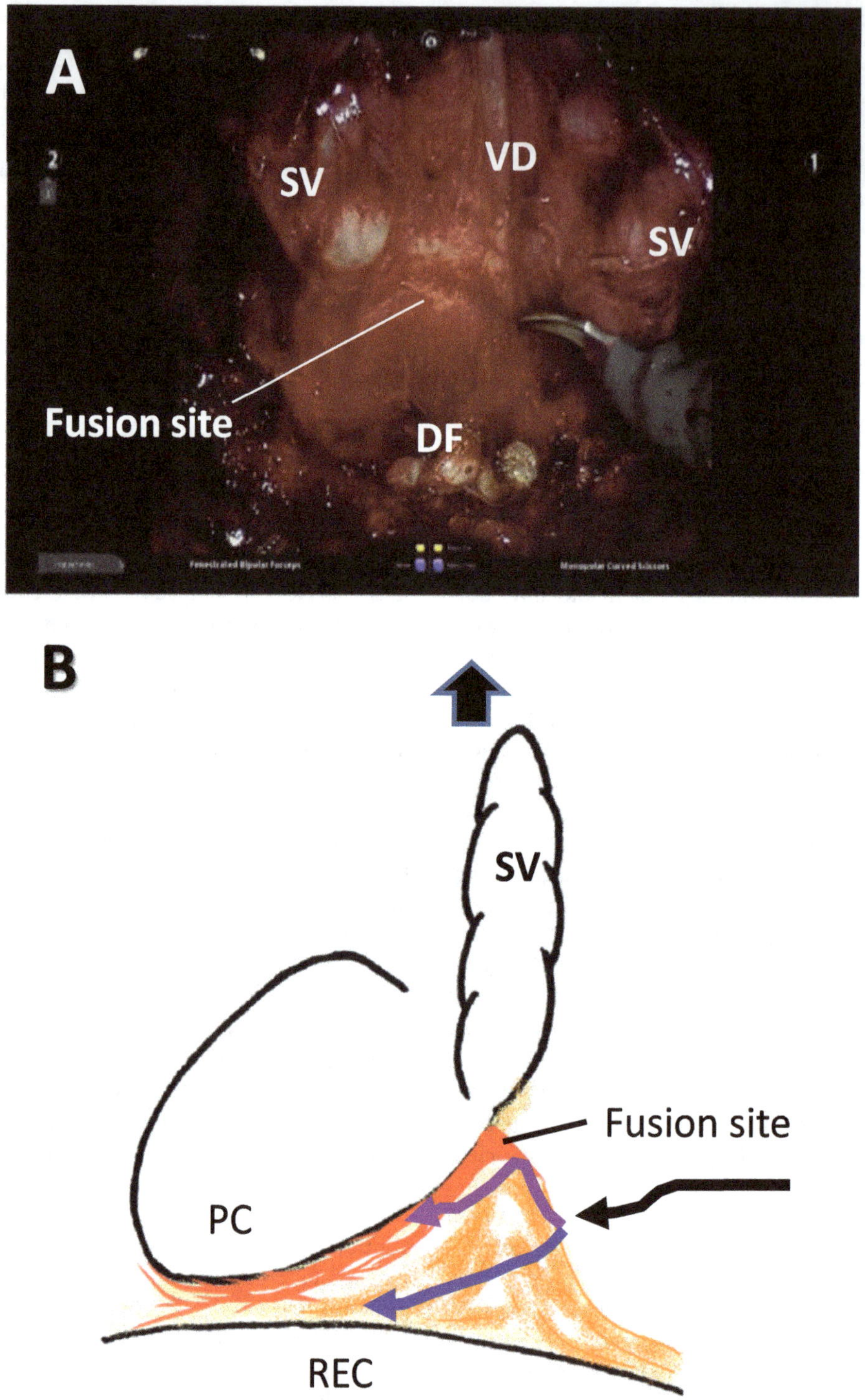

Figure 5 Intraoperative findings **(A)** and schema **(B)** of Denonvilliers' fascia. When the seminal vesicles and vas deferens are pulled ventrally, Denonvilliers' fascia (DF) is observed as a membranous structure, and the fusion site of DF with the prostatic capsule is recognized near the seminal vesicle-prostate junction (Panel **A**). DF between the seminal vesicles and rectum should first be cut at the midline to avoid entering the prostatic capsule (black arrow). After this incision, a mesh-like structure is found behind the posterior aspect of the prostate. With a nerve-sparing procedure, the dissection plane should be as close to the prostate as possible (purple arrow). If there is advanced cancer at the border of the posterior aspect of the prostate, the dissection plane can remain adjusted to the rectal wall (blue arrow). PC: prostatic capsule; REC: rectum; SV: seminal vesicle; VD: vas deferens.

the dissection plane unfolds at the loose connective tissue of DF to the apex. If advanced cancer is present at the border of the posterior aspect of the prostate, the dissection plane should be as close as possible to the rectal wall. This is because the fascial space between the prostate and rectum is not interposed with mesorectal loose tissues in some cases (Figure 5B) [17].

Distal to the fusion site, some DF leaves fuse with the prostatic capsule and/or the fascia propria of the rectum. DF reportedly conglutinates to the prostatic capsule with considerable frequency [4,5], whereas conglutination to the fascia propria of the rectum has not yet been reported, possibly because of difficulty in identification of the latter. During RARP, surgeons should be careful to avoid rectal injury during pre-rectal dissection because leaves of DF sometimes conglutinate to the fascia propria of the rectum.

DF converges on the grossly and histologically demonstrable posterior median raphe of rhabdosphincter and fibers of the RUM extended anteriorly into this fibrous raphe or central tendon of the perineum [20]. Soga et al. [21] reported that DF ends at the rhabdosphincter and the apical portion of the RUM. In our study, at least three specimens were found in which parts of the DF ended at the RUM. Of course, interindividual variations exist in the rhabdosphincter and RUM, and the shape of the rhabdosphincter is not always circular, but can show an omega shape [22]. In older men, the posterior rhabdosphincter is thin or absent in most cases. We suggest that the type of termination of DF depends on the size and shape of the rhabdosphincter and RUM [3].

Some potential limitations to this study should be considered when interpreting our findings. Variations of DF, such as the area in square millimeters and the numbers of leaves, were not evaluated quantitatively, because semiserial sections were used. Similarly, neither prostate size nor volume was evaluated before preparation of specimens for histological examination. Furthermore, because specimens including the rectum were difficult to obtain from young cadavers, no controls for likely changes with age were available.

Conclusions

Site-dependent and interindividual variations in DF were observed in donated elderly male cadavers. All or most DF is fused with the prostatic capsule near the base of the seminal vesicles and some DF is fused with the fascia propria of the rectum posterior to the apex of prostate. Based on our results, surgeons should be aware of variations and search for them to create a suitable dissection plane to avoid iatrogenic positive margins and rectal injury.

Abbreviations

DF: Denonvilliers' fascia; HE: Hematoxylin and eosin staining; LPF: Lateral pelvic fascia; NVB: Neurovascular bundle; RARP: Robot-assisted radical prostatectomy; RUM: Rectourethralis muscle.

Competing interests

The authors declare that they have no competing interests.

Authors' contributions

Conception and design: KM, GM, AKT, and AT. Acquisition of data: KM, NH, SM, and MH. Analysis and interpretation of data: KM, NH, SM, and TS. Drafting of the manuscript: KM, GM, and AT. Critical review of the manuscript for important intellectual content: KM and AT. Statistical analysis: KM and AT. Administrative, technical, or material support: GM. Supervision: AKT. All authors read and approved the final manuscript.

Acknowledgements

We are grateful to the people who donated their bodies after death to Sapporo Medical University for research and education on human anatomy without any economic benefit. We would also like to thank their families for agreeing to the donation, as well as for their patience while waiting for the return of their remains after the study.

Author details

[1]Division of Urology, Department of Surgery, Tottori University Faculty of Medicine, Yonago 683-8504, Japan. [2]Department of Urology, Kobe University Graduate School of Medicine, Kobe, Japan. [3]Division of Internal Medicine, Iwamizawa Kojin-kai Hospital, Iwamizawa, Japan. [4]Department of Urology, Mount Sinai Hospital, New York, NY, USA.

References

1. Tobin C, Benjamin J. Anatomical and surgical restudy of Denonvilliers' fascia. Surg Gynecol Obstet. 1945;80:373–88.
2. Lindsey I, Guy RJ, Warren BF, Mortensen NJ. Anatomy of Denonvilliers' fascia and pelvic nerves, impotence, and implications for the colorectal surgeon. Br J Surg. 2000;87(10):1288–99.
3. Takenaka A, Tewari A. Anatomical basis for carrying out a state-of-the-art radical prostatectomy. Int J Urol. 2012;19(1):7–19.
4. Ayala AG, Ro JY, Babaian R, Troncoso P, Grignon DJ. The prostatic capsule: does it exist? Its importance in the staging and treatment of prostatic carcinoma. Am J Surg Pathol. 1989;13(1):21–7.
5. Villers A, McNeal JE, Freiha FS, Boccon-Gibod L, Stamey TA. Invasion of Denonvilliers' fascia in radical prostatectomy specimens. J Urol. 1993;149(4):793–8.
6. Kiyoshima K, Yokomizo A, Yoshida T, Tomita K, Yonemasu H, Nakamura M, et al. Anatomical features of periprostatic tissue and its surroundings: a histological analysis of 79 radical retropubic prostatectomy specimens. Jpn J Clin Oncol. 2004;34(8):463–8.
7. Kourambas J, Angus D, Hosking P, Chou S. A histological study of Denonvilliers' fascia and its relationship to the neurovascular bundle. Br J Urol. 1998;82(3):408–10.
8. Costello A, Brooks M, Cole O. Anatomical studies of the neurovascular bundle and cavernosal nerves. BJU Int. 2004;94(7):1071–6.
9. Menon M, Shrivastava A, Tewari A, Sarle R, Hemal A, Peabody JO, et al. Laparoscopic and robot assisted radical prostatectomy: establishment of a structured program and preliminary analysis of outcomes. J Urol. 2002;168(3):945–9.
10. Motohashi O, Suzuki M, Shida N, Umezawa K, Ohtoh T, Sakurai Y, et al. Subarachnoid haemorrhage induced proliferation of leptomeningeal cells and deposition of extracellular matrices in the arachnoid granulations and subarachnoid space. Immunhistochemical study. Acta Neurochir (Wien). 1995;136(1-2):88–91.
11. Hayashi T, Kumasaka T, Mitani K, Yao T, Suda K, Seyama K. Loss of heterozygosity on tuberous sclerosis complex genes in multifocal micronodular pneumocyte hyperplasia. Mod Pathol. 2010;23(9):1251–60.
12. Miyake N, Hayashi S, Kawase T, Cho B, Murakami G, Fujimiya M, et al. Fetal anatomy of the human carotid sheath and structures in and around it. Anat Rec (Hoboken). 2010;293(3):438–45.

13. Bertrand MM, Alsaid B, Droupy S, Benoit G, Prudhomme M. Biomechanical origin of the Denonvilliers' fascia. Surg Radiol Anat. 2014;36(1):71–8.
14. Takenaka A, Kawada M, Murakami G, Hisasue S, Tsukamoto T, Fujisawa M. Interindividual variation in distribution of extramural ganglion cells in the male pelvis: a semi-quantitative and immunohistochemical study concerning nerve-sparing pelvic surgery. Eur Urol. 2005;48(1):46–52. discussion 52.
15. Hisasue S, Hashimoto K, Kobayashi K, Takeuchi M, Kyoda Y, Sato S, et al. Baseline erectile function alters the cavernous nerve quantity and distribution around the prostate. J Urol. 2010;184(5):2062–7.
16. Burnett AL, Tillman SL, Chang TS, Epstein JI, Lowenstein CJ, Bredt DS, et al. Immunohistochemical localization of nitric oxide synthase in the autonomic innervation of the human penis. J Urol. 1993;150(1):73–6.
17. Takenaka A, Tewari A, Fujisawa M. Neuro- and fascial anatomy in the male pelvis for robotic radical prostatectomy. Vienna: Medical Robotics; 2008.
18. Menon M, Shrivastava A, Kaul S, Badani KK, Fumo M, Bhandari M, et al. Vattikuti Institute prostatectomy: contemporary technique and analysis of results. Eur Urol. 2007;51(3):648–57. discussion 657-648.
19. Martinez-Pineiro L. Prostatic fascial anatomy and positive surgical margins in laparoscopic radical prostatectomy. Eur Urol. 2007;51(3):598–600.
20. Myers RP, Villers A. Anatomic considerations in radical prostatectomy. In: Kirby RS, Partin AW, Feneley M, Kellogg Parsons J, editors. Prostate Cancer; Principles and Practice, vol. 1. Abingdon: Taylor & Francis; 2006. p. 701–13.
21. Soga H, Takenaka A, Murakami G, Fujisawa M. Topographical relationship between urethral rhabdosphincter and rectourethralis muscle: a better understanding of the apical dissection and the posterior stitches in radical prostatectomy. Int J Urol. 2008;15(8):729–32.
22. Murakami G, Nakajima F, Sato TJ, Tsugane MH, Taguchi K, Tsukamoto T. Individual variations in aging of the male urethral rhabdosphincter in Japanese. Clin Anat. 2002;15(4):241–52.

9

Tadalafil 5 mg once daily for the treatment of erectile dysfunction during a 6-month observational study (EDATE): impact of patient characteristics and comorbidities

Dimitrios Hatzichristou[1], Gianluca d'Anzeo[2*], Hartmut Porst[3], Jacques Buvat[4], Carsten Henneges[5], Andrea Rossi[2], Karim Hamidi[6] and Hartwig Büttner[5]

Abstract

Background: To explore the impact of patient-characteristics and relevant comorbidities on treatment continuation rates, effectiveness, and satisfaction in patients with erectile dysfunction (ED) who started or switched to tadalafil 5 mg once daily (TAD-OaD) at baseline.

Methods: In the EDATE observational study, phosphodiesterase-type-5 (PDE5)-inhibitor pretreated or naïve ED patients who started or switched to TAD-OaD were prospectively followed for 6 months. Time to discontinuation of TAD-OaD was estimated using the Kaplan-Meier product-limit method at Months 2, 4, and 6 in subgroups stratified by age (18 – 65 years and >65 years), PDE5-inhibitor pretreatment, ED-severity (mild, moderate, severe), and presence or absence of relevant comorbidities (BPH, diabetes, CVD, hypertension, dyslipidemia). LSmean change from baseline in International Index of Erectile Function (IIEF) and Erectile Dysfunction Inventory of Treatment Satisfaction (EDITS) scores and associated 95 % CIs were assessed using a mixed-model for repeated measures. Visit, ED etiology, and subgroups were included as fixed-effects.

Results: Overall, 778 patients received prescriptions for initiating or switching to TAD-OaD at baseline. At Month 2, >90 % of patients remained on TAD-OaD, except those aged >65 years (86.7 %) and patients with severe ED (89.0 %). More than 80 % of patients in all subgroups, except those aged >65 years (75.0 %), continued TAD-OaD at Month 6. There was a significant LSmean negative effect on IIEF- EF domain-score improvement for BPH (LSmean effect [95 % CI]: −2.77 [−4.98, −0.55], $p = 0.014$), previous PDE5-inhibitor treatment (−2.13 [−3.33,-0.94], $p < 0.001$), and mild vs moderate ED (-2.00 [−3.54,-0.46], $p = 0.011$); the latter possibly linked with a bigger treatment-effect in those with more severe ED at baseline. The LSmean effect on change in IIEF-EF was significantly positive for diabetes (2.28 [0.64,3.92], $p = 0.007$), most likely because those with diabetes had more severe ED at baseline. For all other parameters, no statistically significant LSmean effects in IIEF-EF changes were observed. No comorbidity or baseline-characteristic except age (18 – 65 years vs >65 years: 11.25 [2.96,19.54], $p = 0.008$) affected changes in EDITS.

(Continued on next page)

* Correspondence: danzeo_gianluca@lilly.com
[2]Medical Advisor Urology, Eli Lilly Italy S.p.A., Via A. Gramsci 731/733, 50019 Sesto Fiorentino, FI, Italy
Full list of author information is available at the end of the article

(Continued from previous page)

Conclusions: Under routine clinical conditions, treatment continuation rate or satisfaction does not seem to be significantly affected by the presence of comorbidities in men who choose ED-treatment with TAD-OaD. The magnitude of treatment effectiveness was affected by certain baseline characteristics and comorbid conditions.

Keywords: Tadalafil, Once daily use, Erectile dysfunction, Comorbidities, Observational study, EDATE

Background

Men with erectile dysfunction (ED) have several comorbid conditions such as cardiovascular disease (CVD) and associated risk factors including diabetes, hypertension, dyslipidemia, smoking, obesity, sedentary lifestyle, and others such as depression, premature ejaculation, lower urinary tract symptoms (LUTS) secondary to benign prostatic hyperplasia (BPH), and overactive bladder [1–4]. In the Men's Attitudes to Life Events and Sexuality (MALES) study, 64 % of the men reported having at least 1 comorbid condition including hypertension (36 %), dyslipidemia (29 %), depression (25 %), CVD (17 %), and diabetes (14 %) [1].

Given these prevalence rates of comorbidities in men with ED, it is important to choose an appropriate treatment that maintains its efficacy and tolerability in the presence of the comorbidities [5]. Oral phosphodiesterase type 5 (PDE5) inhibitors including avanafil, sildenafil, tadalafil, and vardenafil are proven to be safe and effective for managing ED [6–14]. Furthermore, these drugs have demonstrated efficacy in men with ED who have comorbid cardiovascular risk factors including hypertension, dyslipidemia, and/or diabetes [5], and tadalafil once daily (OaD) has shown efficacy in the treatment of BPH/LUTS [15–17].

It has been suggested that appropriate treatment of concomitant ED may help in improving the adherence and management of associated comorbidities, which may eventually decrease healthcare costs and improve the overall health of the affected men [18]. However, some pharmacological drugs used for treating these comorbid conditions have sexual side effects. For example, antihypertensive drugs such as thiazide diuretics increase the risk of ED; 5α-reductase inhibitors, used for treating LUTS linked to symptomatic BPH, are associated with sexual disorders; and α-blockers tamsusolin and silodosin, used for treating BPH, are frequently responsible for ejaculatory disorders like anejaculation and reduced ejaculate volume [19]. This further underscores the significance of choosing an efficacious medication for treating ED in these subpopulations, if required.

The EDATE study was the first multinational, observational study in patients with ED, with or without previous exposure to PDE5 inhibitors, that documented the effectiveness and tolerability of tadalafil 5 mg OaD under routine conditions. The study highlighted that more than 85 % of men who choose to be treated with tadalafil OaD maintained the treatment in the next 6 months [20]. In this article, we present results of secondary analyses for the impact of patient characteristics and relevant comorbidities on treatment continuation rates as well as treatment effectiveness and satisfaction in patients with ED who had started with or switched to tadalafil OaD and were followed for a period of 6 months.

Methods

Patients and study design

EDATE was a prospective, longitudinal, observational study conducted in 59 centres across Germany, France, Italy, and Greece, enrolling patients from November 2011 through June 2012 [20]. Adult male patients who met the investigator's criteria for ED and presented within the normal course of care were eligible to participate if they had decided, in consultation with their physician, to either initiate PDE5 inhibitor treatment for the first time (treatment-naïve) or switch from any previous PDE5 inhibitor taken on-demand. Patients with previous experience with tadalafil OaD were excluded. The study was approved by the Comité de protection des personnes "Nord-Ouest IV", centre hospitalier universitaire, faculté de médecine, pôle recherche, 59045 Lille Cedex, and additional ethical review boards as per individual study site and country requirements (full list provided as Additional file 1). Patients provided written informed consent for data collection, storage, and release of anonymised data.

Assessment and treatment of patients were performed as per routine investigator practice for managing ED. In this article, data from patients who initiated or switched to treatment with tadalafil OaD at baseline (Visit 1) and were followed up longitudinally for up to 6 months (tadalafil OaD cohort) are reported. Post-baseline data were collected at routine visits (Visit 2, Visit 3) within 1 to 3 months and 4 to 6 months after initiation of therapy. Patients who switched or discontinued tadalafil OaD treatment during the observation were followed until the end of the 6-month observation period. A follow-up phone call was made to patients who did not visit within 4 to 6 months after baseline.

Outcome measures

The primary results on the time to treatment discontinuation of tadalafil OaD in men who had initiated or switched to tadalafil OaD at baseline have already been published [20]. The current article includes secondary outcome results on the impact of patients characteristics and comorbidities on time to treatment discontinuation, and on mean changes from baseline to end of observation in the International Index of Erectile Function (IIEF) domain scores [21], and Erectile Dysfunction Inventory for Treatment Satisfaction (EDITS) total score [22].

Statistical analysis

Sample size

A sample size of 250 patients initiating or switching to tadalafil OaD at baseline was planned, based on the primary outcome (continuation rate on tadalafil OaD, estimated to be 50 – 80 % after 6 months of treatment) [20]. Consecutive enrollment was planned to be stopped as soon as either 3,000 patients were enrolled overall, or 600 patients were enrolled in the tadalafil OaD cohort.

Primary analysis

All patients prescribed tadalafil OaD treatment at baseline were included in the analysis. The distribution of time to discontinuation of tadalafil OaD was estimated using the Kaplan-Meier product-limit method. The Kaplan-Meier proportions and associated 95 % confidence intervals (CIs) of patients on tadalafil OaD at Months 2, 4, and 6 were reported for the tadalafil OaD cohort (primary analysis) as well as subgroups stratified by age (18–65 years and >65 years), pretreatment with PDE5 inhibitors, ED severity (mild, moderate, severe), and presence or absence of BPH, diabetes, CVD, hypertension, and dyslipidemia (prespecified subgroup analyses, reported in this manuscript).

An additional, prespecified exploratory analysis was performed to investigate the association between time to discontinuation of tadalafil OaD and selected baseline factors using a Cox proportional hazards model; hazard ratios (HRs) and the corresponding 95 %CIs were reported. The final model included factors associated with treatment discontinuation identified by backward selection (removing those with $p > 0.1$). These included presence of relevant comorbidities, type of physician who initially diagnosed the ED, country, duration of living arrangement, age, ED etiology, ED severity, and work status [20].

Secondary analyses

All patients prescribed tadalafil OaD at baseline were included in the longitudinal analyses. Least-square (LS) mean effects in IIEF domain scores and EDITS total score from baseline to Month 6 were assessed using a mixed model for repeated measures (MMRM), including the following prespecified variables as fixed effects: visit, age (18–65 vs >65 years), pretreatment with PDE5 inhibitors (yes vs no), etiology of ED, ED severity, BPH (yes vs no), diabetes (yes vs no), CVD (yes vs no), hypertension (yes vs no), and dyslipidemia (yes vs no). p-values <0.05 were considered statistically significant and 95 % CIs were produced. Data were analyzed using the SAS 9.2 software (SAS Institute Inc., Cary, NC, USA).

Results

Patient characteristics

Overall, 778 patients received prescriptions for initiating or switching to tadalafil OaD at baseline. The majority of patients were aged 18 to 65 years (76.9 %), had suffered from ED for at least 1 year (63.1 %), and presented with mild to moderate disease at baseline (73.7 %) (Table 1). Most patients (65.6 %) were naïve to PDE5 inhibitor treatment. Baseline IIEF domain scores were similar in PDE5 inhibitor-naïve and pretreated patients (Additional file 2). Over half of the patients (58.4 %) reported having at least 1 comorbid condition. The most commonly reported comorbidities included CVD (34.5 %), hypertension (33.4 %), dyslipidemia (18.5 %), and diabetes (15.9 %). A small proportion of patients reported BPH (6.3 %) and hypogonadism (1.5 %). Approximately 57.1 % of the patients were on at least 1 concomitant medication (Table 1).

Impact of baseline characteristics and comorbidities on continuation rates of tadalafil OaD

At Month 2, Kaplan-Meier estimation revealed that more than 90 % of patients were still on tadalafil OaD, except those aged >65 years (86.7 %) and men with severe ED (89.0 %) (Table 2). More than 80 % of patients in all subgroups, except those aged >65 years (75.0 %) continued tadalafil OaD at Month 6 (Table 2; Additional file 3). Reasons for discontinuation did not differ notably between the older (>65 years) and younger age group (Table 3).

As the majority of patients remained on tadalafil OaD at Month 6, the median time to discontinuation could not be estimated in any of the subgroups. Patients with severe ED had lower treatment continuation rates than those with mild ED or moderate ED, but these were still >80 % at all time points (Additional file 4). The Kaplan-Meier analysis did not suggest any influence of individual comorbidities on treatment continuation rates (Table 2).

These findings were consistent with those from the Cox proportional hazard model evaluating factors associated with time to discontinuation of tadalafil OaD. The risk of discontinuation was significantly decreased among younger vs older patients (HR [95 % CI]: 18–65 vs >65 years: 0.54 [0.30, 0.96], $p = 0.038$). There was no significant effect of disease severity (mild vs moderate ED: 1.26 [0.68, 2.32], $p = 0.462$; severe vs moderate ED: 1.51 [0.95, 2.39], $p = 0.077$), or the presence of relevant comorbidities (presence vs absence of relevant comorbidities, namely,

Table 1 Baseline characteristics of patients starting tadalafil 5 mg OaD ($N = 778$)

Variable	N with data	
Age, years	778	
Median (IQR)		57 (47–65)
18 – 65 years, n (%)		598 (76.9)
Smoking habits, n (%)	775	
Current smoker		148 (19.0)
Former smoker		159 (20.4)
Never smoker		468 (60.2)
Currently drink alcohol, n (%)	775	456 (58.8)
ED severity, n (%)	775	
Mild		160 (20.6)
Moderate		411 (53.0)
Severe		204 (26.3)
Duration of ED symptoms, n (%)	776	
< 3 months		55 (7.1)
3 to <12 months		231 (29.7)
≥ 12 months		490 (63.1)
ED etiology, n (%)	776	
Mixed		343 (44.2)
Organic		240 (30.9)
Psychogenic		145 (18.7)
Unknown		48 (6.2)
With penile defects, n (%)	776	24 (3.1)
With former invasive diagnostic procedure for ED, n (%)	776	150 (19.3)
Non-coital erections, n (%)	771	422 (54.7)
Decreased libido, n (%)	775	310 (40.0)
IIEF-EF at baseline, mean (SD)	776	14.5 (7.06)
EDITS total score at baseline, mean (SD)	178[a]	59.6 (21.27)
Previous treatment, n (%)	777	
PDE5 inhibitor pretreated		267 (34.3)
PDE5 inhibitor-naïve		510 (65.6)
Relevant categories of comorbidities, n (%)	778	
At least 1 comorbidity		454 (58.4)
Cardiovascular disorder		268 (34.5)
Hypertension		260 (33.4)
Dyslipidemia		144 (18.5)
Diabetes		124 (15.9)
Pelvic surgery		89 (11.4)
Benign prostatic hyperplasia		49 (6.3)
Hypogonadism		12 (1.5)
Concomitant medication, n (%)	778	
At least 1 concomitant medication		444 (57.1)
Antihypertensive medication		260 (33.4)
Lipid lowering medication		152 (19.5)
Oral antidiabetic medication		102 (13.1)
Cardiovascular medication		94 (12.1)
α-blockers		58 (7.5)
5α-reductase inhibitors		14 (1.8)

ED, erectile dysfunction, *EDITS* Erectile Dysfunction Inventory of Treatment Satisfaction, *IIEF-EF* International Index of Erectile Function-Erectile Function, *IQR* inter quartile range, *N* number of patients with data, *n* number of patients, *OaD* once a day, *PDE5* phosphodiesterase type 5, *SD* standard deviation
[a]EDITS scores at baseline were collected only in patients pretreated with PDE5 inhibitors

BPH, diabetes, CVD, hypertension, dyslipidemia: 1.27 [0.82, 1.94], $p = 0.287$) in this model.

Impact of patient characteristics and comorbidities on erectile function and treatment satisfaction during treatment with tadalafil OaD

Overall, treatment with tadalafil OaD for 6 months was associated with significant improvement at Visit 2 (1–3 months) and Visit 3 (4–6 months) in all IIEF domain scores, including the IIEF-erectile function (EF) domain ($p < 0.001$ for both visits), as well as the EDITS total score ($p = 0.035$ and $p = 0.028$ for Visits 2 and 3, respectively) (Table 4). Improvements in the mean (standard deviation [SD]) IIEF domain scores and EDITS total score are given in Additional file 5.

MMRM analysis showed that PDE5 pretreatment had a significantly smaller LS mean effect on IIEF-EF ($p < 0.001$), orgasmic function ($p = 0.003$), intercourse satisfaction ($p = 0.003$), and overall satisfaction ($p = 0.001$) domain scores vs no previous PDE5 inhibitor treatment. Mild ED had a significantly smaller LS mean effect on IIEF-EF ($p = 0.011$), sexual desire ($p = 0.029$), and overall satisfaction ($p < 0.001$) domain scores, while severe ED had a significantly increased LS mean effect on the IIEF orgasmic function ($p < 0.001$) domain score relative to moderate ED. The negative effect of BPH on change in IIEF-EF ($p = 0.014$), orgasmic function ($p = 0.044$), and sexual desire ($p = 0.017$) domain scores was statistically significant. Furthermore, diabetes showed a significant positive effect on changes in IIEF-EF ($p = 0.007$), orgasmic function ($p = 0.013$), intercourse satisfaction ($p = 0.030$), and overall satisfaction ($p = 0.009$) domain scores (Table 4).

There were no significant effects for age, ED etiology, CVD, hypertension, or dyslipidemia ($p > 0.05$ for all comparisons) on IIEF domain scores over 6 months of tadalafil OaD treatment. LS mean effects in EDITS total

Table 2 Impact of patient characteristics and comorbidities on the continuation of treatment with tadalafil 5 mg OaD ($N = 778$)

Population	Number of patients with		Patients without events (%), KM estimate [95 % CI]		
	Data	Events	Month 2	Month 4	Month 6
Overall (primary analysis)	773	107	94.0 [92.3,95.7]	88.3 [85.9,90.6]	86.3 [83.7,88.9]
By age					
Age ≤65 years	593	61	**96.2 [94.7,97.8]**	**91.7 [89.4,93.9]**	**89.8 [87.1,92.4]**
Age >65 years	180	46	**86.7 [81.7,91.6]**	**77.3 [71.1,83.5]**	**75.0 [68.5, 81.5]**
By PDE5-I treatment					
PDE5-I naïve	507	71	93.9 [91.8,96.0]	88.5 [85.7,91.4]	86.1 [82.9,89.4]
PDE5-I pretreated	265	36	94.2 [91.4,97.1]	87.6 [83.6,91.7]	86.6 [82.3,90.9]
By disease severity					
Mild ED	160	16	**98.1 [96.0,1.00]**	**94.1 [90.3,97.8]**	89.8 [84.4,95.3]
Moderate ED	407	55	94.8 [92.7,97.0]	88.6 [85.5,91.8]	87.3 [83.9,90.8]
Severe ED	203	36	**89.0 [84.6,93.3]**	**82.8 [77.4,88.2]**	80.8 [75.1,86.5]
By presence of BPH					
BPH present	49	10	91.8 [84.2,99.5]	87.8 [78.6,96.9]	84.9 [74.5,95.3]
BPH absent	724	97	94.1 [92.4,95.9]	88.3 [85.9,90.7]	86.4 [83.7,89.1]
By presence of diabetes					
Diabetes present	123	19	93.4 [88.9,97.8]	85.3 [78.9,91.8]	84.0 [77.2,90.9]
Diabetes absent	650	88	94.1 [92.3,95.9]	88.8 [86.3,91.3]	86.7 [83.9, 89.5]
By presence of CVD					
CVD present	266	41	90.9 [87.4,94.4]	86.8 [82.7,91.0]	84.6 [80.1,89.2]
CVD absent	507	66	95.6 [93.8,97.4]	89.0 [86.2,91.8]	87.2 [84.0,90.3]
By presence of hypertension					
Hypertension present	258	40	91.0 [87.5,94.5]	86.8 [82.6,91.0]	84.6 [79.9,89.2]
Hypertension absent	515	67	95.5 [93.7,97.3]	89.0 [86.2,91.8]	87.2 [84.0,90.3]
By presence of dyslipidemia					
Dyslipidemia present	144	24	91.6 [87.0,96.1]	86.3 [80.6,92.1]	83.5 [77.2,89.9]
Dyslipidemia absent	629	83	94.5 [92.8,96.3]	88.7 [86.2,91.2]	87.0 [84.2,89.8]

Event = Discontinuation of tadalafil OaD
Note: KM estimates for subgroups with non-overlapping CIs at given time points are marked in bold
BPH benign prostatic hyperplasia, *CI* confidence interval, *CVD* cardiovascular diseases, *ED* erectile dysfunction, *KM* Kaplan-Meier, *N* number of patients, *OaD* once a day, *PDE5-I* phosphodiesterase type 5 inhibitor

score were not affected by any comorbidity or baseline characteristic except age ($p = 0.008$) (Table 4).

Safety

No treatment-related serious adverse events were reported during the study. The most frequently reported adverse events included headache (1.3 %), dyspepsia (0.5 %), and a new diagnosis of BPH (0.5 %); no new or unexpected safety signals were observed [20].

Discussion

Currently, there are few observational studies in patients with ED that assess the impact of baseline characteristics and presence of comorbid conditions on PDE5 inhibitor treatment continuation rates. In particular, few existing studies assess treatment satisfaction and effectiveness beyond the IIEF-EF domain. The primary analysis of the EDATE observational study demonstrated high treatment continuation rates (86.3 %) over a period of 6 months in 778 patients with ED who initiated or switched to PDE5 inhibitor treatment with tadalafil OaD at baseline (Additional file 6) [20].

Here in this cohort with high frequency of comorbidities and use of concomitant medications, we found that continuation rates over 6 months of treatment with tadalafil OaD were comparable across subgroups. Furthermore, continuation rates were over 80 % regardless of the presence of comorbidities, pretreatment with PDE5 inhibitors, or ED severity. Even in the subgroup of older patients (>65 years), the continuation rate was 75 % at Month 6. IIEF was affected by some baseline characteristics including ED severity, pretreatment with

Table 3 Reasons for discontinuation of tadalafil OaD treatment by age group

	Number (%) of patients		
	Age ≤65 years $N = 598$	Age >65 years $N = 180$	Overall $N = 778$
Discontinued tadalafil OaD[a]	61 (100.0)	46 (100.0)	107 (100.0)
Reasons			
Lack of efficacy (hardness of erection)	17 (27.9)	16 (34.4)	33 (30.8)
Adverse event	10 (22.5)	12 (26.1)	22 (20.6)
Cost of medication	11 (18.0)	5 (10.9)	16 (15.0)
Didn't want to take a pill every day	7 (11.0)	5 (10.9)	12 (11.2)
Patient discontinued study	7 (11.5)	2 (4.3)	9 (8.4)
Partner's request	2 (3.3)	3 (6.5)	5 (4.7)
Felt that medication controlled his sexual life	2 (4.2)	1 (2.2)	3 (2.8)
Slow onset of action	2 (3.3)	1 (2.2)	3 (2.8)
Lack of efficacy (duration of erection)	1 (1.6)	1 (2.2)	2 (1.9)
Lack of confidence in medication	1 (1.6)	0	1 (0.9)
Non-desired spontaneous erections	1 (1.6)	0	1 (0.9)

N number of patients, *OaD* once a day

[a]Includes all patients with documented end date of tadalafil OaD treatment, irrespective if the patient completed or discontinued the study

PDE5 inhibitors, and the presence or absence of diabetes and BPH. However, treatment satisfaction remained predominantly unaffected by any comorbid condition or baseline characteristic except for age, with patients aged 18–65 years reporting significantly higher satisfaction scores vs those aged >65 years.

In our study, younger patients (18–65 years) had higher chances of continuing tadalafil OaD vs older patients. This finding resonates with that from the DETECT observational study in which age less than 60 years was one of the factors associated with continuation of tadalafil on-demand treatment at 12 months [23]. Similarly, an observational study in Latin America found that persistence and adherence rates for PDE5 inhibitor treatment at 6 months were generally higher in younger men with ED (mean age, 52.3 years vs 54.9 years for non-persistent patients and 52.1 years vs 55.5 years for non-adherent patients) [24]. In a Korean study, the most common reason for discontinuing PDE5 inhibitor treatment given by older men (>70 years) with ED was concerns about the side effects, possibly due to higher prevalence of comorbidities in this subgroup [25].

We observed significant improvement from baseline in all the IIEF domain scores and EDITS total score at the second (1–3 months) and third (4–6 months) visits in the overall tadalafil OaD cohort. In particular, the LS mean IIEF-EF domain score increased by 7.1 points from baseline to 4 to 6 months after initiation of tadalafil OaD, exceeding the minimal clinically important difference (MCID) of 4 points [26]; this observation aligns with the 9.4-point increase observed with tadalafil OaD in a previous randomised controlled trial [27].

We found that PDE5 inhibitor pretreatment had a significant impact on IIEF scores, i.e. pretreated patients showed less improvement during tadalafil OaD treatment compared with treatment-naïve patients, in the domains of EF, orgasmic function, intercourse satisfaction, and overall satisfaction. In the EDATE cohort, 36.7 % of patients switched to tadalafil OaD due to lack of efficacy of previous PDE5 inhibitor treatment [20]. Thus, we believe that some of the patients in the tadalafil OaD cohort who were pretreated with PDE5 inhibitors may have been insufficient responders to any PDE5 inhibitor treatment, leading to a negative effect on their IIEF domain scores. In real-life clinical practice, men with inadequate response to ED treatment will usually keep seeking for a better treatment option to improve their erection. A large observational study in Middle Eastern countries among men with ED receiving tadalafil on-demand ($N = 1,080$) also found significantly higher mean IIEF-EF domain scores in treatment-naïve patients vs those who were pretreated (13.26 vs 9.28; $p < 0.0001$) [28].

ED etiology had no significant effect on IIEF in our study. This is in keeping with findings from an integrated analysis of 6 randomised studies which showed that tadalafil OaD was consistently efficacious across disease etiologies in men with ED [29].

In this study, there were significant effects of ED severity on the IIEF-EF, orgasmic function, sexual desire, and overall satisfaction domains. Mild ED reduced the change from baseline for IIEF-EF, sexual desire, and overall satisfaction, while severe ED meant an increased change in orgasmic function relative to moderate ED. This aligns with findings from an analysis of 6

Table 4 Impact of patient-characteristics and comorbidities on EF and treatment-satisfaction during tadalafil OaD treatment ($N = 778$; MMRM)

	IIEF domain scores ($n = 646$)					EDITS total score ($n = 165$)[a]
	Erectile function	Orgasmic function	Sexual desire	Intercourse satisfaction	Overall satisfaction	
Change from baseline at Visit 2						
LS mean	**+6.17***	**+1.06***	**+0.38***	**+2.70***	**+2.26***	**+14.17***
95 % CI	+4.82 to +7.51	+0.54 to +1.57	+0.03 to +0.74	+2.02 to +3.38	+1.77 to +2.75	+1.00 to +27.34
p-value	<0.001	<0.001	0.034	<0.001	<0.001	0.035
Change from baseline at Visit 3						
LS mean	**+7.11***	**+1.36***	**+0.48***	**+3.18***	**+2.56***	**+14.83***
95 % CI	+5.76 to +8.47	+0.83 to +1.88	+0.12 to +0.84	+2.48 to +3.87	+2.06 to +3.06	+1.64 to +28.02
p-value	<0.001	<0.001	0.010	<0.001	<0.001	0.028
Fixed effects						
Age group (18–65 vs >65 years)						
LS mean effect	+0.45	−0.11	+0.15	+0.20	+0.04	**+11.25***
95 % CI	−0.98 to +1.88	−0.66 to +0.44	−0.23 to +0.53	−0.53 to +0.92	−0.49 to +0.56	+2.96 to +19.54
p-value	0.539	0.707	0.444	0.592	0.896	0.008
PDE5-I pretreatment (yes vs no)						
LS mean effect	**−2.13***	**−0.69***	−0.10	**−0.93***	**−0.74***	+7.11
95 % CI	−3.33 to −0.94	−1.15 to −0.23	−0.41 to +0.22	−1.54 to −0.33	−1.17 to −0.30	−12.5 to +26.74
p-value	<0.001	0.003	0.548	0.003	0.001	0.475
ED etiology						
Psychogenic vs mixed						
LS mean effect	−0.25	+0.17	+0.04	−0.03	+0.06	−4.69
95 % CI	−1.75 to +1.26	−0.41 to +0.75	−0.35 to +0.44	−0.79 to +0.74	−0.49 to +0.62	−15.2 to +5.79
p-value	0.747	0.558	0.825	0.944	0.817	0.378
Organic vs mixed						
LS mean effect	−0.63	−0.17	−0.13	−0.44	−0.39	−1.70
95 % CI	−1.97 to +0.71	−0.69 to +0.34	−0.48 to +0.23	−1.12 to +0.24	−0.88 to +0.10	−9.31 to +5.92
p-value	0.359	0.507	0.479	0.205	0.116	0.661
ED severity (investigator assessment)						
Mild vs moderate						
LS mean effect	−2.00*	−0.06	**−0.45***	−0.56	**−0.97***	−4.52
95 % CI	−3.54 to −0.46	−0.66 to +0.53	−0.86 to −0.05	−1.35 to +0.22	−1.53 to −0.41	−16.4 to +7.35
p-value	0.011	0.833	0.029	0.156	<0.001	0.453
Severe vs moderate						
LS mean effect	+0.99	**+0.93***	−0.21	+0.30	+0.30	+3.99
95 % CI	−0.37 to +2.34	+0.41 to +1.45	−0.57 to +0.15	−0.39 to +0.99	−0.20 to +0.80	−3.37 to +11.35
p-value	0.154	<0.001	0.260	0.395	0.237	0.285
Comorbidities						
BPH (yes vs no)						
LS mean effect	**−2.77***	**−0.87***	**−0.72***	−1.08	−0.52	+5.78
95 % CI	−4.98 to −0.55	−1.73 to −0.02	−1.30 to −0.13	−2.21 to +0.04	−1.34 to +0.29	−8.38 to +19.94
p-value	0.014	0.044	0.017	0.058	0.206	0.421

Table 4 Impact of patient-characteristics and comorbidities on EF and treatment-satisfaction during tadalafil OaD treatment ($N = 778$; MMRM) *(Continued)*

Diabetes (yes vs no)						
LS mean effect	**+2.28***	**+0.81***	+0.06	**+0.92***	**+0.81***	+5.62
95 % CI	+0.64 to +3.92	+0.17 to +1.44	−0.38 to +0.50	+0.09 to +1.76	+0.20 to +1.41	−3.62 to +14.71
p-value	0.007	0.013	0.787	0.030	0.009	0.223
CVD (yes vs no)						
LS mean effect	−1.78	−1.93	0	−0.97	−0.49	+3.48
95 % CI	−7.53 to +3.96	−4.14 to +0.29	−1.52 to +1.52	−3.88 to +1.95	−2.60 to +1.62	−2.70 to +33.97
p-value	0.542	0.088	0.997	0.515	0.648	0.822
Hypertension (yes vs no)						
LS mean effect	+1.62	+1.91	+0.29	+0.77	−0.04	−1.33
95 % CI	−4.14 to +7.39	−0.31 to +4.13	−1.24 to +1.81	−2.16 to +3.69	−2.15 to +2.07	−31.7 to +29.00
p-value	0.580	0.091	0.711	0.606	0.969	0.931
Dyslipidemia (yes vs no)						
LS mean effect	−0.05	−0.19	−0.31	+0.02	−0.17	−4.26
95 % CI	−1.61 to +1.51	−0.79 to +0.41	−0.72 to +0.11	−0.78 to +0.81	−0.74 to +0.41	−13.1 to +4.60
p-value	0.946	0.528	0.145	0.966	0.568	0.343

BPH benign prostatic hyperplasia, *CI* confidence interval, *CVD* cardiovascular disease, *ED* erectile dysfunction, *EDITS* Erectile Dysfunction Inventory of Treatment Satisfaction, *IIEF* International Index of Erectile Function, *LS mean* least-square mean, *MMRM* Mixed Model for Repeated Measures, *N* number of patients, *n* number of patients included in the model, *OaD* once a day, *PDE5-I* phosphodiesterase type 5 inhibitor

[a]EDITS scores at baseline were collected only in patients pretreated with PDE5-I

*95 % confidence interval does not include zero and *p*-value statistically significant (<0.05)

randomised studies of tadalafil 2.5 and 5 mg OaD in patients with ED. Placebo-adjusted LS mean changes in IIEF-EF from baseline for both doses of tadalafil were numerically higher in patients with severe ED (4.6 and 5.8) vs those in patients with mild (2.3 and 4.5) and moderate (4.4 and 5.5) ED [29]. This may be explained by the possibility of greater changes from baseline in patients with more severe disease compared with those with mild or moderate disease. Furthermore, Rosen and colleagues have demonstrated that the MCID in the IIEF-EF domain increases significantly with higher baseline severity of ED ($p < 0.0001$) [26].

We observed a significant impact of reported BPH on IIEF-EF, orgasmic function, and sexual desire domain scores, i.e., the presence of BPH reduced improvement during tadalafil OaD treatment. However, BPH can be accompanied by other comorbidities and the estimated reduction in efficacy from our model is unlikely to define the differences between BPH and non-BPH patients alone. It is worth noting that patients with BPH in our study did show improvement from baseline to Month 6 in unadjusted mean (SD) IIEF-EF domain score (5.7 [6.7]); Additional file 5). However, self-reported prevalence of BPH was small (6.3 %), and a full baseline assessment of LUTS/BPH was not actively performed. Thus, our findings in the small number of patients with BPH should be interpreted with caution.

In our study, diabetes significantly impacted the changes in IIEF domains of EF, orgasmic function, intercourse satisfaction, and overall satisfaction, i.e., patients with diabetes showed more improvement than patients without diabetes. This may have occurred because patients with diabetes had more severe ED at baseline. According to the MALES study, men with diabetes were more likely to perceive their ED to be severe and permanent vs those without diabetes [30]. The efficacy of tadalafil OaD for ED treatment in males with diabetes has been previously evaluated in a placebo controlled, randomised multicentre study, showing statistically significant improvements in the IIEF-EF ($p \leq 0.005$), intercourse satisfaction ($p = 0.033$), and overall satisfaction ($p < 0.001$) domain scores vs placebo [31].

There was no significant effect of CVD, dyslipidemia, and hypertension on any of the IIEF domain scores, similar to results from previous studies. In an integrated analysis of data from 6 randomised controlled trials, patients with ED receiving tadalafil 2.5 and 5 mg OaD experienced IIEF-EF LS mean improvements reaching or exceeding the MCID (≥4) regardless of CVD, diabetes, hypertension, or hyperlipidemia [29]. Furthermore, in an analysis of 11 placebo-controlled randomised studies, tadalafil on-demand significantly improved IIEF EF domain score from baseline ($p < 0.005$ vs placebo) in all subpopulations regardless of age, disease etiology, severity and duration, and presence of comorbid conditions such as diabetes, hypertension, CVD, hyperlipidemia, depression, and BPH [32].

Treatment satisfaction, as assessed by EDITS, was not affected by pretreatment with PDE5 inhibitors, ED etiology, ED severity, or presence of relevant comorbidities in this study. This is consistent with data from a previous randomised study in which patients receiving fixed-dose tadalafil on-demand were significantly more satisfied with their treatment vs placebo ($p < 0.001$) despite high incidence of severe, organic ED and presence of comorbid conditions [33].

Large overall sample size, longitudinal nature, real life setting, and including patients with ED from several countries were important strengths of this study. In addition, to increase the external validity of the study, study sites were selected randomly from a list of investigators who expressed interest in participation and by asking sites to enroll patients consecutively. However, results may still be biased as only sites and investigators with interest were selected. As patients had to pay for their treatment, the study may also be biased towards those with higher education and economic status. The prevalence of comorbidities was based on patient-reported data, and was not confirmed by active baseline assessment by investigators. Thus, results may have been biased by false positive or missed diagnoses, and should be interpreted with caution.

Being an observational study, the patient population within subgroups was not well-defined. The small number of discontinuation events additionally limits the subgroup analysis of time to discontinuation. Nevertheless, this study provides valuable data on the impact of baseline characteristics and presence of comorbidities on continuation rates, and effectiveness and satisfaction of treatment with tadalafil OaD in a naturalistic setting and therefore has implications for everyday clinical practice. Furthermore, ED and CVD have common pathogenic pathways mediated via endothelial dysfunction [34], and it is suggested that tadalafil may potentially provide beneficial effects in patients with coronary artery disease, hypertension, heart failure, pulmonary arterial hypertension, diabetes mellitus, and Raynaud's phenomenon [35].

Conclusions

This observational study found that under routine clinical conditions, the presence of comorbidities did not have any significant impact on treatment continuation rates and treatment satisfaction among men with ED who choose treatment with tadalafil OaD. Continuation rates and treatment satisfaction were comparatively lower in men older than 65 years. Pretreatment with PDE5 inhibitors, ED severity, and presence or absence of diabetes and BPH had an impact on treatment effectiveness; however, age and presence of hypertension, CVD, dyslipidemia, or ED etiology did not affect IIEF in this cohort. These findings have clinical implications for counseling patients with ED, particularly for discussing expectations after PDE5 inhibitor treatment, as comorbidities are common in these patients, especially in older men.

Additional files

Additional file 1: List of ethical review boards.

Additional file 2: IIEF domain scores at baseline in PDE5 inhibitor-naïve and PDE5 inhibitor pretreated patients (*N* = 778).

Additional file 3: Kaplan-Meier estimation in different age groups for time to discontinuation of tadalafil OaD treatment.

Additional file 4: Kaplan-Meier estimation in patients stratified according to severity of erectile dysfunction for time to discontinuation of tadalafil OaD treatment.

Additional file 5: Change of IIEF and EDITS total scores from baseline to Month 6 during treatment with tadalafil OaD - subgroup analysis (*N* = 778; unadjusted data).

Additional file 6: Kaplan-Meier estimation for time to discontinuation of tadalafil OaD treatment.

Abbreviations

BPH: benign prostate hyperplasia; CI: confidence interval; CVD: cardiovascular disease; ED: erectile dysfunction; EDITS: Erectile Dysfunction Inventory of Treatment Satisfaction; EF: erectile function; HR: hazard ratio; IIEF: International Index of Erectile Function; LS mean: least squares mean; LUTS: lower urinary tract symptoms; MCID: minimal clinically important difference; MMRM: mixed model for repeated measures; OaD: once daily; PDE5-inhibitor: phosphodiesterase-type-5 inhibitor; SD: standard deviation.

Competing interests

The study was funded by Eli Lilly and Company, Indianapolis, IN, USA. D. Hatzichristou has received research grants for this study from Eli Lilly and speaker honoraria from Menarini, and reports activities as Advisory Board member for Eli Lilly, Menarini, Medispec and Dornier. H. Porst reports activities as speaker, investigator, and consultant for Eli Lilly and the Menarini/Berlin Chemie group. J. Buvat reports no conflicts of interest. G. d'Anzeo, C. Henneges, A. Rossi, K. Hamidi, and H. Büttner are employees of Eli Lilly and Company, H. Büttner also owns Lilly stock.

Authors' contributions

HB and CH designed the study, the manuscript outline, and provided data interpretation. CH was responsible for the statistical analyses. DH, HP, and JB were study investigators. AR contributed to data interpretation and manuscript outline. HB and CH drafted the manuscript with medical writing support provided by Trilogy Writing and Consulting GmbH. AR, DH, GdA, HP, JB, and KH provided substantial feedback on the draft manuscript. All authors read and approved the final manuscript.

Acknowledgements

We thank all patients who volunteered to participate in this trial and all study investigators for their contribution to data acquisition and patient care. We thank Frank G. Boess, Eli Lilly and Company, for contributing to the design of the study and data interpretation. We thank Julia Branicka, Eli Lilly and Company, for supporting the conduct of the study. We thank Kraig Kinchen for medical advice. We thank Clare Barker, Bruce Basson, Ann Gibb, and Xiao Ni, all from Eli Lilly and Company, for statistical support and for their contributions to the statistical analysis plan. Statistical analyses were programmed by PSI CRO LTD, St. Petersburg, Russia. We thank Karin Helsberg, Ph.D., and Dr Pradnya Kulkarni from Trilogy Writing and Consulting GmbH, Frankfurt, Germany, for providing medical writing services on behalf of Eli Lilly and Company.

Author details
[1]Centre for Sexual and Reproductive Health and 1st Department of Urology, Aristotle University of Thessaloniki, Thessaloniki, Greece. [2]Medical Advisor Urology, Eli Lilly Italy S.p.A., Via A. Gramsci 731/733, 50019 Sesto Fiorentino, FI, Italy. [3]Private Practice of Urology and Andrology, Hamburg, Germany. [4]Centre d'Etude et de Traitement de la Pathologie de l'Appa reil Reproducteur et de la Psychosomatique (CETPARP), Lille, France. [5]Lilly Deutschland GmbH, Bad Homburg, Germany. [6]Eli Lilly and Company, Neuilly sur Seine, France.

References

1. Rosen RC, Fisher WA, Eardley I, Niederberger C, Nadel A, Sand M. Men's Attitudes to Life Events and Sexuality (MALES) Study. The multinational Men's Attitudes to Life Events and Sexuality (MALES) study: I. Prevalence of erectile dysfunction and related health concerns in the general population. Curr Med Res Opin. 2004;20:607–17.
2. Grover SA, Lowensteyn I, Kaouache M, Marchand S, Coupal L, DeCarolis E, et al. The prevalence of erectile dysfunction in the primary care setting: importance of risk factors for diabetes and vascular disease. Arch Intern Med. 2006;166:213–9.
3. Nehra A. Erectile dysfunction and cardiovascular disease: efficacy and safety of phosphodiesterase type 5 inhibitors in men with both conditions. Mayo Clin Proc. 2009;84:139–48.
4. Zaman Huri H, Lian Choo T, Sulaiman CZ, Mark R, Abdul Razack AH. Oral drug treatments in patients with erectile dysfunction and multiple comorbidities: a retrospective observational study. BMJ Open. 2014;4:e005381.
5. Axilrod AC. Phosphodiesterase type 5 inhibitor therapy: identifying and exploring what attributes matter more to clinicians and patients in the management of erectile dysfunction. Curr Med Res Opin. 2007;23:3189–98.
6. Mulhall JP, Burnett AL, Wang R, McVary KT, Moul JW, Bowden CH, et al. A phase 3, placebo controlled study of the safety and efficacy of avanafil for the treatment of erectile dysfunction after nerve sparing radical prostatectomy. J Urol. 2013;189:2229–36.
7. Wang H, Yuan J, Hu X, Tao K, Liu J, Hu D. The effectiveness and safety of avanafil for erectile dysfunction: a systematic review and meta-analysis. Curr Med Res Opin. 2014;30:1565–71.
8. Goldstein I, Lue TF, Padma-Nathan H, Rosen RC, Steers WD, Wicker PA. Oral sildenafil in the treatment of erectile dysfunction. Sildenafil Study Group. N Engl J Med. 1998;338:1397–404.
9. Brock GB, McMahon CG, Chen KK, Costigan T, Shen W, Watkins V, et al. Efficacy and safety of tadalafil for the treatment of erectile dysfunction: results of integrated analyses. J Urol. 2002;168:1332–6.
10. Porst H, Giuliano F, Glina S, Ralph D, Casabé AR, Elion-Mboussa A, et al. Evaluation of the efficacy and safety of once-a-day dosing of tadalafil 5mg and 10mg in the treatment of erectile dysfunction: results of a multicenter, randomized, double-blind, placebo-controlled trial. Eur Urol. 2006;50:351–9.
11. Montorsi F, Aversa A, Moncada I, Perimenis P, Porst H, Barker C, et al. A randomized, double-blind, placebo-controlled, parallel study to assess the efficacy and safety of once-a-day tadalafil in men with erectile dysfunction who are naïve to PDE5 inhibitors. J Sex Med. 2011;8:2617–24.
12. Hellstrom WJ, Gittelman M, Karlin G, Segerson T, Thibonnier M, Taylor T, et al. Vardenafil for treatment of men with erectile dysfunction: efficacy and safety in a randomized, double-blind, placebo-controlled trial. J Androl. 2002;23:763–71.
13. Tsertsvadze A, Fink HA, Yazdi F, MacDonald R, Bella AJ, Ansari MT, et al. Oral phosphodiesterase-5 inhibitors and hormonal treatments for erectile dysfunction: a systematic review and meta-analysis. Ann Intern Med. 2009;151:650–61.
14. Yuan J, Zhang R, Yang Z, Lee J, Liu Y, Tian J, et al. Comparative effectiveness and safety of oral phosphodiesterase type 5 inhibitors for erectile dysfunction: a systematic review and network meta-analysis. Eur Urol. 2013;63:902–12.
15. Giuliano F, Oelke M, Jungwirth A, Hatzimouratidis K, Watts S, Cox D, et al. Tadalafil once daily improves ejaculatory function, erectile function, and sexual satisfaction in men with lower urinary tract symptoms suggestive of benign prostatic hyperplasia and erectile dysfunction: results from a randomized, placebo- and tamsulosin-controlled, 12-week double-blind study. J Sex Med. 2013;10:857–65.
16. Porst H, Roehrborn CG, Secrest RJ, Esler A, Viktrup L. Effects of tadalafil on lower urinary tract symptoms secondary to benign prostatic hyperplasia and on erectile dysfunction in sexually active men with both conditions: analyses of pooled data from four randomized, placebo-controlled tadalafil clinical studies. J Sex Med. 2013;10:2044–52.
17. Donatucci CF, Brock GB, Goldfischer ER, Pommerville PJ, Elion-Mboussa A, Kissel JD, et al. Tadalafil administered once daily for lower urinary tract symptoms secondary to benign prostatic hyperplasia: a 1-year, open-label extension study. BJU Int. 2011;107:1110–6.
18. Scranton RE, Goldstein I, Stecher VJ. Erectile dysfunction diagnosis and treatment as a means to improve medication adherence and optimize comorbidity management. J Sex Med. 2013;10:551–61.
19. Descazeaud A, de La Taille A, Giuliano F, Desgrandchamps F, Doridot G. Negative effects on sexual function of medications for the treatment of lower urinary tract symptoms related to benign prostatic hyperplasia. Prog Urol. 2015;25:115–27.
20. Buvat J, Hatzichristou D, Boess FG, Büttner H, Gehchan N, Henneges C, et al. Continuation and effectiveness of tadalafil once daily during a 6-month observational study in erectile dysfunction: the EDATE study. Int J Clin Pract. 2014;68:1087–99.
21. Rosen RC, Riley A, Wagner G, Osterloh IH, Kirkpatrick J, Mishra A. The international index of erectile function (IIEF): a multidimensional scale for assessment of erectile dysfunction. Urology. 1997;49:822–30.
22. Althof SE, Corty EW, Levine SB, Levine F, Burnett AL, McVary K, et al. EDITS: development of questionnaires for evaluating satisfaction with treatments for erectile dysfunction. Urology. 1999;53:793–9.
23. Roumeguère T, Verheyden B, Arver S, Bitton A, Belger M, Schmitt H. DETECT study investigators. Therapeutic response after first month of tadalafil treatment predicts 12 months treatment continuation in patients with erectile dysfunction: results from the DETECT study. J Sex Med. 2008;5:1708–19.
24. Rubio-Aurioles E, Reyes LA, Borregales L, Cairoli C, Sorsaburu S. A 6 month, prospective, observational study of PDE5 inhibitor treatment persistence and adherence in Latin American men with erectile dysfunction. Curr Med Res Opin. 2013;29:695–706.
25. Kim SC, Lee YS, Seo KK, Jung GW, Kim TH. Reasons and predictive factors for discontinuation of PDE-5 inhibitors despite successful intercourse in erectile dysfunction patients. Int J Impot Res. 2014;26:87–93.
26. Rosen RC, Allen KR, Ni X, Araujo AB. Minimal clinically important differences in the erectile function domain of the International Index of Erectile Function scale. Eur Urol. 2011;60:1010–6.
27. Buvat J, Büttner H, Hatzimouratidis K, Vendeira PA, Moncada I, Boehmer M, et al. Adherence to initial PDE-5 inhibitor treatment: randomized open-label study comparing tadalafil once a day, tadalafil on demand, and sildenafil on demand in patients with erectile dysfunction. J Sex Med. 2013;10:1592–602.
28. El Khiat Y, Ghazi S, Allam A, Khawaja M, Belger M, Tamer M, et al. Psychosocial impact and effectiveness of tadalafil among treatment-naïve and previously-treated men with erectile dysfunction in Saudi Arabia and other Gulf-region countries. Curr Med Res Opin. 2008;24:1965–73.
29. Porst H, Gacci M, Büttner H, Henneges C, Boess F. Tadalafil once daily in men with erectile dysfunction: an integrated analysis of data obtained from 1913 patients from six randomized, double-blind, placebo-controlled, clinical studies. Eur Urol. 2014;65:455–64.
30. Eardley I, Fisher W, Rosen RC, Niederberger C, Nadel A, Sand M. The multinational Men's Attitudes to Life Events and Sexuality study: the influence of diabetes on self-reported erectile function, attitudes and treatment-seeking patterns in men with erectile dysfunction. Int J Clin Pract. 2007;61:1446–53.
31. Hatzichristou D, Gambla M, Rubio-Aurioles E, Buvat J, Brock GB, Spera G, et al. Efficacy of tadalafil once daily in men with diabetes mellitus and erectile dysfunction. Diabet Med. 2008;25:138–46.
32. Lewis RW, Sadovsky R, Eardley I, O'Leary M, Seftel A, Wang WC, et al. The efficacy of tadalafil in clinical populations. J Sex Med. 2005;2:517–31.
33. Carson C, Shabsigh R, Segal S, Murphy A, Fredlund P, Kuepfer C. Trial Evaluating the Activity of Tadalafil for Erectile Dysfunction-United States (TREATED-US) Study Group. Efficacy, safety, and treatment satisfaction of tadalafil versus placebo in patients with erectile dysfunction evaluated at tertiary-care academic centers. Urology. 2005;65:353–9.
34. Jackson G, Rosen RC, Kloner RA, Kostis JB. The second Princeton consensus on sexual dysfunction and cardiac risk: new guidelines for sexual medicine. J Sex Med. 2006;3:28–36.
35. Chrysant SG. Effectiveness and safety of phosphodiesterase 5 inhibitors in patients with cardiovascular disease and hypertension. Curr Hypertens Rep. 2013;15:475–83.

10

Staging lymphadenectomy in patients with localized high risk prostate cancer: comparison of the laparoendoscopic single site (LESS) technique with conventional multiport laparoscopy

Frank Friedersdorff[1*†], Seven Johannes Aghdassi[1†], Ahmed Magheli[1], Maximilian Richter[1], Carsten Stephan[1], Jonas Busch[1], Dirk Boehmer[2], Kurt Miller[1] and T Florian Fuller[1]

Abstract

Background: In patients with localized high-risk prostate cancer awaiting radiation therapy, pelvic lymphadenectomy (PL) is a reliable minimally invasive staging procedure. We compared outcomes after laparoendoscopic single site PL (LESSPL) with those after conventional multiport laparoscopic PL (MLPL).

Methods: A retrospective case-control study was carried out at the authors' center. For LESSPL the reusable X-Cone single port was combined with straight and prebent laparoscopic instruments and an additional 3 mm needlescopic grasper. MLPL was performed via four trocars of different sizes using standard laparoscopic instruments.

Results: Patients who underwent either LESSPL (n = 20) or MLPL (n = 97) between January 2008 and July 2013, were included in the study. Demographic data were comparable between groups. Patients in the LESSPL group tended to be older and had a significantly higher ASA-score. The mean operating time was 172.4 ± 34.1 min for LESSPL and 116.6 ± 40.1 min for MLPL ($P < .001$). During LESSPL, no conversion to MLPL was necessary. An average of 12 lymph nodes per patient was retrieved, with no significant difference between study groups. Postoperative pain scores were similar between groups. The hospital stay was 2.3 ± 0.7 days after LESSPL and 3.1 ± 1.2 days after MLPL ($P = .01$). Two days postoperatively, significantly more patients after LESSPL than after MLPL recovered their normal physical activity ($P < .001$). Six months postoperatively, no complications were registered in the LESSPL group and cosmetic results were excellent.

Conclusions: In the present study, shorter hospitalization and quicker postoperative recovery were major benefits of LESSPL over MLPL. In patients with localized prostate cancer, staging LESS pelvic lymphadenectomy may be a safe alternative to conventional multiport laparoscopy.

Keywords: Laparoscopy, LESS, Single port, Prostate cancer staging

Background

In patients with localized high-risk prostate cancer (T1-T3, PSA ≥20 ng/ml, Gleason score ≥7) suited for radiation therapy, staging lymphadenectomy is recommended by the German Society of Radiooncology (DEGRO; www.degro.org). According to the S3 consensus guidelines of the DEGRO, pelvic lymph node dissection in prostate cancer patients helps to detect systemic disease and may therefore serve as therapeutic decision guidance. A minimum yield of 10 lymph nodes per patient along both external iliac arteries and the obturator fossae are recommended.

Since laparoscopic pelvic lymphadenectomy represents a surgical procedure for merely diagnostic purposes, complications should be infrequent and recuperation should be quick. In recent years, laparoendoscopic single site surgery (LESS) has evolved as an advanced laparoscopic technique. It is based upon the idea of solely

* Correspondence: frank.friedersdorff@charite.de
†Equal contributors
[1]Department of Urology, Charité University Hospital, Charitéplatz 1, 10117 Berlin, Germany
Full list of author information is available at the end of the article

employing one large umbilical port without any additional ports, thus minimizing tissue trauma. LESS was initially described in 1999 [1]. In 2011, Kaouk et al. reviewed more than 1000 urologic LESS cases that had been performed worldwide, mainly in high-volume academic institutions [2]. The application of LESS in urology encompasses a wide range of procedures, including pelvic lymphadenectomy in males with localized high-risk prostate cancer [3-7]. According to a few comparative studies, laparo-endoscopic single-site surgery (LESS) may yield better postoperative outcomes compared with conventional multiport laparoscopic surgery [8-10].

In our department LESS pelvic lymphadenectomy (LESSPL) is carried out with the reusable X-Cone single port platform via the umbilicus (Karl Storz, Tuttlingen, Germany). We hypothesized that patient outcomes after LESSPL, performed with the X-Cone single port are superior to those after multiport laparoscopic pelvic lymphadenectomy (MLPL) performed via four laparoscopic trocars in the lower abdomen.

Methods

All patient enrolled in this single-center retrospective case-control study were screened and followed by the Departments of Urology and Radiation Therapy, Charité University Hospital, Berlin, Germany. Both institutions are members of the Charité Comprehensive Cancer Center, Berlin, Germany. Using our institution's electronic database, a total of 117 patients with localized high-risk prostate cancer, who underwent laparoscopic staging lymphadenectomy before radiation therapy were identified. Between Mai 2011 and July 2013, 20 patients underwent LESS pelvic lymphadenectomy (LESSPL), whereas 97 patients underwent conventional multiport laparoscopic pelvic lymphadenectomy (MLPL) between January 2008 and April 2013. After Mai 2011, MLPL was performed in case the experienced LESS surgeon (T.F.F.) was unavailable.

Postoperative parameters were collected by a standardized questionnaire. After screening for patient privacy issues, the questionnaire and the study were approved by the local Ethics Committee at Charité University Hospital Berlin (EA1/112/12). All patients provided written informed consent for this research study. Written informed patient consent to publish their image was obtained.

Before transfer to the recovery room, all patients were given 0.2 mg fentanyl and 2 g metamizole for early postoperative analgesia. If needed, 1 g paracetamol i.v. was given during the recovery phase. After transfer to the urology ward, metamizole was continued on patient's request. The dosage was weight adapted with a maximum of 4 grams of metamizole per patient per day. Pain on postoperative day 1 was assessed by using the numerical analog scale (NAS) as a pain score: a value of 0 indicating no pain and a value of 10 indicating most severe pain. Full recovery of normal physical activity, defined as the ability to carry out routine daily tasks (eating, ambulating, toileting, bathing and dressing) with no need for pain medications, was evaluated on postoperative day 2. The cosmetic outcome and the incidence of complications were evaluated 6 months postoperatively.

Surgical techniques

Surgical equipment and setup of the reusable X-Cone single port

A detailed description, of the use of the X-Cone single port platform (Karl Storz, Tuttlingen, Germany) has previously been published [10,11]. In brief, LESSPL was performed with both surgeons at the same side of the table and the patient being placed in a supine low lithotomy position. A periumbilical incision was made to reach the abdominal space. The surgeon gently introduced the two L-shaped steel half shells of the X-Cone to form an autostatic X-shaped funnel, measuring 2.5 cm at its narrow end (Figure 1). The X-Cone was sealed with a silicone rubber cap, offering one 14 mm and four 5 mm working channels (Figure 1). From the existing armamentarium of differently shaped and prebent laparoscopic instruments (i.e. Carus, Cuschieri, Leroy) we chose the rigid Carus grasper (S-

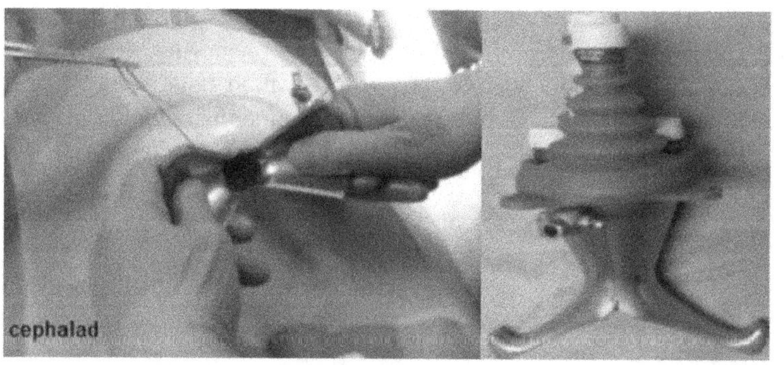

Figure 1 Transumbilical introduction of the two single port half shells (left). X-Cone fully assembled with a reusable silicone cap, providing 5 working channels (right).

portal series, Karl Storz, Tuttlingen, Germany). It was used together with a straight laparoscopic scissors and a 5 mm extra-long 30° telescope (Karl Storz, Tuttlingen, Germany). A straight 3 mm needlescopic grasper (Karl Storz, Tuttlingen, Germany) was routinely used via an additional subumbilical trocar (Figure 2). According to the current nomenclature, adding an extra needlescopic instrument transforms LESS into needlescopic-assisted or hybrid LESS [12].

Surgical steps of hybrid LESS pelvic lymphadenectomy

An experienced urologic laparoscopist (T.F.F.) performed LESSPL. Towards the end of the initial learning curve, a urologic fellow performed LESSPL on one side, whenever appropriate. Cases were then completed by the experienced laparoscopist. On each side a peritoneal incision was used to expose the external iliac vessels and the obturator nerve as important anatomical landmarks. At first, lymphatic tissue along the external iliac artery was mobilized by blunt and sharp dissection. Excellent exposure of the iliac fossa is achieved by static retraction of the lower margin of the external iliac vein using the prebent Carus grasper. All 5 mm instruments including the prebent grasper were inserted transumbilically via the X-Cone. Introduction of an additional 3 mm needlescopic grasper via a subumbilical port (Figure 2) provided triangulation ofinstruments, thus improving maneuverability and safety. All lymphatic tissue along the obturator nerve was carefully dissected and removed using a 5 mm scissors and a 3 mm grasper. After retrieval of the specimen via the umbilical incision, the fascia and skin were closed using absorbable sutures.

Multiport laparoscopic pelvic lymphadenectomy

Fifteen urologic laparoscopists with different levels of expertise performed MLPL. The surgical steps hereof were identical to those described for LESSPL. Two 10 mm and two 5 mm trocars were placed in the lower abdomen (Figure 2). One 10 mm transumbilical trocar was used for the 0° telescope (Karl Storz, Tuttlingen, Germany). Another 10 mm trocar, placed in the midline below the umbilicus, was used for dissection and specimen extraction (Figure 2).

Statistical analysis

SPSS 19.0 for Windows (SPSS Inc.; Chicago IL) was used for statistical analysis. For comparison of means ± standard deviation of continuous variables between the two study groups, the Student's t-test was employed. Frequency data were compared between groups by the chi-square and Fisher's exact test. Two-sided P values were reported. A P-value of less than .05 was considered statistically significant.

Results

Patient characteristics are shown in Table 1. Patients in the LESSPL group tended to be older and had a significantly higher American Society of Anesthesiologists (ASA)-score, suggesting reduced physical fitness. Preoperative oncologic specifications, including the PSA value and Gleason sum, were indicative of high risk prostate cancer in both study groups. In all patients, preoperative metastatic disease was excluded with a negative bone scan.

The average operating time was significantly longer in the LESSPL group (172.1 ± 34.1 min) than in the MLPL

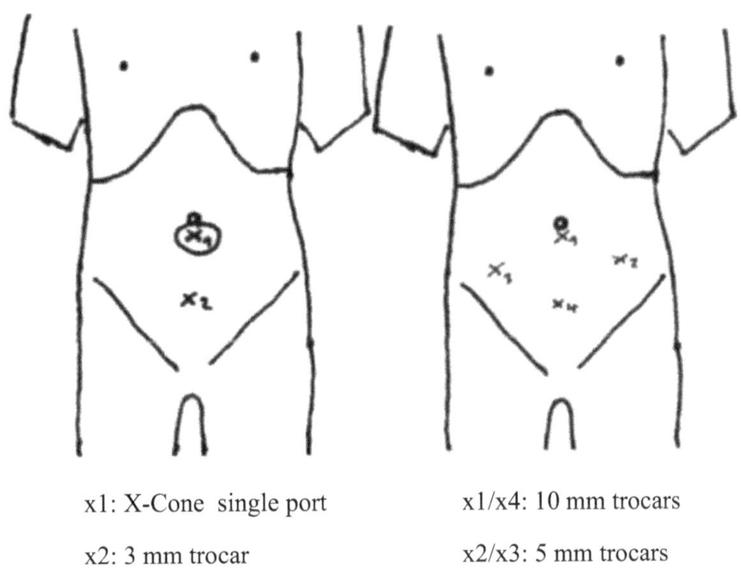

Figure 2 Trocar placement in LESSPL (left) and multiport PL (right).

Table 1 Patient characteristics

	LESSPL (LESS pelvic lymphadenectomy) n = 20	MLPL (Multiport pelvic lymphadenectomy) n = 97	*P* value
Patient age (mean ± SD)	71.8 (±4.2)	69.2 (±5.6)	.06
ASA-Score[a] (mean ± SD)	2.5 (±0.5)	2.1 (±0.6)	.01*
BMI (kg/m^2)	27.3 (±3.4)	27.7 (±4.0)	.70
Preoperative PSA value (ng/ml)	44.7 (±83.5)	32.3 (±56.2)	.50
Gleason sum	7.7 (±0.9)	7.7 (±1.0)	1.0

[a]American Society of Anesthesiologists physical status classification system.
*statistically significant.

group (116.6 ± 40.1 min) ($P < .001$) (Table 2). No conversions from LESSPL to MLPL were necessary and blood loss was minimal in all patients. The average number of retrieved lymph nodes (n =12) and the proportion of patients with positive lymph nodes (31%) was equally distributed among groups.

In the LESSPL group, the length of hospital stay was significantly shorter than in the MLPL group (2.3 ± 0.7 days vs. 3.1 ± 1.2 days; $P = .01$). Pain scores on day 1, tended to be lower in the LESSPL group, but differences did not reach statistical significance: 2.5 ± 2.0 vs. 3.2 ± 1.7, respectively. By day 2, a significantly higher proportion of patients in the LESSPL group than in the MLPL group reported return to normal physical activity (84% vs. 32%; $P < .001$). All patients in the LESSPL group reported full satisfaction with the cosmetic outcome (Figure 3), whereas 95% of patients after MLPL were fully satisfied with cosmesis ($P = .58$).

No intra or postoperative complications occurred in the LESSPL group, whereas 23 out of 75 patients (31%) in the MLPL group experienced complications. In one patient intraoperative bladder injury required intracorporeal suturing and urine drainage for several days. Postoperative complications included chronic abdominal pain, reversible paresthesia of the upper thigh, hematoma, lymphoedema, wound infection (Clavien Grade 1; n =18 patients) and deep vein thrombosis (Clavien grade 2; n =1 patient). One patient with a port site hernia and 3 patients with a lymphocele required surgical intervention (Clavien grade 3; n =4 patients).

Figure 4 shows the evolution of total operating time in 16 selected patients undergoing LESSPL. Operating times are divided into two groups: the experienced laparoscopist's initial LESSPL learning curve and subsequent teaching cases. Four patients were excluded. In one patient the surgery was stopped after a lymph node metastasis was detected upon frozen section. In 3 patients, operating times were prolonged based on technical problems, including $C0_2$ leakage or malfunction of laparoscopic instruments.

Discussion

Trocars used for conventional laparoscopy measure between 5 mm and 12 mm in diameter. The use of multiple trocars in the mid or lower abdomen may leave behind visible scars, thus compromising the cosmetic outcome. Laparoendoscopic single site surgery (LESS) typically uses the umbilicus for insertion of instruments and for specimen extraction via a larger single port. The advantage of the umbilical access is a relatively hidden and thus cosmetically favourable scar, even though the incisional length is longer than that of a conventional 12 mm trocar (Figure 3). According to the literature, umbilical hernias after single port surgery occur in less than 1% of cases [13,14]. In our present LESSPL series, no wound complications occurred within 6 months of follow-up.

Over the past years, LESS has gained popularity in various surgical disciplines. In abdominal surgery, significant clinical benefits of LESS over conventional laparoscopy have not yet been proven [15-17]. In selected adult urologic procedures, i.e. living donor nephrectomy and

Table 2 Postoperative outcomes

	LESSPL (LESS pelvic lymphadenectomy) n = 20	MLPL (Multiport pelvic lymphadenectomy) n = 97	*P* value
Total operating time (min)	172.1 (±34.1)	116.6 (±40.1)	< .001*
No. retrieved lymph nodes per patient	12.5 (±5.1)	12.2 (±6.2)	.87
No. patients with positive nodes	7/20 (35%)	29/97 (30%)	.79
Hospital stay (days)	2.3 (±0.7)	3.1 (±1.2)	.01*
Pain score (NAS) postop. day 1	2.5[a] (±2.0)	3.2[a] (±1.7)	.12
No. patients with full recovery of normal physical activity by postop. day 2	16/19[b] (84%)	24/75[b] (32%)	< .001*
No. patients with complications	0/19[b] (0%)	23/75[b] (31%)	.01*
No. patients fully satisfied with cosmetic result	19/19[b] (100%)	71/75[b] (95%)	.58

[a]numerical analog scale (NAS): 0 = no pain; 10 = most severe pain.
[b]missing data: n =1 patient (LESSPL); n =22 patients (MLPL).
*statistically significant.

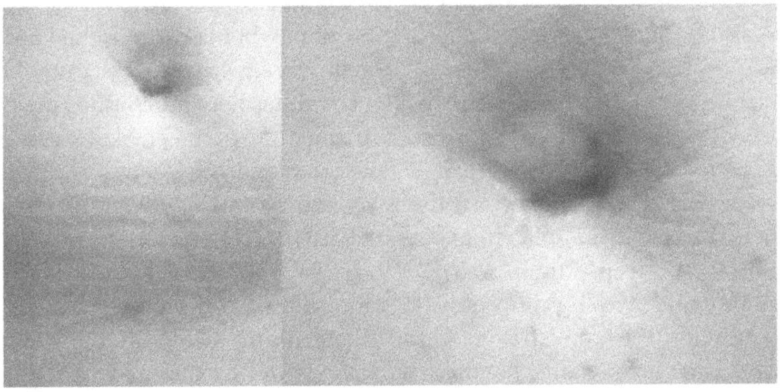

Figure 3 Abdominal scars 6 months after LESSPL.

varicocelectomy, LESS reduced analgesic requirements and accelerated postoperative recovery as compared to conventional laparoscopy [9,10,18]. In staging lymphadenectomy for endometrial cancer, outcome parameters after LESS were comparable to those after conventional multiport laparoscopy [8,19]. One group, however, reported significantly reduced pain scores after LESS surgical staging for endometrial cancer [20].

We herein investigated potential benefits of LESS over conventional laparoscopy for surgical staging in high-risk prostate cancer patients awaiting radiation therapy. For comparison of LESS with conventional multiport laparoscopy we used a monocentric retrospective case-control study in an academic teaching environment. For the first time we showed that, apart from a significantly longer total operating time, the length of hospitalization as well as recovery of normal physical activity after pelvic lymphadenectomy was significantly shorter in the LESSPL group compared with the multiport laparoscopy group (MLPL). Moreover, the incidence of intra and postoperative complications was 0% in the LESSPL group and 30% in the MLPL group within 6 months of follow up. The average yield of pelvic lymph nodes per patient was 12.4, with no statistically significant difference between the two cohorts. In a large study on multiport laparoscopic lymph node dissection for prostate cancer, comparing the extended and modified techniques, authors reported lymph node yields of 17.8 and 9.3, respectively [21]. Given its high efficiency and low morbidity compared with the extended technique, modified laparoscopic pelvic lymphadenectomy, involving the obturator and hypogastric nodes is the preferred method for prostate cancer staging [21].

A total of 15 urologic surgeons with different levels of laparoscopic expertise performed MLPL, whereas only one experienced laparoscopist carried out LESSPL. This may contribute to the lower complication rate observed in the LESSPL group. All complications in the MLPL group were seen after discharge from hospital. It is, therefore, unlikely that longer hospitalization and slower recovery of physical activity early after MLPL may be linked to the higher complication rate in this group. Rather was reduced postoperative pain responsible for quicker recovery and shorter hospitalization in the LESSPL group. Despite a trend in favor of the LESSPL group, differences in postoperative pain scores between groups were not statistically significant. Preoperative physical fitness was assessed by the American Society of Anesthesiologists (ASA)-score. Patients in the LESSPL

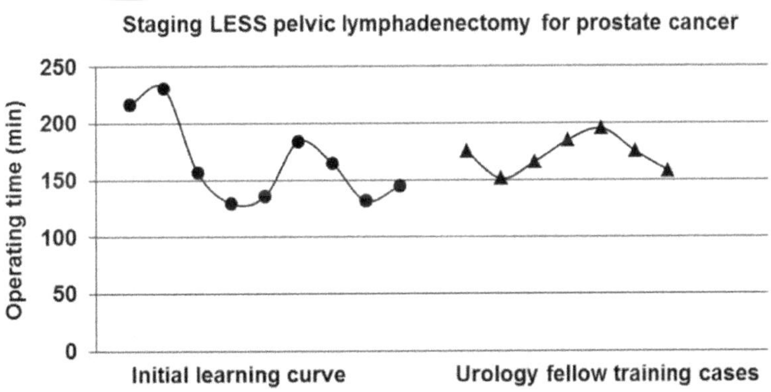

Figure 4 Evolution of total operating time in 16 patients undergoing LESSPL.

group showed quicker postoperative recovery, despite a significantly higher ASA-score, indicative of reduced physical fitness (Table 1).

In a recent article by Liedberg et al. on the benefits of multiport laparoscopic pelvic lymphadenectomy in prostate cancer patients, the incidence of Clavien grade 2 and 3 complications was 10.5% [22]. In comparison, the incidence of Clavien grade 2 and 3 complications in patients who underwent MLPL at our institution was 6%. In the context of the literature, our MLPL group proved to be a valid control group for the comparison with LESSPL. In our present work, no postoperative complications occurred within 6 months after LESSPL. In a series of 15 consecutive LESSPL in males with localized high risk prostate cancer, Schwentner et al. reported on one patient with inadvertent bowel injury, requiring intracorporal suturing [11]. In our view, patient safety should be a major issue in a pure diagnostic staging procedure, especially when a novel minimally invasive technique is used.

In our study, trainee involvement may have contributed to increased operative time, since MLPL and in part also LESSPL, were used to provide laparoscopic training to urology fellows. Recently, Rais-Bahrami et al. proposed that LESS training should be incorporated into the laparoscopic training program of urology residents and fellows. Establishing a credential process for LESS should be strongly considered by accrediting bodies [23].

The lack of triangulation and overcrowding of laparoscopic instruments not only accounts for a slow learning curve in almost all LESS procedures, but may also compromise patient safety. To overcome the lack of triangulation, instruments with flexible tips are increasingly used in single port surgery. In most cases, these instruments are disposable and therefore reduce cost effectiveness of LESS [9,24]. For LESSPL, we favor a totally reusable single port platform (X-Cone, Karl Storz, Tuttlingen, Germany) with conventional straight and rigid prebent laparoscopic instruments. In our view, adding an extra 3 mm port for a needlescopic instrument improves triangulation and surgeon dexterity during LESSPL, without compromising the overall cosmetic outcome (Figure 3). Furthermore, it helps to reduce instrument overcrowding in the single port. According to the current nomenclature, "needlescopic-assisted" LESSPL performed in the present study should correctly be denoted "hybrid LESS" [12].

The majority of LESS platforms currently available on the market use disposable components. In an earlier publication, we estimated cumulative cost of 10 LESS procedures, performed with different single ports, and identified the reusable X-Cone as being the most cost-effective [10]. In their recent publication on different urologic LESS procedures, Schwentner et al. found that LESS nephrectomy performed with the X-Cone is more cost-effective than conventional multiport laparoscopic nephrectomy [11].

Limitations of our present work include the relatively small number of cases in the LESSPL group and the monocentric, retrospective design of the study. The laparoscopic procedures herein described are embedded in an academic training program. Thus, the relatively high number of participating surgeons and the inconsistency of laparoscopic expertise across study groups, i.e. one surgeon performing LESS vs. 15 surgeons performing multiport laparoscopy, represent a bias. Length of hospitalization as an outcome measure could have been biased by the fact that early discharge in the LESSPL group was probably promoted more aggressively by the medical staff than in the MLPL group. However, all patients in the LESSPL group were free to prolong their hospital stay as needed.

Conclusions

In conclusion, our present study demonstrates that staging pelvic lymphadenectomy for prostate cancer, performed by laparoendoscopic single site surgery (LESS) is feasible and safe in the hands of an experienced urologic laparoscopist. Given its reusable components, the X-Cone single port platform is cost-effective. Compared with conventional multiport laparoscopy, LESS offers quicker postoperative recovery of prostate cancer patients awaiting radiation therapy for localized disease. Despite its limitations, our study provides the basis for prospective randomized trials to further evaluate the benefits of LESS in urology and cognate disciplines.

Abbreviations

BMI: Body mass index; LESS: Laparoendoscopic single site; LESSPL: Laparoendoscopic single site pelvine lymphadenectomy; MLPL: Multiport laparoscopic pelvine lymphadenectomy; PL: Pelvine lymphadenectomy; PSA: Prostate specific antigene.

Competing interests

Tom Florian Fuller received a travel grant from Karl Storz Endoscopy. All other authors declare that they have no competing interests.

Author's contribution

Conception and design: FF, SJA, TFF Acquisition of data: FF, SJA, MR Analysis and interpretation of the data: FF, JB, AM, TFF, KM, CS Drafting of the manuscript: FF, SJA, TFF, DB, JB Critical review of the manuscript for important intellectual content: FF, TFF, AM, KM, DB Statistical analysis: FF, SJA Administrative, technical or material support: SJA, MR, CS Supervision: AM, KM, TFF. All authors read and approved the final manuscript.

Acknowledgments

T. F. Fuller received a travel grant from Karl Storz Endoscopy. We thank Mr. C. Portscheller for technical support.

Author details

[1]Department of Urology, Charité University Hospital, Charitéplatz 1, 10117 Berlin, Germany. [2]Department of Radiation Oncology, Charité University Hospital, Berlin, Germany.

References

1. Piskun G, Rajpal S: **Transumbilical laparoscopic cholecystectomy utilizes no incicions outside the umbilicus.** *J Laparoendosc Adv Surg Tech A* 1999, **9:**361–364.
2. Kaouk JH, Autorino R, Kim FJ, Han DH, Lee SW, Yinghao S, Cadeddu JA, Derweesh IH, Richstone L, Cindolo L, Branco A, Greco F, Allaf M, Sotelo R, Liatsikos E, Stolzenburg JU, Rane A, White WM, Han WK, Haber GP, White MA, Molina WR, Jeong BC, Lee JY, Linhui W, Best S, Stroup SP, Rais-Bahrami S, Schips L, Fornara P, *et al*: **Laparoendoscopic single-site surgery in urology: worldwide multi-institutional analysis of 1076 cases.** *Eur Urol* 2011, **60:**998–1005.
3. Gill IS, Canes D, Aron M, Haber GP, Goldfarb DA, Flechner S, Desai MR, Kaouk JH, Desai MM: **Single port transumbilical (E-NOTES) donor nephrectomy.** *J Urol* 2008, **180:**637–641.
4. Canes D, Desai MM, Aron M, Haber GP, Goel RK, Stein RJ, Kaouk JH, Gill IS: **Transumbilical single-port surgery: evolution and current status.** *Eur Urol* 2008, **54:**1020–1029.
5. Goel RK, Kaouk JH: **Single port access renal cryoablation (SPARC): a new approach.** *Eur Urol* 2008, **53:**1204–1209.
6. Escobar PF, Fader AN, Rasool N, Espalliat LR: **Single-port laparoscopic pelvic and para-aortic lymph node sampling or lymphadenectomy development of a technique and instrumentation.** *Int J Gynecol Cancer* 2010, **20:**1268–1273.
7. Hahn HS, Kim YW: **Single-port laparoscopic pelvic lymph node dissection with modified radical vaginal hysterectomy in cervical cancer.** *Int J Gynecol Cancer* 2010, **20:**1429–1432.
8. Hudry D, Cannone F, Houvenaeghel G, Buttarelli M, Jauffret C, Chéreau E, Lambaudie E: **Comparison of single-port laparoscopy and conventional laparoscopy for extraperitoneal para-aortic lymphadenectomy.** *Surg Endosc* 2013, **27:**4319–4324.
9. Lee SW, Lee JY, Kim KH, Ha US: **Laparoendoscopic single-site surgery versus conventional laparoscopic varicocele ligation in men with palpable varicocele: a randomized, clinical study.** *Surg Endosc* 2012, **26:**1056–1062.
10. Friedersdorff F, Aghdassi SJ, Werthemann P, Cash H, Goranova I, Busch JF, Ebbing J, Hinz S, Miller K, Neymeyer J, Fuller TF: **Laparoendoscopic single-site (LESS) varicocelectomy with reusable components: comparison with the conventional laparoscopic technique.** *Surg Endosc* 2013, **27:**3646–3652.
11. Schwentner C, Todenhöfer T, Seibold J, Alloussi S, Aufderklamm S, Mischinger J, Stenzl A, Gakis G: **Cost effective laparoendoscopic single-site surgery with a reusable platform.** *JSLS* 2013, **17:**285–291.
12. Georgiou AN, Rassweiler J, Herrmann TR, Stolzenburg JU, Liatsikos EN, Do EM, Kallidonis P, de la Teille A, van Velthoven R, Burchardt M: **Evolution and simplified terminology of natural orifice transluminal endoscopic surgery (NOTES), laparoendoscopic single-site surgery (LESS), and mini-laparoscopy (ML).** *World J Urol* 2012, **30:**573–580.
13. Park JY, Kim TJ, Kang HJ, Lee YY, Choi CH, Lee JW, Bae DS, Kim BG: **Laparoendoscopic single site (LESS) surgery in benign gynecology: perioperative and late complications of 515 cases.** *Eur J Obstet Gynecol Reprod Biol* 2013, **167:**215–218.
14. Madureira FA, Manso JE, Madureira Fo D, Iglesias AC: **Randomized clinical study for assessment of incision characteristics and pain associated with LESS versus laparoscopic cholecystectomy.** *Surg Endosc* 2013, **27:**1009–1015.
15. Carus T: **Current advances in single-port laparoscopic surgery.** *Langenbecks Arch Surg* 2013, **398:**925–929.
16. Antoniou SA, Koch OO, Antoniou GA, Lasithiotakis K, Chalkiadakis GE, Pointner R, Granderath FA: **Meta-analysis of randomized trials on single-incision laparoscopic versus conventional laparoscopic appendectomy.** *Am J Surg* 2014, **207:**613–622.
17. Buckley FP 3rd, Vassaur H, Monsivais S, Jupiter D, Watson R, Eckford J: **Single-incision laparoscopic appendectomy versus traditional three-port laparoscopic appendectomy: an analysis of outcomes at a single institution.** *Surg Endosc* 2014, **28:**626–630.
18. Autorino R, Brandao LF, Sankari B, Zargar H, Laydner H, Akça O, De Sio M, Mirone V, Chueh SC, Kaouk JH: **Laparoendoscopic single site versus laparoscopic living donor nephrectomy: a systematic review and meta-analysis.** *BJU Int* 2014, [Epub ahead of print].
19. Escobar PF, Frumovitz M, Soliman PT, Frasure HE, Fader AN, Schmeler KM, Ramirez PT: **Comparison of single-port laparoscopy, standard laparoscopy, and robotic surgery in patients with endometrial cancer.** *Ann Surg Oncol* 2012, **19:**1583–1588.
20. Park JY, Kim DY, Suh DS, Kim JH, Nam JH: **Laparoendoscopic single-site versus conventional laparoscopic surgical staging for early-stage endometrial cancer.** *Int J Gynecol Cancer* 2014, **24:**358–363.
21. Stone NN, Stock RG, Unger P: **Laparoscopic pelvic lymph node dissection for prostate cancer: comparison of the extended and modified techniques.** *J Urol* 1997, **158:**1891–1894.
22. Liedberg F, Kjölhede H, Sundqvist P: **Laparoscopic extended pelvic lymphadenectomy for staging can be performed with limited morbidity and short hospital stay in patients with prostate cancer.** *Scand J Urol Nephrol* 2012, **46:**332–336.
23. Rais-Bahrami S, Moreira DM, Hillelsohn JH, George AK, Rane A, Gross AJ, Richstone L: **Contemporary perspectives on laparoendoscopic single-site surgery in urologic training and practice.** *J Endourol* 2013, **27:**727–731.
24. Autorino R, White WM, Gettman MT, Khalifeh A, De Sio M, Lima E, Kaouk JH: **Public perception of "scarless" surgery: a critical analysis of the literature.** *Urology* 2012, **80:**495–502.

11

Simvastatin improves the sexual health-related quality of life in men aged 40 years and over with erectile dysfunction

Daksha Trivedi[1*], David M Wellsted[2], Jade B Collard[2] and Michael Kirby[1]

Abstract

Background: Erectile dysfunction is prevalent in men over 40 years, affecting their quality of life and that of their partners. The aims of this study were:

a) To evaluate the internal reliability of the male erectile dysfunction specific quality of life (MED-QoL) scale and explore its factor structure.
b) To evaluate the effect of simvastatin on subscales of the MED-QoL in men over forty years with erectile dysfunction.

Methods: This is a double blind randomised controlled trial of 40 mg simvastatin or placebo given once daily for six months to men over forty years with untreated erectile dysfunction, who were not at high cardiovascular risk and were not on anti-hypertensive or lipid-lowering medication. 173 eligible men were recruited from 10 general practices in East of England. Data were collected at two points over 30 weeks.
We report on the factor structure of MED-QoL, the internal reliability of the scale and the derived subscales, and the effect of simvastatin on MED-QoL subscales.

Results: An initial analysis of the MED-QoL items suggested that a number of items should be removed (MED-QoL-R). Exploratory factor analysis identified three subscales within the MED-QoL-R which accounted for 96% of the variance, related to feelings of Control, initiating Intimacy, and Emotional response to erectile dysfunction. The alpha value for the revised scale (MED-Qol-R) was >0.95 and exceeded .82 for each subscale. Regression analysis showed that patients in the placebo group experienced a significantly reduced feeling of Control over erectile dysfunction than those in the statin group. Those in the placebo group had significantly lower Emotional response than those in the statin group at the close of trial, but there was no significant treatment effect on Intimacy.

Conclusions: Our revised MED-QoL-R identified three subscales. Secondary analysis showed a significant improvement in sexual health related quality of life, specifically in relation to perception of control and emotional health in men with untreated erectile dysfunction given 40 mg simvastatin for six months.

Keywords: Erectile dysfunction, Statins, Sexual health quality of life, Randomised controlled trial

* Correspondence: d.trivedi@herts.ac.uk
[1]Centre for Research in Primary and Community Care, University of Hertfordshire, Hatfield, UK
Full list of author information is available at the end of the article

Background

Erectile dysfunction (ED) is the consistent inability to achieve or maintain an erection that is sufficient for satisfactory sexual intercourse. Although ED affects sexual and mental health [1,2], the rates of consultation for ED remain low [3,4] and not all patients respond to Sildenafil and other phosphodiesterase inhibitors [5]. We reported the results of a randomised controlled trial (RCT) evaluating the effectiveness and cost effectiveness of simvastatin therapy in men with ED in men with untreated ED, but without significant cardiovascular risk factors [6]. The lipid lowering drug simvastatin was chosen for this study because ED shares risk factors with cardiovascular disease (CVD) [7-11]. It is associated with high total and low density lipoprotein cholesterol [12-14] and endothelial dysfunction.

There is a consensus that ED is either a predictor of future CVD or an early marker of silent atherosclerotic cardiovascular disease [9,10]. Small scale studies have indicated that atorvastatin can reduce ED and improve sexual function [12,15] but to date, there is no evidence to suggest that statins improve sexual health related quality of life in men with untreated ED.

In our previously published trial [6], there was a non-significant change in erectile function due to simvastatin treatment, although patients with more severe ED at baseline showed a larger improvement than patients with mild/moderate ED. However, simvastatin significantly improved the male ED-specific quality of life (MED-QoL), LDL cholesterol and reduced future cardiovascular risk [6]. It remains unclear why the MED-QoL improved significantly with only a small effect on erectile function, as the sexual encounter profile data showed nonsignificant treatment effect on satisfaction or success.

The MED-QoL scale has not been widely used, and there are few publications addressing the measurement of sexual health related quality of life at all using the MED-QoL. Only one paper has published any evidence of the scale reliability or validity using a sample of 69 men [16]. The current analysis aims to evaluate the internal reliability of the MED-QoL scale, its factor structure, and the extent any identified factors show drug related changes.

Methods

This is a secondary analysis of data from a double blind RCT comparing treatment with simvastatin or placebo on ED conducted in ten general practices in the East of England. The study design methods and analysis for the main study have been published previously [6,17]. The study protocol was approved by the Essex 1 Research Ethics Committee and clinical trial authorisation was obtained from the UK Medicines and Healthcare Products Regulatory Agency.

Main trial study design

Patients

173 eligible men aged forty years and over with untreated ED (score < 22 on the IIEF-5 (International Index of Erectile Function)), and no other cardiovascular risk factors were randomised to receive 40 mg simvastatin or placebo once daily for six months. Exclusions were based on participants' medical and drug history and those considered by the GP to be unsuitable, such as significant CVD risk requiring statin treatment.

Study design

Randomization to active simvastatin or placebo was on a 1:1 basis and was computer-generated at the Clinical Trials Co-ordinating Centre. Data were collected at baseline, 3 months and 6 months at assessment visits to the GP clinic. At each visit, participants completed the IIEF-5 questionnaire, the MED-QoL and the EQ-5D [16,18,19]. Sexual encounter profile (SEP) diaries were completed whenever an encounter occurred and were collected at each assessment. All questionnaires were completed by the men at the assessment visits in a private area, and were given support if necessary to clarify any raised issues.

The MED-QoL questionnaire consists of 27 items. All domains assess the effects of erectile dysfunction on the respondents' quality of life. The scale is based on 4 response categories: 'Not at all', 'A little', 'Quite a lot' and 'Very much'. All 27 items in the MED-QoL are listed in Table 1.

Analysis

The primary analysis of the data from this trial has been reported previously [6] using the original MED-QoL questionnaire [16].

Secondary data analysis: MED-QoL scale reliability

A step wise approach was taken to evaluate the reliability and factor structure of the MEDQoL scale. In the first step (item reduction) items were evaluated for low mean and a lack of endorsement, and low item-total correlation. Identified items were examined to evaluate their face validity before removal. In the second step an exploratory factor analysis was undertaken, with Varimax rotation, and assessment of Kaiser-Meyer-Olkin (KMO) sampling adequacy. Several factors (subscales) were identified and the internal reliability of the items for each factor was assessed. Items were again considered for removal if the item-test statistics were weak, the factor loading was < .5 and if the KMO value indicated poor model fit.

This process generated a reduced scale, removing 6 items from the original MED-QoL scale. To avoid confusion we named the revised version the MED-QoL-R. The scores for each item in a subscale were summed and the subscale score normalised (0-100). The identified subscales were

Table 1 Exploratory factor analysis of the MED-QoL

Factor	Item*	Factor 1	Factor 2	Factor 3	Cumulative variance	Alpha	Eigenvalue
1 (Control)	1. I feel sexually frustrated because of my erection difficulties	0.638*	0.100	0.302	0.37	0.82	11.40
	2. My problem makes me feel depressed	0.515*	0.119	0.443			
	3. I feel less of a man because of my problem	0.576*	0.296	0.448			
	4. I've lost confidence in my sexual ability	0.676*	0.349	0.211			
	5. I worry that I won't be able to get or keep up an erection	0.644*	0.294	0.302			
	7. I feel that I have lost control over my erections	0.681*	0.230	0.163			
	10. I worry about the future of my sex life	0.512*	0.417	0.327			
	12. I'm embarrassed about my problem	0.532*	0.236	0.480			
	16. I get less pleasure from life because of my erection problem	0.502*	0.401	0.230			
2 (Intimacy)	11. I've lost pleasure in sex	0.454	0.569*	0.070	0.69	0.85	1.54
	17. I feel guilty about my erection problem	0.219	0.521*	0.478			
	18. I am afraid to "make the first move" with my partner	0.316	0.665*	0.127			
	19. I worry that my partner blames herself for my problem	0.062	0.540*	0.305			
	20. I worry that I'm letting my partner down	0.439	0.547*	0.427			
	21. I worry that I am not satisfying my partner sexually	0.506	0.521*	0.217			
	22. I worry that we are going apart because of my problem	0.257	0.605*	0.265			
	25. I worry that she thinks I don't want her because of my problem	0.194	0.690*	0.300			
3 (Emotion)	6. My erection problem is always on my mind	0.459	0.302	0.506*	0.96	0.86	1.02
	8. I blame myself for my problem	0.205	0.381	0.566*			
	9. I feel angry because of my problem	0.313	0.168	0.676*			
	13. I worry about being humiliated because of my problem	0.263	0.288	0.626*			
Excluded	14. I try to avoid having sex	NA	NA	NA			
	15. I feel different from other men because of my erection problem	NA	NA	NA			
	23. I worry that she is looking for someone else because of my problem	NA	NA	NA			
	24. I feel that she blames me for my erection problem	NA	NA	NA			
	26. I have trouble talking to her about my problem	NA	NA	NA			
	27. My erection problem interferes with my daily activities	NA	NA	NA			
Scale total					.96	.95	

MED-QoL-R: male erectile dysfunction-specific quality of life revised scale. *Item numbers are based on the original MED-QoL scale. Factor analysis with varimax rotation, excluding items 14, 15, 23, 24,26 and 27.

evaluated to determine the extent to which the drug related changes in the total MED-QoL-R scores were determined by particular subscales. Based on CONSORT guidelines, the difference in the subscale scores at close of trial was evaluated for each subscale in turn. A regression model was used in which the outcome was the MED-QoL-R subscale score with treatment arm (statin vs. placebo) as a predictor. The outcome was adjusted for baseline ED severity (and the interaction between severity and arm), baseline testosterone, baseline 10 year cardiovascular risk, and the baseline score for the subscale score. As some of the distributions were positively skewed, log transformation was applied to the data and bootstrapped confidence intervals were estimated (with 3000 replications).

Results

In our trial, 173 patients were randomised, of which 131 patients completed some, and 113 completed all of the study outcome measures [6]. 60 (34%) patients withdrew from randomised treatment, but 18 of these patients continued to complete the QoL measures. The proportion withdrawing did not depend on study arm (χ^2 (1) =0.5, p > 0.05).

Item numbers 15, 23, 24 and 27 of the 27 items had low mean response values (1.60, 1.21, 1.48 & 1.15, respectively), and had few responses in the highest category (<3% 'Very much'), indicative of a lack of endorsement of these items. On this basis these items were removed.

Factor analysis

Following item reduction, the aim was to evaluate the underlying factor structure. An initial factor analysis was computed, excluding items 15, 23. 24 and 27 in order to assess the structure within the scale. Alongside the factor analysis, the Kaiser-Meir-Olkin (KMO) was also computed, assessing sampling adequacy of the overall scale and each item for factor analysis. A low KMO indicates that the item may not be relevant for the model specified and therefore may be a basis to exclude the item. For this model 3 factors with an Eigen value above 1 were found. Following the analysis, it was evident that as well as having a low mean, item 14 and 26 had a low KMO (0.88, 0.83, respectively). As item 14 already had a relatively low mean, it was excluded from analysis alongside items 15, 23,24 and 27 and the factor model was re-evaluated (Table 1).

Reliability

Following factor analysis excluding items 14, 15, 23, 24 and 27, the internal reliability of each subscale was determined using Cronbach's Alpha. Item 26 had low item-test reliability (0.58) compared to the rest of subscale 2 and was therefore removed from analysis. Subsequently, factor analysis with varimax rotation was computed once again, excluding items 14, 15, 23, 24, 26 and 27. The analysis yielded 3-factor model accounting for 96% of the variance (Table 1).

The factor loadings for each item followed a pattern, which we interpreted in the following way: Subscale (factor) 1 tended to belong to items which were related to feelings of control (Control); the items in subscale 2 were concerned with difficulties in initiating intimate contact (Intimacy); and the subscale 3 items were related to emotional response to erectile dysfunction (Emotion). Although there is a lot of overlap in the possible meaning of subscales 1 and 3, the 4 highest loading items on factor 1 are related to feelings of control ([item 1] frustration, [item 4] confidence, [item 5] worry, and [item 7] loss of control with the highest loading) rather than emotion, and we have therefor interpreted the factor in that way.

Regression modelling: effectiveness on MED-QoL-R subscales

Our initial analysis showed that the improvement in IIEF due to statin treatment was not statistically different to placebo, although patients with severe ED at baseline showed a larger change than patients with mild/moderate ED [6]. There was a statistically larger improvement in total MED-QoL score for men on statin compared to placebo (5% change in total scale score vs. 2%, z = 2.09, p = .04), which was higher for men with severe ED (12% change in total scale score vs. 5%, z = 4.52, p < 0.001). In this analysis, using the MED-QoL-R, fitting a regression model on each factor (Control, Intimacy and Emotion) allows for an evaluation of changes in quality of life in relation to the three subscales highlighted in the factor analysis. Due to the distribution of the data, log transformations were applied to the outcome variables and the exponentiated values were obtained to better explain the linear relationship between variables (Table 2).

The regression model showed that for the Control subscale, the level of control over their ED perceived by those in the placebo group is significantly less than those in the statin treatment group at the close of trial (z = -3.15, p < 0.005). Similarly, those in the severe ED group have a significantly lower perception of control than those with mild/moderate ED (z = - 1.97 p = 0.05).

Uniquely for this subscale, an increased number of reported encounters between the couples at mid trial was related to the observed advantage for perceived control in men in the statin arm compared to the control arm. Inclusion of the number of encounters did compromise the number of patients entered into the model (n = 61) but was a strong predictor of the outcome that a decision was made to include the number of encounters in the model. The men excluded from the analysis (n = 47) did not substantially differ from the men included in the analysis (n = 61) on any of the major factors measured (e.g. age, ED severity, treatment arm). For the other two factors (Intimacy and Emotion) including the change in the number of reported encounters from baseline to close made no contribution to the model and was therefore not included.

The regression model fitted to the Intimacy subscale showed that there was no significant effect of treatment arm (z = -0.83 p > 0.05), ED severity (z = 0.66 p > 0.05), baseline testosterone levels (z = -0.05 p > 0.05), baseline cardiovascular risk (z = 1.31 p > 0.05) or an interaction between treatment arm and ED severity (z = 0.14 p > 0.05) on the level of intimacy between the participant and their partners.

Table 2 Regression models evaluating the effect of statin treatment on men with ED (statin vs placebo groups) for each subscale (1-3) of the MED-QoL-R

	N	Proportionate difference between study arms and 95% CI (regression model)		Mean values at close of trial (unadjusted values)	
				Severe ED	Mild/moderate ED
Total MED-QoL-R	109	0.16 (0.01, 0.30)	**Statin**	66.1 (58.1, 74.1)	70.7 (62.4, 78.9)
			Placebo	58.3 (48.5, 68.2)	68.7 (61.6, 75.9)
Feeling of control (Subscale 1)	61#	0.40 (0.24, 0.53)*	**Statin**	60.7 (52.3, 69.2)	67.2 (59.6, 74.9)
			Placebo	51.6 (41.4, 61.9)	63.8 (56.6, 71.1)
Initiating intimacy (Subscale 2)	107	0.08 (0.12, 0.26)	**Statin**	67.3 (58.1, 76.6)	72.8 (63.8, 81.8)
			Placebo	62.7 (51.4, 74.1)	71.5 (64.0, 79.0)
Emotion response (Subscale 3)	104	0.25 (0.05, 0.41)*	**Statin**	75.7 (65.8, 85.5)	74.2 (64.2, 84.1)
			Placebo	64.4 (50.7, 78.0)	74.3 (65.9, 82.6)

MED-QoL-R: Revised male erectile dysfunction-specific quality of life. Column 3 provides the estimated proportionate difference between the study arms (1-exp (model coefficient). Thus 0.4 represents a 40% lower value in the Placebo arm compared to the Statin arm. Regression models (bootstrapped n = 3000) for each subscale were specified with treatment arm, ED severity, arm by severity, and baseline testosterone, cardiovascular risk, and time on treatment as variables.
#The number of patients who completed sufficient SEP Diaries (eg encounters) for inclusion in the analysis was lower than for most other outcomes-however for factor 1 (but not the other factors) the number of reported encounters was a very strong predictor of the outcome, and was therefore included in the model. *p < 0.05.

The regression model for the Emotion subscale showed that those in the placebo group have significantly lower emotional state than those in the statin group ($z = -2.35$ $p = 0.02$) at study close. In general, the mild/moderate patients reported a higher emotional state than those with severe ED ($z = -2.47$ $p = 0.01$). There is a significant interaction between treatment arm and severity ($z = 2.45$ $p = 0.01$) indicating that patients in the severe ED group benefited significantly more from treatment than those in the mild to moderate ED groups.

Discussion

Our initial analysis showed that simvastatin significantly improved the overall sexual health related quality of life (MED-QoL), which was largest for men with severe ED, despite the fact that the effect on erectile function was not significant [6]. We identified three subscales within MED-QOL that accounted for 96% of the variance relating to three quality of life characteristics: feelings of Control, problems initiating Intimacy and Emotion response to ED; named MED-QoL-R. Regression analysis showed that for the Control subscale, those with severe ED had significantly lower perception of control than those with mild to moderate ED. Similarly, those treated with statin had significantly improved perceptions of control at the close of trial than those treated with placebo. Similar results were found for subscale 3 (Emotion–excluding 4 outliers) where those treated with statin had a significantly more positive emotional state at the close of trial than those treated with placebo, although this is demonstrated mostly within the severe ED group. Those with mild to moderate ED had more positive emotional states than those with severe ED. The effect of statins on mood is equivocal [20] and it is possible that emotional improvements are mediated via improvement in ED.

Subscale 2, Intimacy, demonstrated no significant effect of either treatment arm or ED severity on level of intimacy and neither this nor Emotion were influenced by the number of encounters at midtrial. Uniquely, an increased number of reported encounters is a significant contributing factor in the improved perception of control over ED for men treated with simvastatin. This finding supports previous studies which show that more frequent erections improve erectile function, suggesting that men with frequent erections are likely to have better perception of control [21].

Our initial results showed no drug specific effect for SEP erections or satisfaction, although there was an increase in reported satisfaction over time for all participants and patients with mild/moderate ED reported greater satisfaction than those with severe ED. However, simvastatin showed no significant effect on SEP erections or satisfaction or reported frequency of encounters or IIEF severity, although participants attempting intercourse more than once a week on average reported higher IIEF scores at close of trial [6]. Our overall findings suggest that small changes in erectile function can have a significant impact on the sexual health related quality of life. This could be a result of an improvement in both the perception of control and emotional domains, but not a change in perceptions of intimacy.

The MED-QoL scale has previously not been extensively used, or tested for reliability and validity. To our knowledge the number of reported cases is less than 200 in total.

Undertaking an analysis of the reliability and factor structure of the scale, and evaluating drug related changes in the determined subscales from the same data limits the external reliability of the reported analysis. Care needs to be taken in interpreting these results until additional data samples can be collected and evaluated from a different population of men, demonstrating the external reliability of our findings.

Our objective in undertaking this analysis was to further evaluate the reliability and explore the factor structure of the MED-QoL scale, given that this had not been done before, and not reported in an external patient sample. Specifically we did not set out to create a brief measure. The scale created, the MED-QoL-R, has 21 items, and represents the most robust (e.g. reliable) scale suggested by the analysis of our data.

A number of scales to evaluate ED in men have been developed over the past 20 years [22-26]. The choice of the MED-QoL in our trial was based on familiarity of the scale amongst the research team. The current study offers additional evaluation of the MED-QoL in an external patient sample with recognised statistical methods, unlike most other scales developed. By undertaking this study in a sample drawn from a clinical trial of men not otherwise being treated, the analysis provides addition information about the reliability and underlying psychological dimensions of the MED-QoL, and provides a revised version of the scale, the MED-QoL-R.

We may have seen larger changes and more benefit if we had larger study sample, a longer treatment interval and a more potent statin. The total MED-QoL-R scores at close of trial showed that health related quality of life significantly improves when treated with statin than with placebo. Also, as found within the individual subscales, those with mild to moderate ED have significantly higher quality of life than those with severe ED. Overall the results demonstrate that sexual health related quality of life in males with ED is significantly influenced by drug treatment (statin compared to placebo) and by severity of the ED. Specifically, both feelings of control and emotional response to ED highlight this, compared to intimacy which is unaffected by treatment and severity of ED. The study excluded patients with significantly high CVD risk factors for ethical reasons. These were the men most likely to benefit from the intervention. Erectile function measured using the IIEF score defines ED principally in physical terms (hardness, penetration success), but does not take account of wider issues related to intimate relationships, which may or may not be related to cardiovascular health. It is possible that improving cardiovascular health has more general effects on sexual health which leads to improved sexual interactions that are not captured by the IIEF, but are captured by the MED- QoL-R, as seen in this additional analysis of subscales. There are also relationship issues to consider as enrolment in this study and contact with research nurses may have altered the sexual behaviour of these couples, and control as well as emotional health may be important. Research nurses involved in this study reported that relationships can be improved by the involvement of partners in the study. Further research into partner issues relating to sexual dysfunction is required. Routine consultations could include questions on ED as it has a big impact on quality of life of sufferer and partner. There is evidence to suggest that doctors need to support patients' sexual activity as regular intercourse may improve erectile function and quality of life [21]. This is supported by our previous findings of a small positive correlation between frequency of intercourse and IIEF score [6].

Conclusions

We have evaluated the MED-QoL and produced the revised MED-QoL-R with three identified subscales. Our secondary analysis has shown a significant improvement in sexual health related quality of life, specifically in relation to perception of control and emotional health in men with untreated ED given 40 mg simvastatin for six months. In addition our findings further demonstrate that the number of reported encounters may have a positive effect on perception of control over ED for men treated with simvastatin. Therefore, women could also be informed not only about the risks associated with ED and later development of CVD but also about their partners' sexual health related quality of life and to encourage them to attend for medical assessment.

Abbreviations

CVD: Cardiovascular disease; ED: Erectile dysfunction; IIEF-5: International index of erectile function; KMO: Kaiser-Meyer-Olkin; MED-QoL: Male erectile dysfunction specific quality of life; MED-QoL-R: Revised male erectile dysfunction specific quality of life; RCT: Randomised controlled trial; SEP: Sexual encounter profile.

Competing interests

Michael Kirby has received funding for research, advice, lecturing, and conference attendance from Pharmaceutical Industry.

Authors' contributions

MK had the initial idea; DT coordinated the trial and has written the final manuscript. DW and JC have conducted the analysis. All authors have given final approval of this version for publication.

Acknowledgements

The project is funded by the UK National Institute for Health Research 'Research for Patient Benefit' programme (Project Number PB-PG-0107-11391). The UK NHS Research and Development has provided service support; the University of Hertfordshire is the sponsor for the trial. We thank the participants and staff from the following sites that participated in the study: *Hertfordshire surgeries*: St Mary's Courtyard, Manor Street, Sheepcot Medical Centre, Castlegate, Dolphin House, Davenport House, Portmill; *Essex surgeries*: Addison House, John Tasker House, Elizabeth Courtauld, We acknowledge contribution from the study team and colleagues as reported in the previous paper [6].

Disclaimer

This article outlines independent research commissioned by the National Institute for Health Research (NIHR). The views expressed in this article are those of the author(s) and not necessarily those of the NHS, the NIHR or the Department of Health.

Supported in part by a research grant from the investigator-Initiated Study Program of Merck, who kindly supplied the simvastatin and matching placebo free of cost. The views of the investigators are not necessarily that of Merck.

Author details
[1]Centre for Research in Primary and Community Care, University of Hertfordshire, Hatfield, UK. [2]Centre for Lifespan and Chronic Illness Research, University of Hertfordshire, Hatfield, UK.

References

1. Laumann EO, Paik A, Rosen RC: **Sexual dysfunction in the United States prevalence and predictors.** *JAMA* 1999, **281**:537–544.
2. Litwin MS, Nied RJ, Dhanani N: **Health-related quality of life in men with erectile dysfunction.** *J Gen Intern Med* 1998, **13**:159–166.
3. Dunn KM, Croft PR, Hackett GI: **Sexual problems: a study of prevalence and need for health care in the general population.** *Fam Pract* 1998, **15**:519–524.
4. Speel TGW, Van Langen H, Meuleman EJH: **The risk of coronary heart disease in men with erectile dysfunction.** *Eur Urol* 2003, **44**:366–371.
5. Moore RA: **Sildenafil (Viagra) for male erectile dysfunction: a meta-analysis of clinical trial reports.** *BMC Urol* 2002, **2**:6. www.biomedcentral.com/1471-2490/2/6/.
6. Trivedi D, Kirby M, Wellsted DM, Ali S, Hackett G, O'Connor B, van Os S: **Can simvastatin improve erectile function and health-related quality of life in men aged ≥40 years with erectile dysfunction? Results of the erectile dysfunction and statins trial [ISRCTN66772971].** *BJU Int* 2013, **111**:324–333.
7. Sullivan ME, Keoghane SR, Miller MAW: **Vascular risk factors and erectile dysfunction.** *BJU Int* 2001, **87**:838–845.
8. Fung MM, Bettencourt R, Barrett-Connor E: **Heart disease risk factors predict erectile dysfunction 25 years later: the Rancho Bernardo study.** *J Am Coll Cardiol* 2004, **43**:1405–1411.
9. Tikkanen MJ, Jackson G, Tammela T, Assmann G, Palomäki A, Kupari M, Olsson A: **Erectile dysfunction as a risk factor for coronary heart disease: implications for prevention.** *Int J Clin Prac.* 2007, **61**:265–268.
10. Billups KL, Bank AJ, Padma-Nathan H, Katz S, Williams R: **Erectile dysfunction is a marker for cardiovascular disease: results of the minority health institute expert advisory panel.** *J Sex Med* 2005, **2**:40–52.
11. Walczak MK, Lokhandwala N, Hodge MB, Guay AT: **Prevalence of cardiovascular risk factors in erectile dysfunction.** *J Gend Specif Med* 2002, **5**:19–24.
12. Tsunekawa T, Hayashi T, Kano H, Sumi D, Matsui-Hirai H, Thakur NK, Egashira K, Iguchi A: **Cerivastatin, a hydroxymethylglutaryl coenzyme a reductase inhibitor, improves endothelial function in elderly diabetic patients within 3 days.** *Circulation* 2001, **104**:376–379.
13. Saltzman EA, Guay AT, Jacobson J: **Improvement in erectile dysfunction in men with organic erectile dysfunction by correlation of elevated cholesterol levels: a clinical observation.** *J Urol* 2004, **172**:255–258.
14. Feldman HA, Goldstein I, Hatzichristou DG, Krane RJ, McKinlay JB: **Impotence and its medical and psychosocial correlates: results of the Massachusetts male aging study.** *JUrol* 1994, **151**:54–61.
15. Herrmann HC, Levine LA, Macaluso J Jr, Walsh M, Bradbury D, Schwartz S, Mohler ER 3rd, Kimmel SE: **Can atorvastatin improve the response to sildenafil in men with erectile dysfunction not initially responsive to sildenafil? Hypothesis and pilot trial results.** *J Sex Med* 2006, **3**:303–308.
16. Wagner TH, Patrick DL, McKenna SP, Froese PS: **Cross-cultural development of a quality of life measure for Men with erection difficulties.** *Qual Life Res* 1996, **5**:443–449.
17. Trivedi D, Kirby M, Norman F, Przybytniak I, Ali S, Wellsted D: **Can simvastatin improve erectile function and health-related quality of life in men aged > 40 years with erectile dysfunction? Rationale and design of the Erectile Dysfunction and Statins (EDS) Trial [ISRCTN66772971].** *BJU Int* 2011, **108**:1850–1854.
18. Rosen RC, Cappelleri JC, Smith MD, Lipsky J, Pena BM: **Development and evaluation of an abridged, 5-item version of the International Index of Erectile Function (IIEF-5) as a diagnostic tool for erectile function.** *Int J Impot Res* 1999, **11**:319–326.
19. Brooks R, Rabin R, de Charro F (Eds): *The measurement and valuation of health status using EQ-5D: a European perspective: evidence from the EuroQol BIO MED research programme.* Rotterdam: Kluwer Academic Publishers; 2003.
20. While A, Keen L: **The effects of statins on mood: a review of the literature.** *Eur J Cardiovasc Nurs* 2012, **11**:85–96.
21. Koskimäki J, Shiri R, Tammela T, Hakkinen J, Hakama M, Auvinen A: **Regular intercourse protects against erectile dysfunction: tampere aging male urologic study.** *Am J Med* 2008, **121**:592–596.
22. MacDonagh R, Ewings P, Porter T: **The effect of erectile dysfunction on quality of life: psychometric testing of a new quality of life measure for patients with erectile dysfunction.** *J Urol* 2002, **167**:212–217.
23. Costa P, Arnould B, Cour F, Boyer P, Marrel A, Jaudinot EO, Solesse de Gendre A: **Quality of sexual life questionnaire (QVS): a reliable, sensitive and reproducible instrument to assess quality of life in subjects with erectile dysfunction.** *Int J Impot Res* 2003, **15**:173–184.
24. Porst H, Gilbert C, Collins S, Huang X, Symonds T, Stecher V, Hvidsten K: **Development and validation of the quality of erection questionnaire.** *J Sex Med* 2007, **4**:372–381.
25. Gutiérrez P, Hernández P, Sanz E, Cardenosa O, Mas M: **Further psychometric validation of the sexual life quality questionnaire for men with erectile dysfunction and their partners on a modified spanish language version.** *J Sex Med* 2009, **6**:2698–2706.
26. Latini DM, Penson DF, Colwell HH, Lubeck DP, Mehta MM, Henning JM, Lue TF: **Psychological impact of erectile dysfunction: validation of a new health related quality of life measure for patients with erectile dysfunction.** *Clinical Urol* 2002, **168**:2086–2091.

12

Virus encoded circulatory miRNAs for early detection of prostate cancer

Jayoung Kim[1,2,3*], Seok Joong Yun[4] and Wun-Jae Kim[4*]

Abstract

Background: Prostate cancer (PCa) is the most commonly diagnosed cancer and kills about 28,000 American men annually. Although progress has been made in understanding the molecular features of different forms of the disease, PCa is considered incurable when it becomes resistant to standard therapies. Prostate specific antigen (PSA) test has been a gold standard of diagnosis for PCa, however, it can result in lead to the unnecessary biopsies and treatment of indolent cancers due to the low specificity. Thus, the limitations of PSA screening for PCa have prompted much focus on strategies how to enhance the accuracy of PSA for distinction between aggressive and indolent cancers.

Discussion: Studies of miRNAs in PCa patients have suggested differentially expressed miRNAs between healthy controls and those with PCa, providing potential biomarker candidates using body fluids including urine and blood. Virus infection has been considered to associate with PCa incidence. Virus infected PCa cells may shed extracellular vesicles and communicate with neighboring cells, which were not infected yet, however, no mechanistic approaches were performed to understand the biology. The miRNAs composition in the shedding extracellular vesicles, and its role in PCa are completely undefined. In the near future, new insights to connect between the viral derived miRNAs and PCa progression might provide an opportunity to diagnose, risk prediction and therapeutic strategies.

Summary: The goal of this debate article is to provide a short review on miRNAs, virus infection and viral encoded miRNAs in PCa, with a primary focus on circulating miRNAs as potential non-invasive biomarkers for PCa patients.

Keywords: miRNAs, Virus, Extracellular vesicles, Prostate cancer

Background

Prostate cancer (PCa) remains one of the most commonly diagnosed malignant tumor in men and the second leading cause of death from cancer [1–3]. Several new drugs including Radium-223, Cabazitaxel, Sipuleucel-T, Abiraterone, and Enzalutamide have shown significantly improved survival in castration-resistant metastatic disease (CRPC) patients in Phase 3 trials [4–8]. For early detection of PCa, urologists rely on serum prostate-specific antigen (PSA) testing or digital rectal examination (DRE) [9]. Serum PSA testing has successfully achieved a dramatic increase of PCa detection, however, PSA testing has a low specificity because an increase of PSA level is not a PCa-specific event. Serum PSA levels are also elevated in men with benign prostatic hyperplasia and prostatitis. Limitations of DRE for the early detection derived from its low accuracy and the dependence on highly trained clinicians. Such a lack of PCa-specific early detection tool leads to create unnecessary biopsies or severe treatments for indolent PCa [2]. Development of methods of prebiopsy risk stratification and more simple, noninvasive, sufficiently sensitive and specific tests for PCa diagnosis would allow the stratification of PCa patients who are at the very early stage of disease [1, 10]. Current efforts to improve the accuracy of PSA and develop new biomarkers for PCa may hold the promise of improving the screening, diagnosis, and monitoring of prostate cancer. PCA3, a non-coding and large chain RNA that is significantly overexpressed in PCa compared to non-tumorous prostate cells, was introduced as a biomarker for PCa to show high sensitivity (52 % to 58 %) and specificity (72 % to 87 %) [11–16]. The US FDA approved PCA3 as a risk assessment tool for PCa to guide prostatic biopsy

* Correspondence: Jayoung.Kim@cshs.org; wjkim@chungbuk.ac.kr
[1]Departments of Surgery and Biomedical Sciences, Cedars-Sinai Medical Center, 8700 Beverly Blvd., Davis Room 5071, Los Angeles, CA 90048, USA
[4]Department of Urology, Chungbuk National University College of Medicine, 62 Kaeshin-dong, Heungduk-gu, Cheongju 361-763, Republic of Korea
Full list of author information is available at the end of the article

among men with negative previous prostate biopsies. Urinary PCA3 assay combined with TMPRSS2:ERG is reported to improve the diagnostic accuracy [17, 18]. Recently reported studies suggested that these requirements could be fulfilled using the diagnostic approach based on analysis of urine, which has become the future for non-invasive biomarker testing [10, 19].

This brief debate article is to discuss ad seek to characterize the circulating microRNAs (miRNAs) in urine with regard to PCa. We aim to provide our audience the current knowledge, in particular, focused on clinical implication as a liquid biopsy with a clinically satisfactory degree of sensitivity and specificity.

Discussion

MicroRNAs in prostate cancer

What are microRNAs?

Small non-coding microRNA (miRNA) molecules are known as post-transcriptional regulators involved in the regulation of gene and protein expression by interfering in the post-transcriptional level, resulting in the degradation and translation inhibition of mRNAs. Approximately more than 2,000 mature human miRNAs have been reported so far. These miRNAs are short (19–24 nt) and low molecular weight RNAs. miRNAs are derived from hairpin-like precursor transcripts (pre-miRNAs) and taken out of nucleus by a mediator protein, exportin 5. Pre-miRNA is then cleaved by Dicer (a ribonuclease III enzyme) to excise the mature miRNAs in the form of siRNA-like duplexes and asymmetrical assembling of the mature miRNA strands. Since miRNAs interact with multiple messenger RNAs by binding the pairing of bases of the mRNAs and repress target gene expression, and regulate mRNA cleavage and mRNA decay initiated by the miRNA-guided rapid deadenylation, miRNAs have a wide variety of functions contributing to various pathological conditions including prostate cancer [20].

How miRNAs are connected with PCa development and progression cancer?

Many of miRNAs play roles in cell proliferation and apoptosis processes, thus miRNA expression profiles can be considered as useful biomarkers monitoring many types of cancer progression and treatment responses [21]. Previous studies have suggested several miRNA biomarker candidates associated with PCa [22]. miR-548c-3p was found significantly overexpressed in CRPC. Expression levels of miR-548c-3p negatively correlated with recurrence-free survival. miR-375 was significantly downregulated in 83.5 % of PC patients compared to BPH controls. Metastatic CRPC patients with chemotherapy-resistant had the higher miR-21 levels compared with those with hormone dependent primary PCa. A combined diagnostic testing of miR-21 and PSA could stratify patients effectively. miR-21 was introduced as one of miRNAs of a multiple diagnostic profile, which includes miR-21,miR-141, and miR-221. miR-141 was independently identified as a biomarker of CRPC. Another combination panel of PSA and expression levels of let-7c, miR-30c, miR-141, and miR-375 was suggested as diagnostic biomarkers for PCa screening outperforming the PSA testing alone. Some PCa-specific miRNAs were identified from mouse PCa model. A set of 46 miRNAs in the serum of transgenic mice with advanced adenocarcinoma PCa were identified. Among those, miR-141, miR-298, and miR-375 were found to be elevated in the serum of metastatic CRPC patients. In particular, miR-141 and miR-375 showed a correlation with disease outcome. Diagrammatic representation of miRNAs associated with PCa is shown in Fig. 1.

What can be the target genes or pathways of miRNAs in PCa?

In the accumulated literature the roles of miRNAs in the pathobiology of PCa were found in cell cycle, apoptosis, epithelial to mesenchymal transition (EMT) and

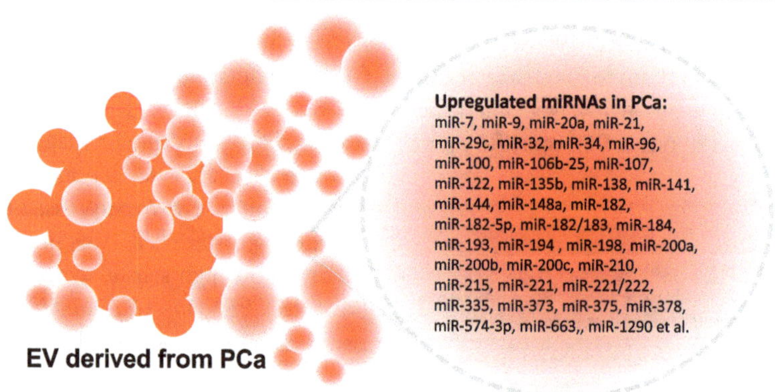

Fig. 1 miRNAs upregulated in PCa

mesenchymal to epithelial transition (MET) states, invasion and metastasis, PCa stem cell, and androgen receptor (AR) pathway. PTEN-PI3 Kinase-AKT, EGFR and AR pathways are considered as the most important signaling pathways in PCa. Upregulation of miR-221/-222 in PCa suggest a mechanistic link to PCa since miR-221/-222 plays a role in AR pathway regulation, c-kit, PTEN, and TIMP3 et al. miR-124 was characterized to have a direct targeting of AR thereby inducing down-regulation of miR-125b and up-regulation of p53. When miR-125b is suppressed miR-125b effectors (p52, Puma, Bak1, and p14ARF) were downregulated. The regulation of miR-125b on apoptotic proteins (mitochondrial cytochrome C and Caspase-3) and NCOR2 (a co-repressor of AR) was well known. Another PCa-associated miRNA, miR-let-7c regulates AR pathway and involves in the conversion of hormone dependent PCa to CRPC.

Urinary microRNAs as prostate cancer biomarkers

Several cancer-associated miRNAs were found in circulating body fluids such as urine, which make it possible to develop non-invasive biomarkers mainly due to their ease of access and stability. Only few studies for PCa-associated miRNA in urine were reported. Five of the miRNAs that were differentially quantified in PCa patients compared to controls (miR-107, miR-574-3p, miR375, miR200b and miR-141) were successfully quantified in urine of men with cancer, which were much higher in PCa patients than that of healthy volunteers. Such reports provide evidence that circulating miRNAs might be a next-generation biomarker and contribute to cancer screening in non-invasive liquid biopsy. Two additional promising miRNAs, miR-141 and miR-375 were found in the patient blood. In particular, data from this study showed that metastatic PCa patients have approximately 50 fold higher miR-141 levels, compared to the healthy individuals.

Virus infection and prostate cancer

Among the various viruses, herpes virus is one of the viruses most commonly related to carcinogenesis. Several epidemiological studies evaluated the association between herpes virus infection and prostate cancer risk, although results were inconsistent. Herpes virus plays an important role in the pathogenesis of cancer via the inhibition of cell apoptosis and stimulation of DNA synthesis, which may ultimately lead to PC. Previous meta-analysis indicated that infection by herpes simplex virus type 2 (HSV-2) or human herpesvirus 8 (HHV-8) may be associated with a higher prostate cancer risk. However, there has not been a study to elucidate the potential mechanism of HSV-2 infection underlying viral PC carcinogenesis. A potential link between HPV infection and PCa risk was attempted to study the causal role of HPV-16 in prostate carcinogens. A significant increase of PCa risk related with HPV-16 infection was observed. However, this is still contradictory since other epidemiological studies could not find same association [23–25]. Therefore, an elaborate and comprehensive demonstration of the association between herpes virus infection and prostate cancer risk is of significance [24]. Further investigations and large-sample studies are required to and the relationship between herpes virus infection and prostate cancer risk.

Our recent findings demonstrated the overexpression of herpes virus-encoded miRNAs in urine samples from prostate cancer patients, compared to those of control subjects [19]. Interestingly, hsv1-miR-H18 and hsv2-miR-H9-5p detected in urine samples showed better diagnostic performance than tPSA levels in patients within the PSA grey zone. A recent meta-analysis showed that HSV infection is associated with an increased PCa risk, however, it remains puzzling how these two particular vir-miRNAs contribute to PCa. To better understand the biological contribution of hsv1-miR-H18 and hsv2-miR-H9-5p to PCa, the geographic distribution, gender difference and socioeconomic variation of virus infection and their possible impact on prostate cancer should be considered to investigate (Fig. 2).

Viral miRNAs circulating through biofluids

Viruses also encode their own sets of miRNAs, which they use to control the expression of either the host's genes and/or their own. In the past few years' evidence of the presence of cellular miRNAs in extracellular human body fluids such as serum, plasma, saliva, and urine has been accumulated [26, 27]. Furthermore, it has been also demonstrated that miRNAs secreted by virus-infected cells are transferred to and act in uninfected recipient cells [19].

The first viral-encoded miRNAs was found in cells infected with EBV [27, 28]. The majority of natural viruses found to encode miRNAs. In DNA viruses (such as herpes virus, polyomavirus, ascovirus, baculovirus, iridovirus, and adenovirus families), a DNA component to replication cycle can exploit the initiating host miRNA biogenesis machinery in the nucleus, where they replicate and cause long-term persistent infections. Among DNA viruses, which account for the majority of known virus-encoded miRNAs, 95 % of viral miRNAs known today are of herpes virus origin. However, little has been identified about the role of circulating miRNAs from the virus-infected cells.

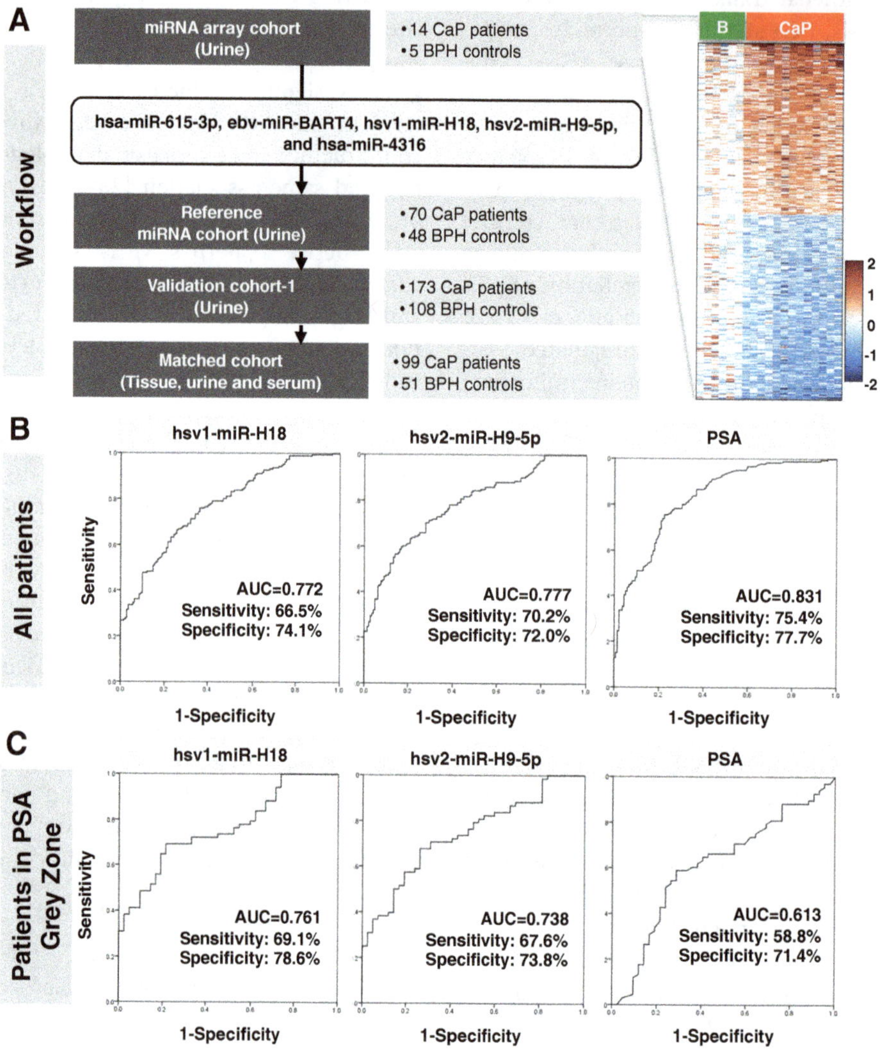

Fig. 2 Diagnostic performance of urinary hsv1-miR-H18 and hsv2-miR-H9-5p compared with serum PSA levels (published data) [19]. **a** Overview of the study design. A heatmap representing miRNA microarray data suggested that miRNA signature segregates PCa from BPH controls (right). **b** ROC curves for all patients. **c** ROC curves for patients only within the PSA grey zone (3–10 ng/ml)

Extracellular vesicles and their biological role of EV in prostate cancer

Cells can release different types of vesicles, which have been difficult to categorize in a definitive manner. The transmission of vesicles from cancer cells to other cell types has been the subject of intensive studies in recent years. It is a process that can make it possible a sophisticated form of cellular communication through the delivery of highly complex and dynamic cargo. As a delivery vehicle between cells, extracellular vesicles (EV) have been considered as a molecular cargo mediating a communication between cells in the microenvironment. Although EV were originally considered to be a means for exclusion of garbage molecules from cells, it is now clear that EV alter signaling pathways and have a biological influence in neighboring cells [29]. Also, since EV have the bioactivity of their molecular cargo and can be readily isolated from multiple biological fluids (e.g., urine, serum, plasma, pleural effusion, saliva), EV has been considered as a non-invasive biomarker candidate [30–32].

There are multiple types of EV, the small sealed membrane vesicles that are produced from cells differing in size, biology, contents, and secretory mechanisms. Exosomes and microparticles (MPs) are two distinct groups of EV. Exosomes are originated from the inward budding of the limiting membrane of multivesicular bodies (MVBs), while MPs are in bigger size vesicles formed by the outward membrane budding. Vesicles that are produced from cells during cell death are apoptotic bodies.

It is known that PCa patients had higher levels of urinary exosomes than the healthy donors. The membranes of exosomes are resistant to the osmeolytic and proteolytic activity of urine, indicating that exosomes are quite stable in urine. PC cell-derived EV can deliver various genetic factors such as nucleic acids, including DNA, mRNA, miRNA, and small non-coding RNAs, as well as oncoproteins and metabolites, leading to the horizontal transfer of oncogenic information to neighboring immune cells, vessel cells, or cancer cells [33, 34]. EV-mediated RNA transfer provides benefits as a communicasome [35–37]. However, little is known how EV-mediated transfer of these molecules enters into recipient cells, and how specific miRNA species can be sorted into EV. Our series of publications in this field suggest that EV shedding can influence on microenvironment of PCa by modulating immune cell proliferation and activation [38].

EV influence immune response in prostate cancer

Role of immune response caused/mediated by miRNA was suggested by a series of studies showing that EV-derived miRNAs participate in the regulation of inflammatory responses. A recent report from our group demonstrated that EV derived from amoeboid phenotype of prostate cell may influence the immune response of the tumor microenvironment. A tritiated thymidine (^{3}H-thymidine) incorporation assay revealed that EV contain miRNAs (e.g., miR-125a), which are transferred to tumor microenvironment leading to proliferative inhibition of immune cells. Other interesting findings suggest immune response may be mediated by miRNAs regulating Toll-like receptors (TLRs), which play an important role in immune response and inflammation including tissue repair and tissue injury-induced inflammation. In PCa cell lines, several miRNAs (e.g., has-miR-29b, -29c, -148b, and -152) were upregulated by TLR3 activation, leading to antitumoral effects on PCa. EV derived from dendritic cells contain miR-155 (a promoter of inflammatory responses) and miR-146a (a mediator of immune suppression), which are known as important players to regulate inflammation, alter the gene expression of inflammation related targets and reprogramm the response to endotoxin [39, 40].

EV released from virus-infected cells

In virology field, biology of extracellular vesicles are well understood compared to cancer mainly because virus should be enveloped to be released from infected host. The accumulating evidence suggests that viruses, such as retroviruses, hepatitis C virus, herpes simplex virus, Epstein-Barr virus, Coxsackie virus B3 (CVB3), utilize the cellular vesiculation pathway for budding and assembly, immune evasion, and intercellular communication. It is also well known that many virally infected cells secrete vesicles (most of cases, exosomes) containing various viral proteins and genetic materials such as RNAs. Studies on herpes simplex virus-infected cells demonstrated that virus communicate via vesicles. In the case of Epstein-Barr virus, recent reports suggested that herpes virus utilizes exosomes, one kind of extracellular vesicles, as a mechanism of cell-to-cell communication and transfers signaling competent proteins and functional miRNAs to uninfected neighbor cells. For example, exosomes released from infected cells have been shown to contain co-receptors for HIV, which can enhance virus entry into cells. Proteins in the secreted exosomes from virus-infected cells can induce apoptosis in CD4 T cells, and contribute innate immune response.

EV as cargoes to deliver viral miRNAs

EV-mediated communication would allow the virus to respond to the cellular microenvironment. Virus-infected cells continuously shed and transfer EV to uninfected neighboring cells. Throughout EV shedding and secretion to extracellular space, the virus-encoded miRNAs were delivered to other cells, leading to alteration of miRNA-mediated gene repression and intercellular communication. Thus, the presence of viral-encoded miRNAs in EV suggests that virus-infected cells perturb gene expression in the surrounding tissue, resulting in destruction of the immune system. Exosomes secreted from HIV-infected alveolar macrophages have been identified to carry viral miRNA (vir-miRNA) such as vmiR88, vmiR99, and vmiR-TAR. It has not been clearly identified how vir-miRNA composition is decided and recruited to EV. Vir-miRNAs might have a role in cancer initiation by blocking of major tumor suppressors (e.g., p53) or acceleration of cancer development by evading cellular immune response (e.g., mi17-92).

These findings still raise a number of exciting questions. Does virus-infected prostate cells secrete miRNAs using EV as a cargo? What are the target genes of the abundantly secreted viral miRNAs? Are extracellular vesicles shed only in the absence of viral replication? Is there any evidence for functional miRNA delivery in vivo? If so, what's the biological mechanism? In addition, the detail mechanism is currently lacking whether virus infection promotes miRNAs sorting into EV, or whether this secretion is a selective and specific process.

Conclusions

In PCa biomarker development, the greatest unmet need remains: a biomarker that stratifies men at risk of aggressive PCa or a biomarker that identify the early stage of patients who need active surveillance, eventually leading to a reduction of unnecessary interventions. Although miRNAs might have many useful clinical applications for patients with PCa, many additional studies are warranted to clarify their function and regulation during tumorigenesis and tumor progression. The studies to determine the role of circulating miRNAs during PCa progression would have the potential that PCa patients can be molecularly stratified based on their miRNAs profile in urine samples. In addition, the studies could uncover important clues about underlying disease mechanisms.

Urine analyses have great potential to be adapted in clinical practice, based on its non-invasiveness. Identification of non-invasive clinical indicators of PCa would be one of the most important advances achievable in this field. Our current mechanistic understanding of shedding vesicle biology and function, especially in the context of virus infection and communication with host, is not mature enough. Identification of potential candidates of the circulating miRNAs signature in patient urine samples would have significant implications for an alternative and/or supportive diagnostic tool for PCa.

Unnecessary diagnostic procedures would be minimized for patients with early stage of PCa, contributing to the easier diagnostic assessment and to the reducing associated public health and economic burden to patients. In addition, the studies to understand role and biology of the circulating miRNAs have significant clinical relevance to public health since it will improve accuracy of predicting patient survival, identifying responsiveness candidates of PCa patients. Furthermore, we envision that this study will also provide the mechanistic data to address the long-term goal of the PCa field identifying new treatments tailoring more specific and effective therapies for PCa, thus it holds great promise for the treatment of high risk PCa patients.

Abbreviations

PCa: Prostate cancer; CRPC: Castration-resistant metastatic disease; PSA: Prostate-specific antigen; DRE: Digital rectal examination; miRNAs: MicroRNAs; EMT: Mesenchymal transition; MET: Mesenchymal to epithelial transition; AR: Androgen receptor; HSV-2: Herpes simplex virus type 2; HHV-8: Human herpesvirus 8; EV: Extracellular vesicles; MPs: Microparticles; MVBs: Multivesicular bodies; CVB3: Coxsackie virus B3.

Competing interests

The authors have stated that they have no conflicts of interest.

Authors' contributions

JK, SY and WK participated in the design of the study and performed the analysis of references. JK and WK supervised study design and led obtaining funding. JK drafted the manuscript, and SY and WK participated critical revision of the manuscript. All authors read and approved the final manuscript.

Acknowledgements

This work was supported by the National Research Foundation of Korea (NRF) grant funded by the Korea government (MSIP) (No. NRF-2014R1A2A1A09006983), the Ministry of Education, Science and Technology (2012R1A1A4A01008753 and 2013R1A1A2004740) (to W-J.K.), NIH grants 1R01DK100974-01, DoD W81XWH-15-1-0415, U24 DK097154, NIH NCATS UCLA CTSI UL1TR000124, IMAGINE NO IC Research Grant, the Steven Spielberg Discovery Fund in Prostate Cancer Research Career Development Award, Interstitial Cystitis Association (ICA) Pilot Grant, and a Fishbein Family IC Research Grant by ICA, New York Academy of Medicine; Boston Children's Hospital Faculty Development (to J.K.).

Author details

[1]Departments of Surgery and Biomedical Sciences, Cedars-Sinai Medical Center, 8700 Beverly Blvd., Davis Room 5071, Los Angeles, CA 90048, USA. [2]Departments of Medicine, University of California, Los Angeles, CA, USA. [3]Department of Surgery, Harvard Medical School, Boston, MA, USA. [4]Department of Urology, Chungbuk National University College of Medicine, 62 Kaeshin-dong, Heungduk-gu, Cheongju 361-763, Republic of Korea.

References

1. Attard G, Parker C, Eeles RA, Schroder F, Tomlins SA, Tannock I, et al. Prostate cancer. Lancet. 2015.
2. Behesnilian AS, Reiter RE. Risk stratification of prostate cancer in the modern era. Curr Opin Urol. 2015;25(3):246–51.
3. Siegel RL, Miller KD, Jemal A. Cancer statistics, 2015. CA Cancer J Clin. 2015;65(1):5–29.
4. Hoy SM. Abiraterone acetate: a review of its use in patients with metastatic castration-resistant prostate cancer. Drugs. 2013;73(18):2077–91.
5. McGann S, Horton ER. Radium-223 dichloride: a novel treatment option for castration-resistant prostate cancer patients with symptomatic bone metastases. Ann Pharmacother. 2015;49(4):469–76.
6. Mukherji D, Omlin A, Pezaro C, Shamseddine A, de Bono J. Metastatic castration-resistant prostate cancer (CRPC): preclinical and clinical evidence for the sequential use of novel therapeutics. Cancer Metastasis Rev. 2014;33(2–3):555–66.
7. Vuong W, Sartor O, Pal SK. Radium-223 in metastatic castration resistant prostate cancer. Asian J Androl. 2014;16(3):348–53.
8. Zustovich F, Fabiani F. Therapeutic opportunities for castration-resistant prostate cancer patients with bone metastases. Crit Rev Oncol Hematol. 2014;91(2):197–209.
9. Smith RA, Manassaram-Baptiste D, Brooks D, Doroshenk M, Fedewa S, Saslow D, et al. Cancer screening in the United States, 2015: a review of current American cancer society guidelines and current issues in cancer screening. CA Cancer J Clin. 2015;65(1):30–54.
10. Trock BJ. Circulating biomarkers for discriminating indolent from aggressive disease in prostate cancer active surveillance. Curr Opin Urol. 2014;24(3):293–302.
11. Birnbaum JK, Feng Z, Gulati R, Fan J, Lotan Y, Wei JT, et al. Projecting benefits and harms of novel cancer screening biomarkers: a study of PCA3 and prostate cancer. Cancer Epidemiol Biomarkers Prev. 2015;24(4):677–82.
12. Day JR, Jost M, Reynolds MA, Groskopf J, Rittenhouse H. PCA3: from basic molecular science to the clinical lab. Cancer Lett. 2011;301(1):1–6.
13. Hessels D, Klein Gunnewiek JM, van Oort I, Karthaus HF, van Leenders GJ, van Balken B, et al. DD3(PCA3)-based molecular urine analysis for the diagnosis of prostate cancer. Eur Urol. 2003;44(1):8–15. discussion 15–16.
14. Loeb S. Prostate cancer: Predicting prostate biopsy results–PCA3 versus phi. Nat Rev Urol. 2015;12(3):130–1.
15. Marks LS, Fradet Y, Deras IL, Blase A, Mathis J, Aubin SM, et al. PCA3 molecular urine assay for prostate cancer in men undergoing repeat biopsy. Urology. 2007;69(3):532–5.
16. Wei JT, Feng Z, Partin AW, Brown E, Thompson I, Sokoll L, et al. Can urinary PCA3 supplement PSA in the early detection of prostate cancer? J Clin Oncol. 2014;32(36):4066–72.
17. Sidaway P. Prostate cancer: Urinary PCA3 and TMPRSS2:ERG reduce the need for repeat biopsy. Nat Rev Urol. 2015.
18. Tomlins SA, Day JR, Lonigro RJ, Hovelson DH, Siddiqui J, Kunju LP, et al. Urine TMPRSS2:ERG Plus PCA3 for Individualized Prostate Cancer Risk Assessment. Eur Urol. 2015.
19. Yun SJ, Jeong P, Kang HW, Kim YH, Kim EA, Yan C, et al. Urinary MicroRNAs of prostate cancer: virus-encoded hsv1-miRH18 and hsv2-miR-H9-5p could Be valuable diagnostic markers. Int Neurourol J. 2015;19(2):74–84.
20. Ayub SG, Kaul D, Ayub T. Microdissecting the role of microRNAs in the pathogenesis of prostate cancer. Cancer Genet. 2015.
21. Lin XJ, Chong Y, Guo ZW, Xie C, Yang XJ, Zhang Q, et al. A serum microRNA classifier for early detection of hepatocellular carcinoma: a multicentre, retrospective, longitudinal biomarker identification study with a nested case–control study. Lancet Oncol. 2015;16(7):804–15.
22. Korzeniewski N, Tosev G, Pahernik S, Hadaschik B, Hohenfellner M, Duensing S. Identification of cell-free microRNAs in the urine of patients with prostate cancer. Urol Oncol. 2015;33(1):16 e17-22.

23. Heidegger I, Borena W, Pichler R. The Role of Human Papilloma Virus in Urological Malignancies. Anticancer Res. 2015;35(5):2513–9.
24. Ge X, Wang X, Shen P. Herpes simplex virus type 2 or human herpesvirus 8 infection and prostate cancer risk: A meta-analysis. Biomed Rep. 2013;1(3):433–9.
25. Caini S, Gandini S, Dudas M, Bremer V, Severi E, Gherasim A. Sexually transmitted infections and prostate cancer risk: a systematic review and meta-analysis. Cancer Epidemiol. 2014;38(4):329–38.
26. Meckes Jr DG, Shair KH, Marquitz AR, Kung CP, Edwards RH, Raab-Traub N. Human tumor virus utilizes exosomes for intercellular communication. Proc Natl Acad Sci U S A. 2010;107(47):20370–5.
27. Qi P, Han JX, Lu YQ, Wang C, Bu FF. Virus-encoded microRNAs: future therapeutic targets? Cell Mol Immunol. 2006;3(6):411–9.
28. Qureshi A, Thakur N, Monga I, Thakur A, Kumar M. VIRmiRNA: a comprehensive resource for experimentally validated viral miRNAs and their targets. Database (Oxford). 2014;2014.
29. Minciacchi VR, Freeman MR, Di Vizio D. Extracellular vesicles in cancer: exosomes, microvesicles and the emerging role of large oncosomes. Semin Cell Dev Biol. 2015;40:41–51.
30. Hessels D, Schalken JA. Urinary biomarkers for prostate cancer: a review. Asian J Androl. 2013;15(3):333–9.
31. Webber J, Yeung V, Clayton A. Extracellular vesicles as modulators of the cancer microenvironment. Semin Cell Dev Biol. 2015;40:27–34.
32. Kim J, Morley S, Le M, Bedoret D, Umetsu DT, Di Vizio D, et al. Enhanced shedding of extracellular vesicles from amoeboid prostate cancer cells: potential effects on the tumor microenvironment. Cancer Biol Ther. 2014;15(4):409–18.
33. Hessvik NP, Sandvig K, Llorente A. Exosomal miRNAs as Biomarkers for Prostate Cancer. Front Genet. 2013;4:36.
34. Greening DW, Gopal SK, Mathias RA, Liu L, Sheng J, Zhu HJ, et al. Emerging roles of exosomes during epithelial-mesenchymal transition and cancer progression. Semin Cell Dev Biol. 2015;40:60–71.
35. Tetta C, Ghigo E, Silengo L, Deregibus MC, Camussi G. Extracellular vesicles as an emerging mechanism of cell-to-cell communication. Endocrine. 2013;44(1):11–9.
36. Yanez-Mo M, Siljander PR, Andreu Z, Zavec AB, Borras FE, Buzas EI, et al. Biological properties of extracellular vesicles and their physiological functions. Journal of extracellular vesicles. 2015;4:27066.
37. Yoon YJ, Kim OY, Gho YS. Extracellular vesicles as emerging intercellular communicasomes. BMB Rep. 2014;47(10):531–9.
38. Choi DY, You S, Jung JH, Lee JC, Rho JK, Lee KY, et al. Extracellular vesicles shed from gefitinib-resistant nonsmall cell lung cancer regulate the tumor microenvironment. Proteomics. 2014;14(16):1845–56.
39. Alexander M, Hu R, Runtsch MC, Kagele DA, Mosbruger TL, Tolmachova T, et al. Exosome-delivered microRNAs modulate the inflammatory response to endotoxin. Nat Commun. 2015;6:7321.
40. Galli R, Paone A, Fabbri M, Zanesi N, Calore F, Cascione L, et al. Toll-like receptor 3 (TLR3) activation induces microRNA-dependent reexpression of functional RARbeta and tumor regression. Proc Natl Acad Sci U S A. 2013;110(24):9812–7.

13

Partial Segmental Thrombosis of the Corpus Cavernosum (PSTCC) diagnosed by contrast-enhanced ultrasound

Stephanie Sauer[1], Jan P Goltz[2], Tobias Gassenmaier[1], Andreas S Kunz[1], Thorsten A Bley[1], Detlef Klein[1] and Bernhard Petritsch[1*]

Abstract

Background: Partial segmental thrombosis of the corpus cavernosum (PSTCC) is a rare disease predominantly occurring in young men. Cardinal symptoms are pain and perineal swelling. Although several risk factors are described in the literature, the exact etiology of penile thrombosis remains unclear in most cases. MRI or ultrasound (US) is usually used for diagnosing this condition.

Case presentation: We report a case of penile thrombosis after left-sided varicocele ligature in a young patient. The diagnosis was established using contrast-enhanced ultrasound (CEUS) and was confirmed by contrast-enhanced magnetic resonance imaging (ceMRI). Successful conservative treatment consisted of systemic anticoagulation using low molecular weight heparin and acetylsalicylic acid.

Conclusion: PSTCC is a rare condition in young men and appears with massive pain and perineal swelling. In case of suspected PSTCC utilization of CEUS may be of diagnostic benefit.

Keywords: Penile thrombosis, Corpus cavernosum, Priapism, Contrast-enhanced ultrasound, MRI

Background

Partial segmental thrombosis of the corpus cavernosum (PSTCC) is a rare disease predominantly occurring in young men [1]. Priapism (prolonged and painful penile erection) must be discerned from actual thrombosis of the corpus cavernosum [2]. PSTCC is characterized by thrombosis that most often is unilateral andlocated in the proximal part of the corpus cavernosum. Cardinal symptoms are massive pain and perineal swelling [3]. The etiology of penile thrombosis remains unclear. Several risk factors are described in the literature [2-6]. In most patients an excellent outcome is achieved with conservative treatment [7,8].

MRI or ultrasound (US) are usually used for diagnosis [9]. This report describes the use of contrast-enhanced ultrasound (CEUS) for assessment of penile thrombosis.

* Correspondence: Petritsch_B@ukw.de
[1]University Hospital Würzburg, Institute of Diagnostic and Interventional Radiology, Oberdürrbacher Str. 6, 97080 Würzburg, Germany
Full list of author information is available at the end of the article

Case presentation

A 23-year-old male was admitted to our university hospital with severe pain and a history of progressive perineal swelling over a period of two weeks. His medical history was non-contributory except a left-sided varicocele ligature performed six years ago. No sexual trauma, dysuria or urethral discharge was reported by the patient. Excessive bicycle riding, masturbation, marijuana or cocaine consumption as well as recent long distance flights were negated.

Physical examination confirmed the absence of priapism. A firm, fixed and extremely painful mass was palpable at the proximal penis. The complete blood count, electrolytes, coagulation profile, CRP and urine analysis were unremarkable.

Gray-scaled ultrasound (Siemens Acuson S2000, Siemens Sector Healthcare, Erlangen, Germany) combined with color Doppler of the penis using a 6 MHz transducer (Siemens 6C1 HD, Siemens Sector Healthcare, Erlangen, Germany) revealed an elongated hypoechogenic mass (Figure 1, arrow) with irregular hyperechogenic internal

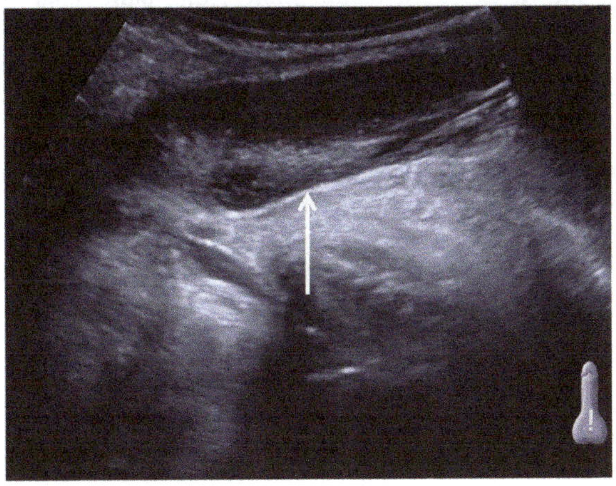

Figure 1 Ultrasound scan (longitudinal axis) of the right corpus cavernosum. Arrow shows thrombus in the proximal part.

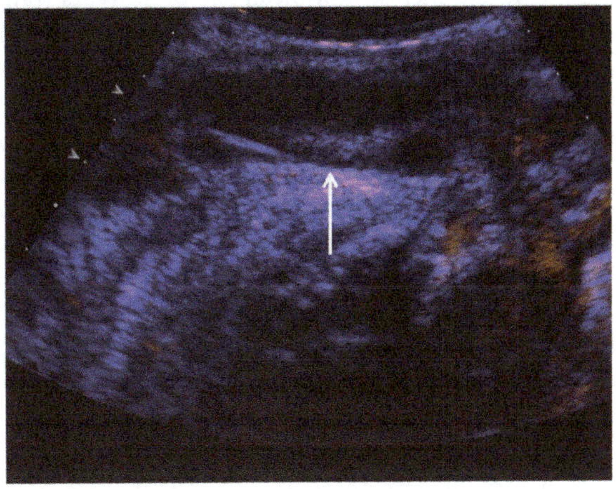

Figure 3 Contrast-enhanced ultrasound shows lack of perfusion and confirms the diagnosis of PSTCC (arrow).

echoes. Color Doppler ultrasound demonstrated absence of flow within the inhomogeneous mass (Figure 2, arrow).

Contrast-enhanced ultrasound (Acuson Sequoia with 4 MHz transducer, Siemens Sector Healthcare, Erlangen, Germany; 1.2 ml SonoVue®, Bracco Imaging, Milano, Italy) revealed a lack of contrast enhancement in the hypoechogenic mass. This was interpreted as segmental thrombosis of the corpus cavernosum (Figure 3, arrow).

For confirmation of this diagnosis a MRI study (1.5 T Siemens Avanto, Siemens Sector Healthcare, Erlangen, Germany) of the pelvis was performed. Transversal T2-weighted images of the pelvis showed a hypointense thrombus of the right proximal corpus cavernosum (Figure 4a, white arrow). T1-weighted fat saturated transversal scans after intravenous contrast medium injection (Gadovist®, Bayer HealthCare AG, Leverkusen, Germany) revealed an intermediate signal and a lack of contrast uptake in the right proximal corpus cavernosum (Figure 4b, black arrow) consistent with sub-acute partial segmental thrombosis of the corpus cavernosum.

Conservative treatment was initiated and consisted of anticoagulation with low molecular weight heparin (Enoxaparin 40 mg once daily) and acetylsalicylic acid (100 mg once daily).

Discussion

Partial segmental thrombosis of the corpus cavernosum (PSTCC) is a rare urological disease which primarily

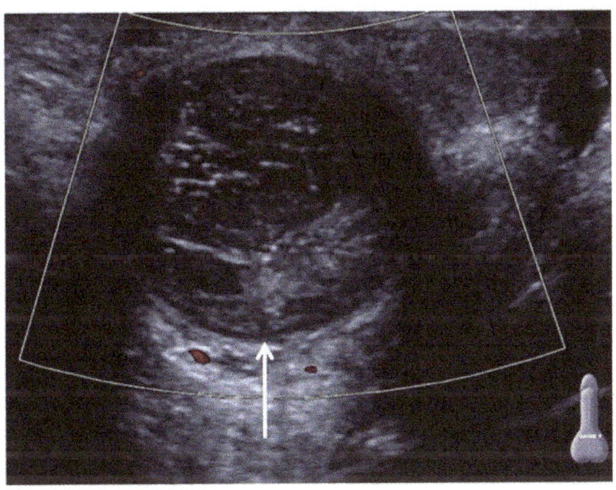

Figure 2 Color Doppler ultrasound (transversal axis) of the proximal penis. Arrow shows absence of flow in the thrombus.

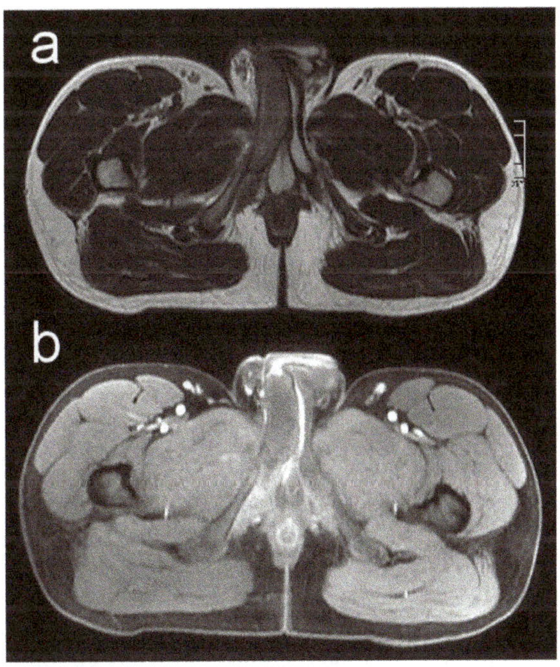

Figure 4 Transversal T2-weighted (a) and fat saturated T1-weighted (b) MRI images through the basis of the penis. Arrows show thrombosis of the right proximal corpus cavernosum.

occurs in young men with a mean age of 30 years (range 18–59 years) [1]. Differential diagnoses include inflammatory processes as well as solid tumors [10].

PSTCC's etiology is poorly understood. Although several risk factors have been described, the exact etiology still remains unclear. Recently Ilicki et al. [1] postulated a two-hit model in which first a transverse membrane, dividing the corpus into a proximal and distal portion, and second a triggering event (microtrauma) is required for the emergence of corpus cavernosum thrombosis. In the presented case no solid membrane as a potentially flow-limiting factor was identified, neither in CEUS nor in MRI. Such membranes may predestinate the emergence of PSTCC but their presence may not be mandatory.

Risk factors for development of PSTCC include haematological abnormalities (sickle cell disease, leukemia, homocysteinemia), abuse of alcohol or drugs (marijuana, cocaine), hypercoagulability associated with malignancy and long distance flights as well as microtrauma after coitus or extended cycling [1-6].

Imaging

Standard imaging modalities include color coded duplex sonography, MRI and CT imaging. The benefits of contrast enhanced MRI have been demonstrated by several authors [1,2,6,11]. In recent years, CEUS has been found to be a cost- efficient alternative in diagnosis of organ and soft tissue pathologies, especially in patients with contraindications for MRI.

This case report outlines the utility of CEUS as an additional cost-saving diagnostic tool for assessment of PSTCC, especially in patients with contraindications for MRI.

Treatment

The first cases of PSTCC were described in 1976 [12]. At that time surgical treatment was the method of choice. Nowadays, as in this case, conservative treatment with systemic anticoagulation appears to be an excellent and reliable therapeutic option. Recent literature shows that all patients treated conservatively have maintained erectile function [5,7,8,13]. Surgery is reserved for patients in whom conservative management fails [5].

Conclusions

PSTCC is a rare condition that predominantly occurs in young men and is accompanied with massive pain and perineal swelling. There are several risk factors described, including abuse of alcohol or drugs, hypercoagulability associated with malignancy and long distance flights as well as microtrauma after coitus or extended bicycle riding. CEUS may be of diagnostic benefit if one suspects PSTCC. Larger studies are warranted to verify this hypothesis. Conservative treatment with systemic anticoagulation has shown excellent results concerning pain relief and erectile dysfunction.

Consent

Written informed consent was obtained from the patient for publication of this case report and any accompanying images. A copy of the written consent is available for review by the Editor of this journal.

Abbreviations

PSTCC: Partial segmental thrombosis of the corpus cavernosum; ceMRI: Contrast-enhanced magnetic resonance imaging; CEUS: Contrast-enhanced ultrasound.

Competing interests

The authors declare that they have no competing interests.

Authors' contributions

SS and DK performed CEUS. JPG and BP evaluated MRI. BP mainly coordinated the development of the manuscript. TG and ASK assisted in both imaging modalities and helped to design, coordinate and draft the manuscript. TAB as well as JPG advanced the manuscript by revising it critically for important intellectual content. All authors read and approved the final manuscript.

Acknowledgements

This publication was funded by the German Research Foundation (DFG) and the University of Würzburg in the funding programme Open Access Publishing.

Author details

[1]University Hospital Würzburg, Institute of Diagnostic and Interventional Radiology, Oberdürrbacher Str. 6, 97080 Würzburg, Germany. [2]University Hospital Schleswig-Holstein, Campus Lübeck, Clinic for Radiology and Nuclear Medicine, Ratzeburger Allee 160, 23538 Lübeck, Germany.

References

1. Ilicki J, Krauss W, Andersson S-O: **Partial segmental thrombosis of the corpus cavernosum: a case report and a review of the literature.** *Urology* 2012, 79:708–712.
2. Goeman L, Joniau S, Oyen R, Claes H, Van Poppel H: **Idiopathic partial thrombosis of the corpus cavernosum: conservative management is effective and possible.** *Eur Urol* 2003, **44:**119–23.
3. Blaut S, Schneider M, Zschuppe E, Günl U, Steinbach F: **Partial unilateral penile thrombosis of corpus cavernosum due to hyperhomocysteinemia. Case report and references.** *Urologe A* 2008, **47:**748–52.
4. Schneede P, Schmeller N, Müller-Lisse UG, Reiser MF, Hofstetter AG: **Partial priapism. Case report and review of the literature of diagnostic and therapeutic measures.** *Urologe A* 1999, **38:**179–83.
5. Lewis JH, Javidan J, Keoleian CM, Shetty SD: **Management of partial segmental priapism.** *Urology* 2001, **57:**169.
6. Horger DC, Wingo MS, Keane TE: **Partial segmental thrombosis of corpus cavernosum: case report and review of world literature.** *Urology* 2005, **66:**194.
7. Kimball DA, Yuh WT, Farner RM: **MR diagnosis of penile thrombosis.** *J Comput Assist Tomogr* 1988, **12:**604–7.
8. Thiel R, Kahn T, Vögeli TA: **Idiopathic partial thrombosis of the corpus cavernosum.** *Urol Int* 1998, **60:**178–80.
9. Pegios W, Rausch M, Balzer JO, Wolfram M, Bentas W, Jonas D, Vogl TJ: **MRI and color-coded duplex sonography: diagnosis of partial priapism.** *Eur Radiol* 2002, **12:**2532–5.
10. Gentile G, Broccoli A, Brunocilla E, Schiavina R, Borghesi M, Romagnoli D, Bianchi L, Derenzini E, Agostinelli C, Franceschelli A, Colombo F, Zinzani PL: **An isolated penile mass in a young adult turned out to be a primary marginal zone lymphoma of the penis. A case report and a review of literature.** *Anticancer Res* 2013, **33:**2639–42.

11. Patel RP, Mucksavage P, Ramchandani P, Hanno PM, Malkowicz SB: **Idiopathic partial thrombosis of the corpus cavernosum.** *Urology* 2010, **76:**1373–4.
12. Hillis RS, Weems WL: **Priapism: an unusual presentation.** *J Urol* 1976, **116:**124–5.
13. Ptak T, Larsen CR, Beckmann CF, Boyle DE: **Idiopathic segmental thrombosis of the corpus cavernosum as a cause of partial priapism.** *Abdom Imaging* 1994, **19:**564–6.

Comparison of the simplified International Index of Erectile Function (IIEF-5) in patients of erectile dysfunction with different pathophysiologies

Zhengyan Tang[1†], Dongjie Li[2†], Xiaobo Zhang[2], Lu Yi[3], Xiangsheng Zhu[4], Xiangyang Zeng[5] and Yuxin Tang[6*]

Abstract

Background: The simplified International Index of Erectile Function (IIEF-5) is a convenient, reliable and validated diagnostic tool for erectile dysfunction (ED). However, few studies focused on IIEF-5 in ED patients with different pathophysiological causes. ,We aim to compare the IIEF-5 score among ED patients with specific pathophysiologies in this study.

Methods: The IIEF-5 score of 3,327 ED patients (median age 39 years) was analyzed. The primary causes of ED were determined by comprehensive diagnostic procedures in the urology/andrology clinics in five training hospitals. Patients with uncertain pathophysiologic cause were excluded.

Results: 176 patients were excluded, 3151 patients with ED history between 0.5 year and 20 years, were enrolled. The causes of ED was classified as psychogenic (59.2%), vasoculogenic (21.3%), neurogenic (4.1%), anatomical/structural (2.8%), hormonal (7.1%) or drug-induced (5.5%). A significant difference was detected in the median IIEF-5 score between psychogenic ED and organic ED (15 (IQR 13, 17) versus 12 (IQR 9.5, 14.5), $P < 0.001$). There was no significant difference of IIEF-5 scores among the organic groups ($P = 0.073$), or between arteriogenic and venogenic groups (13 (IQR 10.5, 15.5) versus 13 (IQR 11–15), $P = 0.912$ (adjusted $\alpha = 0.017$)). However, the median IIEF-5 score of those with a mixed vascular cause was the lowest among vasculogenic patients (11 (IQR 8.5-13.5), scores for the three groups: $P = 0.003$.).

Conclusions: The IIEF-5 scores of men with psychological ED are higher than those with organic causes, but there is no difference among patients with different organic pathophysiologies. Our data indicate that IIEF-5 is not a definitive diagnostic tool to discriminate the pathophysiological causes of ED.

Keywords: Erectile Dysfunction, Pathophysiology, Psychogenic, Organic, IIEF-5

Background

Erectile dysfunction (ED) is defined as the inability to achieve and maintain an erection sufficient to permit satisfactory sexual intercourse [1,2]. A high prevalence of ED has been reported in many studies, and the situation could be even worse in the coming years, particularly in developing countries [3,4]. Although the release of phosphodiesterase type 5 inhibitors (PDE5-i) highly improved the treatment of ED patients with almost all kinds of pathophysiological causes, the high discontinuation rate of PDE5 inhibitors make it still essential to seek the causes for disease diagnosis and treatment [2,5-7].

The pathophysiology of ED includes vasculogenic, neurogenic, hormonal, anatomical, drug-induced and psychogenic causes in nature [8]. Identifying the pathophysiology of ED can significantly help to assess the modifiable risk factors and other medical conditions [9,10]. Furthermore, assessing the causes of ED is essential to cure patients with some certain types of ED [11].

The International Index of Erectile Function (IIEF) and the simplified International Index of Erectile Function (IIEF-5) are widely used, validated, self-administered questionnaires, and havebeen demonstrated to be high degree of sensitivity and specificity to ED [12-14]. Serkan

* Correspondence: mmcct@126.com
†Equal contributors
[6]Department of Urology, The Third Xiangya Hospital of Central South University, Changsha, Hunan, China
Full list of author information is available at the end of the article

Deveci et al. used the Doppler ultrasonography (DUS) to evaluate the ability of the IIEF differentiating different pathophysiologies of ED [15]. However, they concluded that the IIEF is not completely accurate in differentiating between organic and psychogenic ED. In addition, several studies [16-18] have confirmed that there is no significant difference in the IIEF or IIEF-5 scores among patients with specific vascular causes (i.e. arterial insufficiency, vascular leakage and mixed disorder).

However, few investigations about the differences in IIEF-5 among patients with all different pathophysiology have been reported. It is still unclear whether the IIEF-5 is capable of diagnosing the cause of ED. The present study aimed to evaluate the ability of the IIEF-5 to differentiate among all different pathophysiology of ED, according to standard comprehensive diagnostic procedures [8,19].

Methods

We investigated consecutive patients with established ED in the urology or andrology clinics from three university affiliated hospitals (Xiangya Hospital, the Second Xiangya Hospital, and the Third Xiangya Hospital, Central South University) and two training hospitals (the First People's Hospital of Chenzhou, the Central Hospital of Xiangtan) from January 2006 to January 2010. All subjects provided written informed consent. The project was organized by the Third Xiangya hospital, Central South University, and it was approved by the ethics committee of each institution. All protocols were reviewed and approved by the ethics committee of the Third Xiangya hospital, Central South University.

All patients (n = 3327) complained of the inability to achieve and/or maintain erection of sufficient rigidity and duration to permit satisfactory sexual performance. The patients completed the IIEF-5 at doctor's office. Then they underwent independent evaluations by an experienced urologist or andrologist. The diagnostic steps and classification were based on EAU guidelines on erectile dysfunction (update March 2005) [8]. A detailed medical and sexual history was obtained and a physical examination was performed in all patients. Physical examination included the assessment of genitourinary, endocrine, vascular, and neurologic systems. A fasting glucose and lipid profile screen was performed if not assessed in the previous 12 months. Further laboratory testing included a morning sample of total testosterone and additional tests were determined when relevant cause was suspected. Patients with abnormal responses to examinations or tests were referred for specific tests (e.g. nocturnal penile tumescence and rigidity, NTPR).

The most primary cause was judged on the basis of the above-mentioned comprehensive diagnostic procedures. For example, they could be diagnosed as hormonal ED, when the patients with low sexual desire, abnormal physical examination (e.g. small testes, reduced body hair, gynecomastia), low testosterone level, or other related hormone abnormalities (e.g. LH, E_2, PRL, TSH, T3, T4). A patient will be diagnosed as psychogenic ED if no organic cause was detected, whereas he was suffered with mental disorders including performance anxiety, a strained relationship, psychological stress, lack of sexual arousability, and overt psychiatric disorders such as depression and schizophrenia (see Additional file 1).

176 subjects were excluded from this study due to the following reasons: (1) cause could not be determined by above procedures; (2) patients had two or more causes that are equally predominant; (3) patients were not willing to accept further investigations.

The severity of ED was evaluated using IIEF-5, and was classified into 4 levels based on the scores: severe (5–7), moderate (8–11), mild to moderate (12–16), and mild (17–21) [13].

Statistical analysis

Qualitative variables were described by frequency, percentages, mean, and 95% confidence intervals. Nonparametric test was utilized: (1) Spearman correlations were used to assess the association between individual variables; (2) quantitative data of two individual samples were evaluated by Wilcoxon rank sum test; (3) multiple samples were evaluated by Kruskal-Wallis H test. Comparison between categorical variables was performed using chi-square test. Data analysis was performed using the SPSS 17.0 software (SPSS, Chicago, USA). The significance level was set at $P = 0.05$, and it was adjusted to 0.017 (0.05/3 = 0.017) for pairwise comparisons among the three vasculogenic subgroups (arteriogenic, venogenic, mixed vascular).

Results

The median age of the enrolled subjects (n = 3,151) was 39 (interquartile range, 29.5-48.5) years, with a range from 19 to 70 years.

The primary causes of ED were psychogenic (1866 patients, 59.2%) and organic (1285 patients, 40.8%) respectively. The pathophysiological causes of organic ED were vasculogenic (52.1%, 670/1285), neurogenic (10.0%, 129/1285), anatomical/structural (6.9%, 89/1285), hormonal (17.4%, 224/1285), and drug-induced (13.5%, 173/1285), respectively.

The IIEF-5 scores of patients with different primary causes were presented in Figure 1. The median IIEF-5 score of these subjects was 14 (interquartile range, 11.5, 16.5). A significant difference in the mean IIEF-5 score was observed between the subjects with psychogenic ED and those with organic ED ($P = 0.000$) (Table 1). Moreover, although there was a significant difference

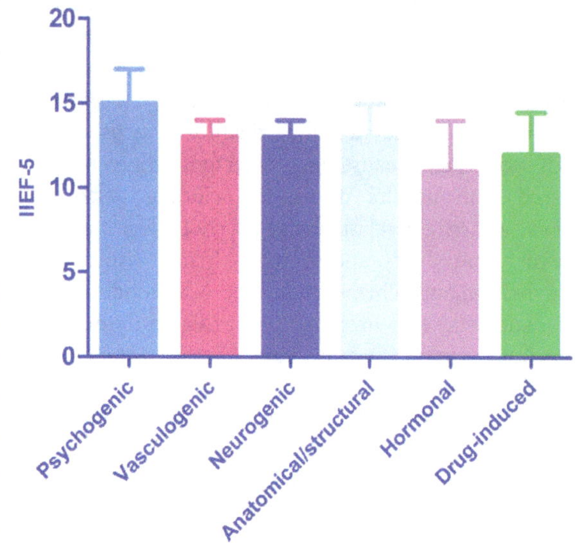

Figure 1 The IIEF-5 scores of 3,151 patients with different pathophysiologic causes. Error bar: interquartile range. Kruskal-Wallis H test for all groups, all organic groups (except for psychogenic): P = 0.000, and P = 0.073, respectively.

in the IIEF-5 scores among all groups (P = 0.000), no significant difference was identified in patients with organic causes (P = 0.073).

The distribution of ED severity in different pathophysiologic causes was presented in Table 2. Moreover, as indicated in Figure 2, the ED severity increased with age. A significant correlation was found between age and IIEF score.

The severity and age distribution of patients with various vasculogenic ED was shown in Table 3 and Table 4 , respectively. A significant difference was detected among the different vascular causes, the ED severity of patients with mixed vascular was higher than those with either arteriogenic or venogenic cause, but no difference was found between arteriogenic and venogenic causes (13 vs 13, P = 0.912 (adjusted α = 0.017)).

Patients' median duration of ED was 2 years (interquartile range, 0.5-3.5). There were significant differences in the duration among patients from each pathophysiology (Kruskal-Wallis H test for all groups, all groups (except for psychogenic), all organic groups (except for psychogenic and unknown): P = 0.000, P = 0.000, and P = 0.000, respectively). Meanwhile, the IIEF-5 score was negatively correlated with ED duration (rs = −0.189, P = 0.000, Spearman correlations). Furthermore, a significant difference in duration was detected among patients with three vascular causes (P = 0.046), but no significant difference in duration was found among arbitrary vascular causes (arteriogenic versus venogenic, arteriogenic versus mixed, venogenic versus mixed, P = 0.538, 0.019, and 0.027 respectively (adjusted α = 0.017).

Table 1 Age distribution and median IIEF-5 scores of patients with different primary pathophysiologic causes

Primary causes	<40 year	≥40 year	Overall	Median IIEF (IQR)
Psychogenic	1145 (66.4)	721 (50.6)	1866 (59.2)	15 (13, 17)
Organic	580 (33.6)	705 (49.4)	1285 (40.8)	12 (9.5, 14.5)
Total	1725	1426	3151	14 (11.5, 16.5)

IQR, interquartile range. Data in parentheses are percentages of different age, unless otherwise noted.
Age: χ^2 test for psychogenic versus organic: Pearson Chi-square = 80.858, P < 0.001.
IIEF-5: Wilcoxon rank sum test for psychogenic versus organic: P < 0.001.

Discussion

ED is a serious and growing public health problem. The prevalence of ED increased with age [20]. In most countries, a large proportion of patients visiting outpatient clinics were older than 40 years [21,22]. However, our results indicated that the number of young (<40 years) ED patients were more than ones over 40 years (Table 1). Similar results were also obtained in several studies of Chinese ED patients [23,24]. In a 5-year survey in 11 cities in China, Liu et al. found that most patients were younger than 50 years old (75.7% in 2003 and 74.5% in 2008) [23]. Another study in older (>40 years) patients in Beijing also showed that only 27.4% of them recognized ED as a disease, and just 12.1% visited their doctors [24]. These were likely associated with more conservative culture in China [10,25].

ED has serious effects on men's physical and mental health [26,27]. According to different pathogenic mechanisms, ED has usually been classified as psychogenic, organic (ie, neurogenic, hormonal, vasculogenic, anatomic/structural, or drug-induced), or mixed psychogenic and organic causes [8,28]. If ED is longstanding, this may build patient's own world of fear, anxiety, worry, depression and distress around his disorder [29,30]. Hence, the mixed form is generally regarded as the most common category in most studies [2,31]. In this study, we also found that nearly half of subjects have combined different causes. Their combined causes are not necessarily the same with each other. Hence, it is not conducive to analyze the ED causes if this large number of patients all just classified as "the mixed form". Therefore, the primary causes of subjects were studied in this investigation to avoid confusion in patients with mixed causes. The primary cause was determined by an experienced urologist or andrologist according to the comprehensive diagnostic procedures (for details see Methods and Additional file 1). It has been confirmed that the comprehensive procedures are superior in establishing the causes of ED [19,32]. Under some circumstances doctors could not draw a clear distinction between the primary cause and the minor cause. These cases (176/3327, 5.3%) were excluded from present investigation. This proportion was similar to a study by Hatzichristou et al. (78/1276, 6.1%) [19].

Table 2 Patient severity and primary pathophysiologic cause erectile dysfunction

Cause	Severe	Moderate	Mild to moderate	Mild	OR (95% CI)	P Value
Psychogenic	17 (0.9)	356 (19.1)	859 (46.0)	634 (34.0)	1.00 (reference)	
Vasculogenic	83 (12.4)	225 (33.6)	281 (41.9)	81 (12.1)	1.29 (1.19-1.38)	0.000
Neurogenic	17 (13.2)	45 (34.9)	54 (41.9)	13 (10.1)	1.27 (1.17-1.39)	0.000
Anatomical/structural	8 (9.0)	26 (29.2)	42 (47.2)	13 (14.6)	1.25 (1.15-1.37)	0.000
Hormonal	17 (7.6)	111 (49.6)	81 (36.2)	15 (6.7)	1.23 (1.14-1.34)	0.000
Drug-induced	15 (8.7)	70 (40.5)	74 (42.8)	14 (8.1)	1.30 (1.19-1.41)	0.000
Overall	157 (5.0)	833 (26.4)	1391 (44.1)	770 (24.4)		

OR, odds ratio; CI, confidence interval. Data in parentheses are percentages, unless otherwise noted. Adjusted OR (for age) was measured by the ratio of sicker patients (severe and moderate, IIEF-5 scores of which are between 5 and 11, versus mild to moderate and mild, IIEF-5 scores of which are between 12 and 21) in every groups. The psychological ED group (IIEF-5 (5–11) / IIEF-5 (12–21)) was put as reference. CI, confidence interval.

IIEF-5 is a brief, validated, multidimensional, self-administered tool to assess erectile function [13,33]. Rosen RC, et al. believed that there are still many potential areas for future research on the IIEF [34]. For example, the IIEF may not be completely accurate in differentiating among various sub-groups [34,35].

The aim of this study was to assess the difference among all the different pathophysiologies of ED in IIEF-5 by analysing a multicenter, large sample of ED patients using the comprehensive procedures. Previous studies have compared the IIEF or IIEF-5 between organic and psychogenic ED, or between arteriogenic and cavernosal ED. Serkan Deveci et al. compared the IIEF scores with the results of flow dynamics analysis, using the penile duplex Doppler ultrasonography (DUS) in 112 patients. They found that the IIEF was not completely accurate in differentiating between organic and psychogenic ED, but have potential ramifications for evaluating the baseline severity of ED in trials of erectogenic agents. All patients with venogenic cause (4/4) were all categorized as severe ED according to IIEF score, and none of the patients (0/16) with venous leak (including venogenic cause and mixed vascular cause) had mild ED. However, more than a fifth (6/28) of the men with normal erectile haemodynamics also were classified as severe ED [15]. Melman A, et al. used the Rigiscan results to assess the ability of the IIEF-6 in 32 consecutive patients. Similarly, no significant correlation was found between NPTR data and IIEF-6 score. They concluded that the IIEF-6 is unable to differentiate between various causes of ED [35].

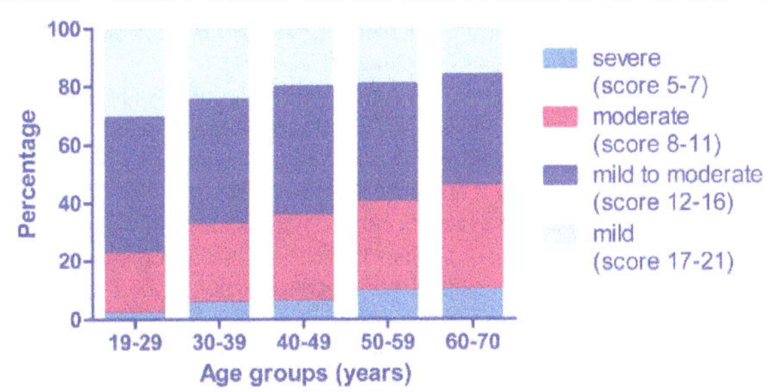

Figure 2 Severity of ED increased with age. Spearman correlations for 3151 patients: rs = −0.198, P = 0.000.

In addition, several studies [16-18] also suggestted that there is no significant difference in the IIEF or IIEF-5 scores among patients with specific vascular causes (i.e. arterial insufficiency, vascular leakage and mixed disorder). Our data indicated that not only there is no significant difference between arteriogenic and venogenic cause in IIEF-5, but also these causes have a similar severity distribution (Table 3). Hence, all these results conducted that IIEF-5 is not accurate in distinguishing the specific causes of vasculogenic ED.

Further, in the current study, although we found a statistical difference among all different pathophysiologies in IIEF-5 (P = 0.000), no significant difference were found among all kinds of organic causes (P = 0.067 or P = 0.073 (except for unknown)) (Figure 1). Hence, the main difference in IIEF-5 was between psychogenic and all other causes. So the IIEF-5 did not statistically differentiate the specific organic causes of ED as determined by evidence-based testing by the comprehensive diagnostic procedures, but it had potential ramifications for the evaluation of whether the patients were psychological origin.

Table 3 Comparison of the severity of patients with different vascular causes according to IIEF-5

Vascular cause n (%)	Severe	Moderate	Mild to moderate	Mild	Median IIEF (IQR)
Arteriogenic	34 (12.9)	80 (30.4)	115 (43.7)	34 (12.9)	13 (10.5, 15.5)
Venogenic	34 (10.5)	106 (32.8)	141 (43.7)	42 (13.0)	13 (11–15)
Mixed vascular	15 (17.9)	39 (46.4)	25 (29.8)	5 (6.0)	11 (8.5-13.5)
Overall	83 (12.4)	225 (33.6)	254 (41.9)	85 (12.1)	13 (11, 15)

IQR, interquartile range. Data in parentheses are percentages, unless otherwise noted. Severity distribution: χ^2 test for all groups, all groups (except for mixed vascular): Pearson Chi-square = 14.351, P = 0.026; Pearson Chi-square = 0.984, P = 0.805 (adjusted α = 0.017), respectively. IIEF-5: Kruskal-Wallis H test for all groups: P = 0.003. Wilcoxon rank sum test for arteriogenic versus venogenic: P = 0.912 (adjusted α = 0.017).

Table 4 Age and specific causes of vasculogenic ED

Vascular cause n (%)	19-29	30-39	40-49	50-59	60-70	Median age (IQR)
Arteriogenic	63 (24.0)	43 (16.3)	114 (43.3)	35 (13.3)	8 (3.0)	40 (32, 48)
Venogenic	81 (25.1)	94 (29.1)	108 (33.4)	34 (10.5)	6 (1.9)	39 (31.5-46.5)
Mixed vascular	11 (13.1)	22 (26.2)	32 (38.1)	16 (19.0)	3 (3.6)	41 (35–47)
Overall	155 (23.1)	159 (23.7)	254 (37.9)	85 (12.7)	17 (2.5)	40 (32.5, 47.5)

IQR, interquartile range. Data in parentheses are percentages, unless otherwise noted. Age distribution: χ^2 test for all groups, all groups (except for mixed vascular): Pearson Chi-square = 30.416, P = 0.000; Pearson Chi-square = 19.24, P = 0.001 (adjusted α = 0.017), respectively. Age: Kruskal-Wallis H test for all groups: P = 0.003. Wilcoxon rank sum test for arteriogenic versus venogenic: P = 0.04 (adjusted α = 0.017).

Our study has several limitations. Firstly, it is not population based. However, the patients seeking treatment at clinics were not chosen on purpose. Rather, they were consecutive patients who were diagnosed with erectile dysfunction by urologist/andrologist. Although these results could not represent the epidemiological characteristics in ED population, it could be more useful for clinical urologists/andrologists. Secondly, all information was recorded by the physicians, thus, self-reported questionnaire (except for IIEF-5) for patients is lacking. This could have resulted in information loss, particularly regarding the demographic characteristics. Thirdly, the contribution of the relational factors (e.g. the types of drugs that can induce ED) in patients were less evaluated, which should be enhanced in follow-up. Finally, an objective, quantitative criteria for judging primary pathophysiology are lacking. Hence, the identification of primary pathophysiological cause depends in part on the physician's judgment, which means inevitable subjectivity. However, this subjective bias could be reduced by basing the identification on uniform guidelines in the diagnostic procedures. We also plan to use statistical methods (e.g. discriminant analysis) to narrow this bias in further research.

Conclusions

This multicenter study was conducted in a large sample of ED patients seeking treatment at clinics. It indicated that the age of Chinese outpatients with ED was younger than other countries. Moreover, no significant difference in IIEF-5 scores was observed among ED patients with different organic pathophysiologies. Therefore, IIEF-5 was not completely sufficient to distinguish the ED pathophysiology, and it should be used with caution.

Additional file

Additional file 1: Self-developed diagnostic criteria for primary pathophysiological cause of ED (based on EAU guidelines on erectile dysfunction [8]).

Abbreviations

IIEF-5: The simplified International Index of Erectile Function; ED: Erectile dysfunction; IQR: Interquartile range; PDE5-i: Phosphodiesterase type 5 inhibitors; DUS: Doppler ultrasonography; NTPR: Nocturnal penile tumescence and rigidity; OR: Odds ratio; CI: Confidence interval.

Competing interests

All the authors declare that they have no financial competing interests.

Authors' contributions

YT participated in the conception and design of entire study; ZT performed the data acquisition, and helped to draft the manuscript;,DL performed the statistical analysis, and coordination and helped to draft the manuscript; XbZ helped to draft the manuscript. LY, performed the data acquisition; XsZ performed the data acquisition; XyZ performed the data acquisition; All authors read and approved the final manuscript.

Acknowledgment

We thank Jiada Li, Ph.D., Xueru Mu, and Jay Mei, M.D., Ph.D. for editorial assistance with our manuscript.

Funding

The work described in this article is supported by Hunan Provincial Innovation Foundation For Postgraduate (Grant No. CX2012B089).

Author details

[1]Department of Urology, Xiangya Hospital of Central South University, Changsha, Hunan 410013, China. [2]Department of Geriatric Urology, Xiangya Hospital of Central South University, Changsha, Hunan 410013, China. [3]Department of Urology, The Second Xiangya Hospital of Central South University, Changsha, Hunan, China. [4]Department of The Andrology, Central Hospital of Xiangtan, Xiangtan, Hunan, China. [5]Department of Urology, The First People's Hospital of Chenzhou, Chenzhou, Hunan, China. [6]Department of Urology, The Third Xiangya Hospital of Central South University, Changsha, Hunan, China.

References

1. NIH Consensus Conference: Impotence: **NIH consensus development panel on impotence.** *JAMA* 1993, **270:**83–90.
2. Shamloul R, Ghanem H: **Erectile dysfunction.** *Lancet* 2013, **381:**153–165.
3. Corona G, Lee DM, Forti G, O'Connor DB, Maggi M, O'Neill TW, Pendleton N, Bartfai G, Boonen S, Casanueva FF, Finn JD, Giwercman A, Han TS, Huhtaniemi IT, Kula K, Lean ME, Punab M, Silman AJ, Vanderschueren D, Wu FC, EMAS Study Group: **Age-related changes in general and sexual health in middle-aged and older men: results from the European Male Ageing Study (EMAS).** *J Sex Med* 2010, **7:**1362–1380.
4. Ayta IA, McKinlay JB, Krane RJ: **The likely worldwide increase in erectile dysfunction between 1995 and 2025 and some possible policy consequences.** *BJU Int* 1999, **84:**50–56.
5. Padma-nathan H, Eardley I, Kloner RA, Laties AM, Montorsi F: **A 4-year update on the safety of sildenafil citrate (Viagra).** *Urology* 2002, **60:**67–90.
6. Son H, Park K, Kim SW, Paick JS: **Reasons for discontinuation of sildenafil citrate after successful restoration of erectile function.** *Asian J Androl* 2004, **6:**117–120.
7. Seftel AD: **Challenges in oral therapy for erectile dysfunction.** *J Androl* 2002, **23:**729–736.
8. Wespes E, Amar E, Hatzichristou D, Hatzimouratidis K, Montorsi F, Pryor J, Vardi Y: **Guidelines on erectile cysfunction: European association of urology.** 2005.

9. Corona G, Mannucci E, Schulman C, Petrone L, Mansani R, Cilotti A, Balercia G, Chiarini V, Forti G, Maggi M: **Psychobiologic correlates of the metabolic syndrome and associated sexual dysfunction.** *Eur Urol* 2006, **50**:595–604.
10. Li D, Jiang X, Zhang X, Yi L, Zhu X, Zeng X, Guo X, Tang Y: **Multicenter pathophysiologic investigation of erectile dysfunction in clinic outpatients in China.** *Urology* 2012, **79**:601–606.
11. Hatzimouratidis K, Amar E, Eardley I, Giuliano F, Hatzichristou D, Montorsi F, Vardi Y, Wespes E, European Association of Urology: **Guidelines on male sexual dysfunction: erectile dysfunction and premature ejaculation.** *Eur Urol* 2010, **57**:804–814.
12. Rosen RC, Riley A, Wagner G, Osterloh IH, Kirkpatrick J, Mishra A: **The international index of erectile function (IIEF): a multidimensional scale for assessment of erectile dysfunction.** *Urology* 1997, **49**:822–830.
13. Rhoden EL, Teloken C, Sogari PR, Vargas SC: **The use of the simplified International Index of Erectile Function (IIEF-5) as a diagnostic tool to study the prevalence of erectile dysfunction.** *Int J Impot Res* 2002, **14**:245–250.
14. Rosen RC, Althof SE, Giuliano F: **Research instruments for the diagnosis and treatment of patients with erectile dysfunction.** *Urology* 2006, **68**:6–16.
15. Deveci S, O'Brien K, Ahmed A, Parker M, Guhring P, Mulhall JP: **Can the international index of erectile function distinguish between organic and psychogenic erectile function?** *BJU Int* 2008, **102**:354–356.
16. Kassouf W, Carrier S: **A comparison of the international index of erectile function and erectile dysfunction studies.** *BJU Int* 2003, **91**:667–669.
17. Chen B, Lu YN, Han YF, Huang XY, Hu K, Wang YX, Huang YR: **IIEF-5 cannot be used as a tool for differential diagnosis of vasculogenic erectile dysfunction.** *Zhonghua Nan Ke Xue* 2007, **13**:118–121.
18. Blander DS, Sanchez-Ortiz RF, Broderick GA: **Sex inventories: can questionnaires replace erectile dysfunction testing?** *Urology* 1999, **54**:719–723.
19. Hatzichristou D, Hatzimouratidis K, Bekas M, Apostolidis A, Tzortzis V, Yannakoyorgos K: **Diagnostic steps in the evaluation of patients with erectile dysfunction.** *J Urol* 2002, **168**:615–620.
20. Akkus E, Kadioglu A, Esen A, Doran S, Ergen A, Anafarta K, Hattat H, Turkish Erectile Dysfunction Prevalence Study Group: **Prevalence and correlates of erectile dysfunction in Turkey: a population-based study.** *Eur Urol* 2002, **41**:298–304.
21. Tariq SH, Haleem U, Omran ML, Kaiser FE, Perry HM, Morley JE: **Erectile dysfunction: etiology and treatment in young and old patients.** *Clin Geriatr Med* 2003, **19**:539–551.
22. Corona G, Mannucci E, Mansani R, Petrone L, Bartolini M, Giommi R, Mancini M, Forti G, Maggi M: **Aging and pathogenesis of erectile dysfunction.** *Int J Impot Res* 2004, **16**:395–402.
23. Liu DF, Jiang H, Hong K, Zhao LM, Ma LL, Zhu JC: **[Epidemiological changes of ED patients: investigations in 11 Chinese cities during the past 5 years].** *Zhonghua Nan Ke Xue* 2009, **15**:724–726.
24. Jiang H, Bai Q, Hong K, Xu QQ, Zhu JC: **[Study on the knowledge of and attitude to sexual dysfunction in aged men].** *Zhonghua Nan Ke Xue* 2005, **11**:752–754.
25. Wong SY, Leung JC, Woo J: **Sexual activity, erectile dysfunction and their correlates among 1,566 older Chinese men in Southern China.** *J Sex Med* 2009, **6**:74–80.
26. Laumann EO, Paik A, Rosen RC: **Sexual dysfunction in the United States: prevalence and predictors.** *JAMA* 1999, **281**:537–544.
27. Althof SE: **Quality of life and erectile dysfunction.** *Urology* 2002, **59**:803–810.
28. Lue TF: **Erectile dysfunction.** *N Engl J Med* 2000, **342**:1802–1813.
29. Dean RC, Lue TF: **Physiology of penile erection and pathophysiology of erectile dysfunction.** *Urol Clin North Am* 2005, **32**:379–395.
30. Corona G, Mannucci E, Lotti F, Boddi V, Jannini EA, Fisher AD, Monami M, Sforza A, Forti G, Maggi M: **Impairment of couple relationship in male patients with sexual dysfunction is associated with overt hypogonadism.** *J Sex Med* 2009, **6**:2591–2600.
31. Caskurlu T, Tasci AI, Resim S, Sahinkanat T, Ergenekon E: **The etiology of erectile dysfunction and contributing factors in different age groups in Turkey.** *Int J Urol* 2004, **11**:525–529.
32. Davis-Joseph B, Tiefer L, Melman A: **Accuracy of the initial history and physical examination to establish the etiology of erectile dysfunction.** *Urology* 1995, **45**:498–502.
33. Ponholzer A, Temml C, Mock K, Marszalek M, Obermayr R, Madersbacher S: **Prevalence and risk factors for erectile dysfunction in 2869 men using a validated questionnaire.** *Eur Urol* 2005, **47**:80–86.
34. Rosen RC, Cappelleri JC, Gendrano N: **The International Index of Erectile Function (IIEF): a state-of-the-science review.** *Int J Impot Res* 2002, **14**:226–244.
35. Melman A, Fogarty J, Hafron J: **Can self-administered questionnaires supplant objective testing of erectile function? A comparison between the International Index Of Erectile Function and objective studies.** *Int J Impot Res* 2006, **18**:126–129.

15

Five-point Likert scaling on MRI predicts clinically significant prostate carcinoma

Taisuke Harada[2], Takashige Abe[1*], Fumi Kato[2], Ryuji Matsumoto[1], Hiromi Fujita[3], Sachiyo Murai[1], Naoto Miyajima[1], Kunihiko Tsuchiya[1], Satoru Maruyama[1], Kohsuke Kudo[2] and Nobuo Shinohara[1]

Abstract

Background: To clarify the relationship between the probability of prostate cancer scaled using a 5-point Likert system and the biological characteristics of corresponding tumor foci.

Methods: The present study involved 44 patients undergoing 3.0-Tesla multiparametric MRI before laparoscopic radical prostatectomy. Tracing based on pathological and MRI findings was performed. The relationship between the probability of cancer scaled using the 5-point Likert system and the biological characteristics of corresponding tumor foci was evaluated.

Results: A total of 102 tumor foci were identified histologically from the 44 specimens. Of the 102 tumors, 55 were assigned a score based on MRI findings (score 1: $n = 3$; score 2: $n = 3$; score 3: $n = 16$; score 4: $n = 11$ score 5: $n = 22$), while 47 were not pointed out on MRI. The tracing study revealed that the proportion of >0.5 cm^3 tumors increased according to the upgrade of Likert scores (score 1 or 2: 33 %; score 3: 68.8 %; score 4 or 5: 90.9 %, χ^2 test, $p < 0.0001$). The proportion with a Gleason score >7 also increased from scale 2 to scale 5 (scale 2: 0 %; scale 3: 56.3 %; scale 4: 72.7 %; 5: 90.9 %, χ^2 test, $p = 0.0001$). On using score 3 or higher as the threshold of cancer detection on MRI, the detection rate markedly improved if the tumor volume exceeded 0.5 cm^3 (<0.2 cm^3: 10.3 %; 0.2-0.5 cm^3: 25 %; 0.5-1.0 cm^3: 66.7 %; 1.0 < cm^3: 92.1 %).

Conclusions: Each Likert scale favobably reflected the corresponding tumor's volume and Gleason score. Our observations show that "score 3 or higher" could be a useful threshold to predict clinically significant carcinoma when considering treatment options.

Background

In the treatment of prostate carcinoma, one of the major disadvantages of preoperative MRI is the lack of a standardized reporting system. Sometimes, the report may be written in a narrative manner, making it difficult to compare studies from different centers. Recently, the European Society of Urogenital Radiology recommended the use of the MR Prostate Imaging Reporting and Data System (PI-RADS) [1], and the Prostate Diagnostic Imaging Consensus Meeting panel proposed using 5-point Likert scaling [2]. Regarding the 5-point Likert scaling, it was the most commonly used method in previous clinical studies [3–5]. In order to promote widespread use of the 5-point Likert scaling system in daily clinical practice, we consider that studies comparing the probability of cancer scaled using the 5-point Likert system and the biological characteristics of correspondig tumor foci should be accumulated, and the results should be shared among surgeons and radiologists as a common language.

In the present study, in order to gain further insight into the association between tumor-foci characteristics and the 5-point Likert score, we performed a detailed comparison between all small cancerous foci on whole-mount histopathology and radiological findings according to 5-point Likert scaling using the recent 3.0-Tesla multiparametric MRI.

Methods

The study protocol was approved by the institutional review board of Hokkaido University Hospital, and patient consent was not deemed necessary because data were

* Correspondence: takataka@rf6.so-net.ne.jp
[1]Department of Urology, Hokkaido University Graduate School of Medicine, North-15, West-7, North Ward, Sapporo 060-8638, Japan
Full list of author information is available at the end of the article

obtained from medical charts and patient identifying information was anonymized before analysis.

Patients

Between June 2009 and April 2013, 80 patients with localized prostate carcinoma underwent laparoscopic radical prostatectomy (LRP). Of these, 56 patients underwent 3.0-Tesla multiparametric MRI before surgery. Excluding 12 patients due to a lack of dynamic contrast-enhanced (DCE) MRI ($n = 5$), susceptibility artifacts on diffusion- weighted imaging (DWI) ($n = 4$), or sequence differences ($n = 3$), the final study population consisted of 44 patients. No prior radiation therapy and/or androgen deprivation therapy was performed in our cohort.

MRI technique

MRI was performed before biopsy in 6 patients, and the interval between biopsy and MRI was a median of 99 days (range: 27–855) in the remaining 38 patients.

Patients underwent MRI with a 3.0-T scanner (Achieva 3.0-T TX series R3.21; Philips Medical Systems, Best, the Netherlands) and a pelvic phased-array coil (32-channel SENSE Torso/Cardiac Coil). No endorectal coil was used. The slice thickness of all the sequences was 3 mm. The following MR sequences were obtained: axial T1-weighted image (T1WI), axial T2-weighted image (T2WI), axial, sagittal, and coronal fat-suppressed T2WI, axial DWI, and DCE MRI. DCE MRI was performed in the axial plane with one pre-contrast and four post-contrast dynamic series after the intravenous administration of gadolinium-based contrast material at a dose of 0.1 mmol per kilogram body weight and subsequent flushing with standardized 20-mL saline. The apparent diffusion coefficient (ADC) values were calculated from two DWI scans acquired with b = 0 and 2,000 s/mm2, and ADC maps were then rebuilt by calculating the ADC values in each pixel of each slice. In the present study, we did not perform any bowel preparation, or administer any agent to suppress bowel peristalsis.

Image analysis

For this retrospective analysis, all MR images were reviewed in consensus by two radiologists with 13 and 5 years' experience in prostate MRI. Both readers were aware that the patients had prostate cancer documented by biopsy and had undergone LRP, but were blind to all other clinical data. On pre-contrast DCE MRI, high-signal-intensity areas were considered hemorrhagic after prostate biopsy. On T2WI, a finding suggesting prostate cancer was defined as a hypointense area in the prostate compared to the adjacent parenchyma, excluding an area of hemorrhage. In the case of a wedge-shaped hypointense area without a mass effect around the adjusting prostatic tissue, we suspected chronic prostatitits rather than prostatic cancer, considering the results of other sequences together. On DWI, it was defined as a focal hyperintense area at b = 2,000 s/mm^2 of DWI, with a low focal ADC value compared to that of the adjacent normal parenchyma on ADC mapping. On DCE-MRI, it was defined as an early enhancing area in the prostate compared to adjacent normal parenchyma. In the case of biopsy–related hemorrhage, we tried to identify an enhanced lesion by carefully comparing pre and post images. The likelihood of the presence of prostate cancer was determined based on an overall combination of the findings from T2WI, DWI, and DCE-MRI using a Likert scale between 1 and 5 (1, very low level of suspicion; 2, low level of suspicion; 3, equivocal; 4, cancer probable; 5, definitely cancer).

Pathology

Following LRP, the specimens were fixed overnight in 10 % neutral buffered formaldehyde. After staining of the surface, each specimen was cut into transverse 5-mm-thick slices, vertical to the dorsorectal surface, and the apex and base were sagittally sectioned. After pathological evaluation, all tumor foci were mapped on the macroscopic photographs. For all LRP specimens, the primary and secondary Gleason grades as well as the combined Gleason score were recorded. The T-category was defined according to the 2009 TNM classification.

For the present study, tumor areas in the macroscopic photographs were traced and measured using computer planimetry software (Image J, free software). If the distance between two tumor foci was greater than 5 mm, they were considered separate. The tumor volume was calculated by multiplying the total tumor surface area by the section thickness (5 mm). For analysis, a shrinkage factor of 1.15 was considered [6]. When the Gleason score in each focal lesion had not been described in the original pathological report, we evaluated it (HF). Thereafter, tracing based on pathological mapping and MRI findings was performed jointly by three of the authors (TH, TA, and FK; Fig. 1).

Statistical analysis

Analyses were performed with JMP® version 11 (SAS Institute, Japan). We used the χ^2 test to compare categorical characteristics among the groups. Univariate and multivariate logistic regression analyses were used to indentify characteristics associated with the visibility of cancerous lesions on 3-Tesla MRI. A p-value <0.05 was considered significant.

Results

Clinical and pathological characteristics of the 44 patients were as follows: mean age, 67.1 years, median age, 68

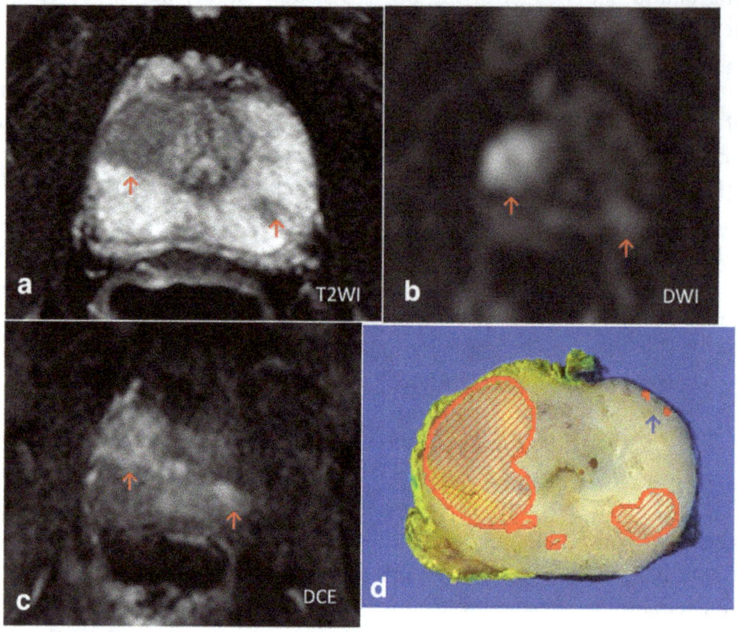

Fig. 1 A 74-year-old patient with a PSA level of 16.08 ng/mL. A T2-weighted image (T2WI) demonstrates decreased signal intensity lesions in both lobes (**a**). These lesions show a focally increased signal intensity on diffusion-weighted (DWI, **b**) and dynamic contrast-enhanced (DCE, **c**) MRI. Using the five-point Likert scale, the two readers assigned a score of 5 to both lesions. On the other hand, the small tumor foci pointed out by the blue arrow in the histology (**d**) was not pointed out on MRI reading

years (range: 52–77); median PSA, 6.91 ng/mL (range: 1.75–37.6); median time between MRI and LRP, 10 days (range: 1–164). Thirty-one patients were in stage pT2 and 13 in pT3. Regarding the node status, all patients showed pN0. Table 1 summarizes the characteristics of tumor foci. A total of 102 tumor foci were identified histologically from the 44 LRP specimens. The median tumor volume was 0.386 cm^3 (range: 0.0023–14.0) after shrinkage correction. The Gleason score distribution was 6 in 49, 7 in 40, and 8–9 in 13.

Table 1 Summary of characteristics of tumor foci

Tumor location, n	
Peripheral zone	85
Central/Transition zone only	17
Tumor volume, cm^3	Median, 0.386 (range, 0.0023–14.0)
Tumor volume distribution, n	
<0.2 mL	39
0.2–0.5	16
0.5–1.0	9
>1.0	38
Gleason score distribution, n	
6	49
7	40
8–9	13

Of the 102 tumors, 55 were assigned a score based on MRI findings (score 1: $n = 3$; score 2: $n = 3$; score 3: $n = 16$; score 4: $n = 11$ score 5: $n = 22$) and 47 were not pointed out on MRI. Figure 2 shows a mosaic plot of the relationship between the tumor volume and each assigned Likert score. The proportion of >0.5 cm^3 tumors increased with the upgrade of Likert scores (score 1 or 2: 33 %; score 3: 68.8 %; score 4 or 5: 90.9 %, χ^2 test, $p < 0.0001$). The median tumor volume according to each scale was 0.459 cm^3 (range: 0.0696–0.597) for scale 1, 0.267 cm^3 (range: 0.0558–0.954) for scale 2, 0.816 cm^3 (range: 0.0023–5.79) for scale 3, 1.53 cm^3 (range: 0.332–7.93) for scale 4, and 2.34 cm^3 (range: 0.065–14.0) for scale 5. Figure 3 shows a mosaic plot of the relationship between the Gleason score and each assigned Likert score. The proportion with a Gleason score >7 also increased from score 2 to score 5 (scale 2: 0 %; scale 3: 56.3 %; scale 4: 72.7 %; scale 5: 90.9 %, χ^2 test, $p = 0.0001$).

On the other hand, 95 areas were pointed out and scaled on image review by the 2 radiologists. Tracing between pathological mapping and MRI findings revealed that 10 areas pointed out on MRI were overlapping on pathological mapping. Of the 85 non-overlapping areas, the positive predictive value for the diagnosis of cancer according to each score was 20 % (2/10) for score 1, 23.5 % (4/17) for score 2, 75 % (15/20) for score 3, 73.3 % (11/15) for score 4, and 95.7 % (22/23) for score 5. The positive predictive value was 82.8 % (48/58) for score >3.

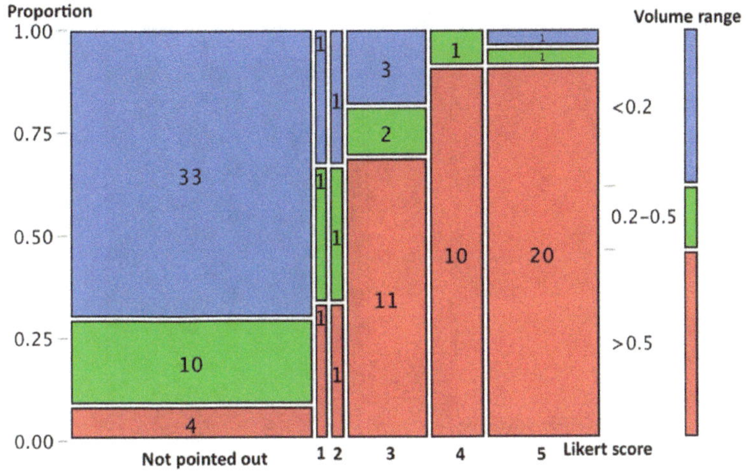

Fig. 2 Mosaic plot of relationship between tumor volume and each assigned Likert score. The proportion of >0.5 cm^3 tumors increased according to the upgrade of Likert scores (χ2 test, $p < 0.0001$)

Based on our current observations, the assigned scores of 3–5 were treated as visible cancerous lesions on MRI in the subsequent analyses. Figure 4 shows a mosaic plot regarding tumor visibility on MRI in accordance with the tumor volume. After the tumor volume exceeded 0.5 cm^3, the detection rate on MRI markedly improved (0.5–1.0 cm^3: 6/9, 66.7 %, 1.0 < cm^3: 35/38, 92.1 %). Overall, the sensitivity for cancer detection was 87.2 % (41/47) for tumors larger than 0.5 cm^3. Table 2 shows the results of multivariate analysis to identify the characteristics associated with visibility on 3-T MRI. The tumor volume and Gleason sum were significant factors on univariate analysis. In the multivariate model, only the tumor volume remained significant.

Discussion

The usefulness of MRI for imaging prostate carcinoma has already been recognized [7]. On the other hand, most radiologists would agree that the diagnosis and localization of carcinoma are not always easy due to coexisting hyperplasia, prostatitis, or bleeding, and it is sometimes difficult to fill in medical records in a "black or white" manner. Recently, two scoring systems were recommended: PI-RADS and the Likert scale. The PI-RADS system uses multi-parametric techniques including T2-weighted imaging, DCE MRI, and DWI, and a score from one to five is given according to each variable [1]. Therefore, total scores range from 3 to 15, and a threshold of 8 or greater, or 9 or greater, has been used as a cutoff for cancer detection in previous studies [8, 9]. Regarding

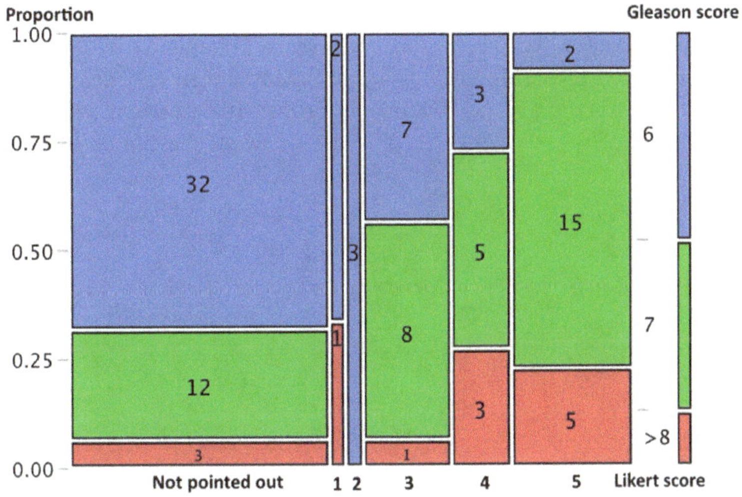

Fig. 3 Mosaic plot of relationship between Gleason score and each assigned Likert score. The proportion of Gleason score >7 also increased from scale 2 to scale 5 (χ2 test, $p = 0.0001$)

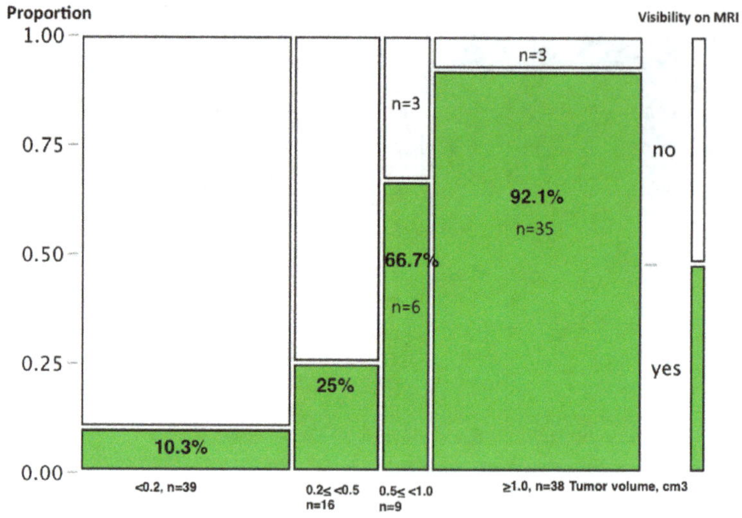

Fig. 4 Mosaic plot of relationship between tumor visibility on 3-Tesla MRI and range of tumor volume

the Likert system, a rating from 1 to 5 was assigned based on the overall impression of MRI findings, and a threshold of 3 or higher was typically used in previous studies [3–5]. In the present study, we performed a close comparison between all small cancerous foci on whole-mount histopathology and radiological findings according to 5-point Likert scaling using the recent 3.0-Tesla multiparametric MRI. We observed that the proportion of >0.5 cm^3 tumors increased according to the upgrade of Likert scores (score 1 or 2: 33 %; score 3: 68.8 %; score 4 or 5: 90.9 %, χ^2 test, $p < 0.0001$), and the proportion of those with Gleason score >7 also increased from score 2 to score 5 (score 2: 0 %; score 3: 56.3 %; score 4: 72.7 %; 5: 90.9 %, χ^2 test, $p = 0.0001$). Our observations confirmed that a threshold of 3 or higher is very helpful for clinicians when considering the possibility of significant cancer, denoting >0.5 cm^3 or Gleason score >7 tumors. Although we did not assess PI-RADS data or inter-observer variability in scoring, Renard-Penna et al. reported favorable interobserver agreement between the Likert scale ($\kappa = 0.80$) and PI-RADS system ($\kappa = 0.73$) [8].

Regarding detectability on MRI according to the cancer volume, Ikonen S et al. previously reported that, with the use of endorectal coil 1.5-T MRI (T2-weighted), the rate of detecting carcinoma foci smaller than 5 mm was 5 %, but it was 89 % for those larger than 10 mm [10]. Roethke MC et al. reported similar results, whereby they were able to visualize 0/56 lesions with a size of <0.3 cm (0 %), 4/116 (3 %) between 0.3 and 0.5 cm, 22/169 (13 %) between 0.5 and 1 cm, 61/136 (45 %) between 1 and 2 cm, and 50/56 (89 %) >2 cm using endorectal coil 1.5-T MRI (T2-weighted) [11]. Villers et al. also reported that sensitivity, specificity, and positive and negative predictive values for cancer detection by 1.5-T pelvic phased-array coil MRI were 90, 88, 77, and 95 %, respectively, for foci larger than 0.5 cc [12]. In the present study, the positive predictive value for a diagnosis of cancer based on MRI findings was 75 % (15/20) for score 3, 73.3 % (11/15) for score 4, and 95.7 % (22/23) for score 5. Using a threshold of 3 or greater to indicate probable cancer, the detection rate on MRI markedly improved (0.5–1.0 cm^3: 6/9, 66.7 %, 1.0 < cm^3: 35/38, 92.1 %) when the tumor foci volume exceeded 0.5 cm^3.

Table 2 Logistic regression analysis of analysis of factors associated with visibility on 3-T MRI

		Univariate analysis		Mutivariate analysis	
Variables analyzed	No. of tumor foci	Odds ratio (95 % CI)	*p*-value	Odds ratio (95 % CI)	*p*-value
Age	102	1.03 (0.976–1.10)	0.266		
PSA	102	1.01 (0.957–1.07)	0.647		
Tumor location					
Central/Transition zone only	17	0.954 (0.329–2.73)	0.929		
Peripheral zone	85	1			
Tumor volume	102	8.53 (3.85–24.3)	<0.0001	9.24 (3.60–31.8)	<0.0001
Gleason sum	102	3.47 (1.89–7.06)	<0.0001	0.871 (0.321–2.24)	0.778

Overall, sensitivity for cancer detection was 87.2 % (41/47) for tumors larger than 0.5 cm^3, and the positive predictive value was 82.8 % (48/58) for score >3. Multivariate analysis identified only the tumor volume as being significantly correlated with visibility on MRI. Because 1 cm in diameter represents a sphere of 0.5 cm^3, we consider that, although the detection limit of small foci was the same as that using endorectal coil or pelvic phased-array coil 1.5-T MRI, modern 3.0-Tesla multiparametric MRI offers a more sophisticated image of the prostate and can clearly visualize most tumors larger than 0.5 cm^3. In other words, 3.0-Tesla can identify clinically significant disease in terms of a tumor volume >0.5 cm^3. In contrast, it can barely detect tumors with a volume of less than 0.5 cm^3 regardless of the Gleason score. In the current study, an endorectal coil was not used, and we, therefore, did not generate data on how an endorectal coil can aid in tumor depiction. Previously, Park BK et al. and Sosna J et al. reported that 3.0-T pelvic phased-array MRI could produce an image equivalent to 1.5-T endorectal MRI [13, 14]. Kim BS et al. also reported that the staging ability was not significantly different between 3.0-T pelvic phased-array MRI and 3.0-T endorectal coil MRI [15]. In contrast, Turkbey et al. recently reported that the combined use of a nonendorectal coil and an endorectal coil led to the detection of more cancerous foci than the sole use of a nonendorectal coil [16]. At present, we consider that patients' discomfort and the additional cost are drawbacks to the use of an endorectal coil, and preoperative evaluation with a nonendorectal coil would be more acceptable universally in daily clinical practice.

As described above, the positive predictive value for a diagnosis of cancer based on MRI findings was 75 % (15/20) for score 3, 73.3 % (11/15) for score 4, and 95.7 % (22/23) for score 5. Conversely, 10 lesions assigned a score >3 (3: $n = 5$; 4: $n = 4$; 5: $n = 1$) were false-positive findings on MRI. After the analysis, we convened a meeting with the pathologists to discuss the cause of these false-positive findings, and found that the most frequent histological finding was inflammation ($n = 7$), and abscess formation was also noted in one case (data not shown). It would be optimal to perform MRI before prostate biopsy to minimize these artifacts. It has been established that an interval of at least eight weeks is needed to minimize artifacts due to prostate biopsy [17]. Regarding the 6 foci greater than 0.5 cm^3 which were missed on MRI (Fig. 3), a strong background due to hemorrhage ($n = 1$), an anterior TZ location ($n = 1$), an apex location ($n = 1$), and islet distribution of small foci ($n = 3$) may have compromised visualization on MRI. Regarding the relationship between the tumor location and MRI visibility, previous studies showed the lack of additional benefit of DCE-MRI and the difficulty of cancer detection in the transition zone [18, 19]. In the present study, as shown in Table 2, although the tumor location was not associated with visibility on 3-T MRI, our sample size was too small to draw a definitive conclusion, and we agree that the co-existing prostatic hyperplasia might compromise cancer detection in the transition zone.

Our study has several potential limitations. Firstly, this was a small retrospective study. There was a selection bias in that only patients undergoing prostatectomy were enrolled. As described above, because all MR images were reviewed in consensus by two radiologists during a single session, we do not have data on inter- or intraobserver variability of the Likert scale. The lack of an endorectal coil may have influenced our observations. Furthermore, in cases undergoing MRI evaluation after biopsy, post-biopsy hemorrhage might have resulted in difficulty of tumor detection. It remains unknown whether the results would be reproducible in a different institute with a reader with a different experience level. Further validation studies are warranted to evaluate whether a scoring system including a Likert scale can become a common language among physicians treating prostate carcinoma patients in daily clinical practice.

Conclusion

Each Likert scale well reflected the corresponding tumor's volume and Gleason score. Our observations show that "scale 3 or higher" could be a useful threshold to predict clinically significant carcinoma when considering treatment options.

Abbreviations

LRP: Laparoscopic prostatectomy; DCE-MRI: Dynamic contrast-enhanced MRI; DWI: Diffusion-weighted imaging; ADC: Apparent diffusion coefficient.

Competing interests

The authors declare that they have no competing interests.

Authors' contributions

TH and TA drafted the manuscript. FK and TH reviewed the MRI findings. RM and HF collected the pathological data. SM, KT, and NM performed volume analysis. TA and SM carried out statistical analysis. NS and KK revised the manuscript. All authors read and approved the final manuscript.

Author details

[1]Department of Urology, Hokkaido University Graduate School of Medicine, North-15, West-7, North Ward, Sapporo 060-8638, Japan. [2]Department of Diagnostic and Interventional Radiology, Hokkaido University Hospital, Sapporo, Japan. [3]Department of Surgical Pathology, Hokkaido University Hospital, Sapporo, Japan.

References

1. Barentsz JO, Richenberg J, Clements R, Choyke P, Verma S, Villeirs G, et al. European Society of Urogenital R: Esur prostate mr guidelines 2012. Eur Radiol. 2012;22:746–57.

2. Dickinson L, Ahmed HU, Allen C, Barentsz JO, Carey B, Futterer JJ, et al. Scoring systems used for the interpretation and reporting of multiparametric mri for prostate cancer detection, localization, and characterization: Could standardization lead to improved utilization of imaging within the diagnostic pathway? J Magn Reson Imaging. 2013;37:48–58.
3. Katahira K, Takahara T, Kwee TC, Oda S, Suzuki Y, Morishita S, et al. Ultra-high-b-value diffusion-weighted mr imaging for the detection of prostate cancer: Evaluation in 201 cases with histopathological correlation. Eur Radiol. 2011;21:188–96.
4. Kitajima K, Kaji Y, Fukabori Y, Yoshida K, Suganuma N, Sugimura K. Prostate cancer detection with 3 t mri: Comparison of diffusion-weighted imaging and dynamic contrast-enhanced mri in combination with t2-weighted imaging. J Magn Reson Imaging. 2010;31:625–31.
5. Vargas HA, Akin O, Franiel T, Mazaheri Y, Zheng J, Moskowitz C, et al. Diffusion-weighted endorectal mr imaging at 3 t for prostate cancer: Tumor detection and assessment of aggressiveness. Radiology. 2011;259:775–84.
6. Jonmarker SVA, Lindberg A, Hellström M, Egevad L. Tissue shrinkage after fixation with formalin injection of prostatectomy specimens. Virchows Arch. 2006;449:297–301.
7. Turkbey B, Mani H, Shah V, Rastinehad AR, Bernardo M, Pohida T, et al. Multiparametric 3t prostate magnetic resonance imaging to detect cancer: Histopathological correlation using prostatectomy specimens processed in customized magnetic resonance imaging based molds. J Urol. 2011;186:1818–24.
8. Renard-Penna R, Mozer P, Cornud F, Barry-Delongchamps N, Bruguiere E, Portalez D, et al. Prostate imaging reporting and data system and likert scoring system: Multiparametric mr imaging validation study to screen patients for initial biopsy. Radiology. 2015;275:458–68.
9. Rosenkrantz AB, Kim S, Lim RP, Hindman N, Deng FM, Babb JS, et al. Prostate cancer localization using multiparametric mr imaging: Comparison of prostate imaging reporting and data system (pi-rads) and likert scales. Radiology. 2013;269:482–92.
10. Ikonen S, Kärkkäinen P, Kivisaari L, Salo JO, Taari K, Vehmas T, et al. Magnetic resonance imaging of clinically localized prostatic cancer. J Urol. 1998;159:915–9.
11. Roethke MC, Lichy MP, Jurgschat L, Hennenlotter J, Vogel U, Schilling D, et al. Tumorsize dependent detection rate of endorectal mri of prostate cancer–a histopathologic correlation with whole-mount sections in 70 patients with prostate cancer. Eur J Radiol. 2011;79:189–95.
12. Villers A, Puech P, Mouton D, Leroy X, Ballereau C, Lemaitre L. Dynamic contrast enhanced, pelvic phased array magnetic resonance imaging of localized prostate cancer for predicting tumor volume: Correlation with radical prostatectomy findings. J Urol. 2006;176:2432–7.
13. Park BKKB, Kim CK, Lee HM, Kwon GY. Comparison of phased-array 3.0-t and endorectal 1.5-t magnetic resonance imaging in the evaluation of local staging accuracy for prostate cancer. J Comput Assist Tomogr. 2007;31:534–8.
14. Sosna J, Pedrosa I, Dewolf WC, Mahallati H, Lenkinski RE, Rofsky NM. Mr imaging of the prostate at 3 tesla: Comparison of an external phased-array coil to imaging with an endorectal coil at 1.5 tesla. Acad Radiol. 2004;11:857–62.
15. Kim BS, Kim TH, Kwon TG, Yoo ES. Comparison of pelvic phased-array versus endorectal coil magnetic resonance imaging at 3 tesla for local staging of prostate cancer. Yonsei Med J. 2012;53:550–6.
16. Turkbey B, Merino MJ, Gallardo EC, Shah V, Aras O, Bernardo M, et al. Comparison of endorectal coil and nonendorectal coil t2w and diffusion-weighted mri at 3 tesla for localizing prostate cancer: Correlation with whole-mount histopathology. J Magn Reson Imaging. 2014;39:1443–8.
17. Qayyum ACF, Lu Y, Olpin JD, Wu L, Yeh BM, Carroll PR, et al. Organ-confined prostate cancer: Effect of prior transrectal biopsy on endorectal mri and mr spectroscopic imaging. AJR Am J Roentgenol. 2004;183:1079–83.
18. Junker D, Quentin M, Nagele U, Edlinger M, Richenberg J, Schaefer G, et al. Evaluation of the pi-rads scoring system for mpmri of the prostate: A whole-mount step-section analysis. World J Urol. 2014;33:1023–30.
19. Rosenkrantz AB, Kim S, Campbell N, Gaing B, Deng FM, Taneja SS. Transition zone prostate cancer: Revisiting the role of multiparametric mri at 3 t. AJR Am J Roentgenol. 2015;204:W266–272.

Interpositional substitution of free vas deferens segment autografts in rat

Teoman Cem Kadioglu[1*], Peter D Temple-Smith[2] and Graeme Southwick[3]

Abstract

Background: Insufficient vas length for performing a tension-free vasovasostomy is a problem occasionally encountered by microsurgeons. Herein we evaluated utilization of a non-vascularized vas deferens autograft in a rat model.

Methods: Segments of isolated vas deferens, 2.5 cm in length, were used as bilateral autografts in 15 rats. Each autograft was implanted between the two transected ends of vas deferens using end-to-end anastomosis. Fertility, sperm motility, and graft survival was evaluated and compared with the control group.

Results: At the end of the 3 months, 9/15 (60%) rats were able to breed successfully and 24 (80%) vas grafts were patent and viable. Large granulomata developed at the proximal anastomosis sites in 6 (20%) autografts that failed. Unilateral minimal fluid leakage was observed in 6 (20%) of the proximal (testicular end) anastomosis sites in those rats that were able to breed. Histological evaluations demonstrated that graft survival was associated with mild to severe changes in the structure of the vas autograft. On semen analysis 76% of the sperms in the experimental group had forward motility compared to 78% in the control group ($p > 0.05$).

Conclusions: Vas autograft can successfully be performed in a rat model with ultimate breeding capability.

Keywords: Vas deferens, Autograft, Microsurgery, Fertility, Histology, Spermatozoa

Background

The vas deferens is a thick-walled, muscular duct that forms the distal extension of the ductus epididymidis and transmits spermatozoa and seminal fluids from the epididymis and seminal vesicles to the ejaculatory duct [1]. While vas deferens is a target for vasectomy [2], one of the most popular methods of male contraception, it also serves as an important focus in the surgical treatment of obstructive azoospermia [3,4]. Advances in microsurgical techniques during the past 30 years have improved the accuracy and success of vas-to-vas and vasoepididymal anastomoses. New modifications, such as the use of biomaterials/sealants, laser soldering, absorbable and nonabsorbable stents, new intussusception vasoepididymostomy (VE) anastomotic techniques, and robotics, are currently under investigation [5-8].

Due to these technical advancements, recent data indicate that microsurgery appears more cost-effective than percutaneous 'Testicular Sperm Extraction' (TESE) and 'Micro Epididimal Sperm Aspiration' (MESA) for the treatment of obstructive azoospermia when considering the impact of indirect costs [9]. A tension-free microanastomosis is the key to patency and is often difficult to achieve in some patients because previous surgery has decreased the available length of the vas deferens bilaterally. In a previous study, we developed a technique in rabbits using 1-cm vascularized segments of the vas deferens to bridge selected regions of the epididymis [10]. Based on the results of this study, we reasoned that vas segments could be used in selected clinical situations as autografts. However, due to the anatomical difficulties of retaining a vascular pedicle in human vas segments, an animal model was required to examine the possibility of using free vas autografts in a manner similar to the use of autografts in vascular surgery [11,12]. Although vascular autografts are now in routine clinical use, few attempts

* Correspondence: teoman@istanbul.edu.tr
[1]Department of Urology, Istanbul School of Medicine, University of Istanbul, 34365 Istanbul, Turkey
Full list of author information is available at the end of the article

have been made to use vas autografts in experimental or clinical situations [1].

The aim of this study is to develop a rat model for vas autograft microsurgery and further examine the survival and function of the free vas autografts. Changes in the interpositional polarity of the vas segment, which were previously believed to interfere with sperm survival and transport in the vas bridge procedure [7], were re-examined using this rat model. Histological evaluation of the vas grafts and comparative fertility assessment of experimental and control groups were performed at three months after surgery as measures of the success of the model.

Methods

The experiments described in this paper were conducted with the approval of the Monash University Department of Anatomy Ethics Committee and under the national animal in experimentation guidelines on the care and use of animals of the National Health and Medical Research Council of Australia. Also, Animal Research: Reporting In Vivo Experiments (ARRIVE) guidelines for reporting animal studies were adhered.

Animals

Fifteen mature male Sprague–Dawley rats (90 days old) were used for vas autograft surgery, and ten unoperated males served as controls. These animals were later mated with 30 female rats (two females: one male) to assess fertility (see "Fertility assessment" below).

Surgical procedures

Following the induction of general anesthesia using sodium pentobarbital (Nembutal 60 mg/ml, intraperitoneal), a 1-cm low, ventral, midline incision was used to expose

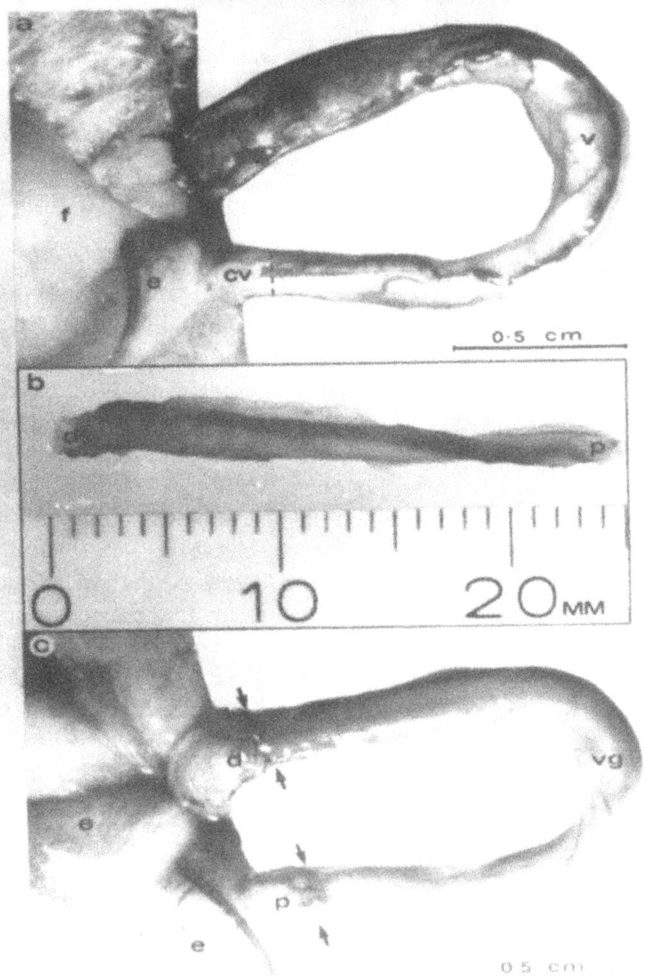

Figure 1 Vas autograft microsurgical procedure in the rat. (a) Vas preparation prior to transaction showing a loop of exposed intact straight vas (v) with transaction sites marked (dashed lines). e, epididymis; f, epididymal fat pad; cv, convoluted vas. **(b)** Isolated 2.5 cm vas segment prepared for use as an autograft. Note the increasing diameter from proximal (p) to distal (d), which is associated with the increasing thickness of the smooth muscle layers. **(c)** Vas autograft (vg) in position after microsurgery showing the proximal (p) and distal (d) lines of 10/0 sutures along each anastomosis site.

the abdominal viscera. The testes and spermatic cords were delivered into the surgical field through the inguinal canals using gentle scrotal pressure to expose the vasa deferentia. A 2.5 cm segment of the right vas was gently freed from the surrounding tissues from the junction of the convoluted and straight vas distally (Figure 1a). Major vessels at the proximal and distal points of transection of the vas were cauterized with microforceps using bipolar cautery, and the vas, along with its associated neurovascular supply, was then severed with microscissors. The same procedure was applied to the distal end of the dissected portion of the vas to produce a 2.5-cm isolated vas segment for use as an autograft (Figure 1b). Care was taken to preserve the integrity of the testicular blood supply. Prior to excising the autograft, the deferential vessels were cauterized immediately proximal and distal to the proposed graft site. The graft segment was detached from the vas using microscissors and placed in Ringer's solution at room temperature. The ischemic time in cold Ringer's solution was less than 20 minutes. A similar segment from the left vas deferens was then excised for cross-grafting. The free portion of the right vas was then interposed as an autograft between the transected ends of the left vas. The proximal and distal anastomoses were performed under 9-25× magnification using a single layer of five full-thickness 10–0 monofilament nylon sutures (Figure 1c). These sutures were placed equidistant around the vas to ensure an exact approximation of the lumen at each end of the autograft and the two severed ends of the vas. The left

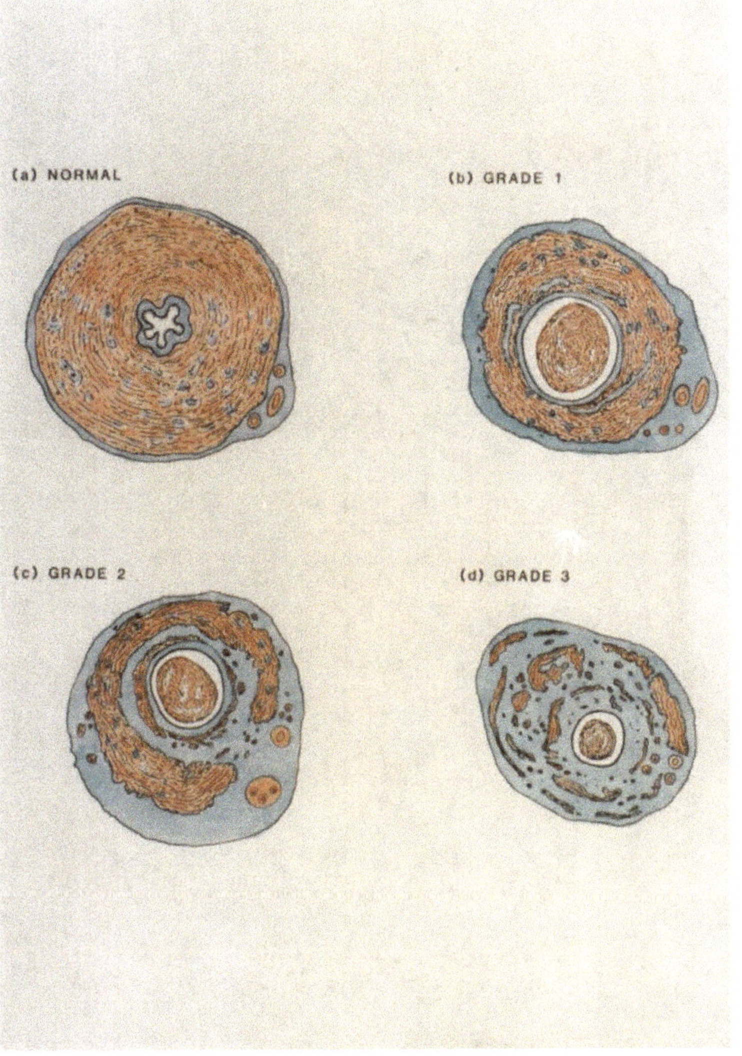

Figure 2 Grading system. (a) Grade 0: Control vas graft; normal histology. **(b)** Grade 1: Loss of stellate lumen but maintenance of periluminal smooth muscle continuity. **(c)** Grade 2: Reduction in mass and progressive fibrosis of the longitudinal and circular smooth muscle causing discontinuity of muscle layers. **(d)** Grade 3: Smooth muscle layers are largely replaced by fibrous tissue surrounded by a revascularizing, thickened adventitia.

vas and its associated testis and epididymis were then returned to the scrotum. The same procedure was performed on the right using the contralateral vas segment and the midline ventral incision was closed in a two-layer fashion using 6–0 nylon sutures for the body wall and 6–0 silk sutures for the skin.

The polarity of the vas autografts was reversed in a sub-group of five rats, such that the proximal end of the autograft was anastomosed to the distal end of the *in situ* vas, and the distal end of the graft was joined to the proximal *in situ* vas.

Fertility assessment

On the 20th postoperative day, two mature female rats were placed in the cage of each male rat. The abdomens of these females were gently palpated daily for evidence of pregnancy. At the first sign of pregnancy in either female, both female rats were isolated from their male consort. The first of the two female rats showing evidence of pregnancy by palpation of the abdomen was followed carefully throughout gestation. At the time of littering, the date and the number of offspring were noted. The date of conception was then calculated based on the 21-day gestational period for rats.

Control animals were exposed to females at the same time when the experimental rats were evaluated for establishment of pregnancies.

Three months after cross-grafting, those males that were unsuccessful in establishing a pregnancy were separated from their female consorts for autograft evaluation. A

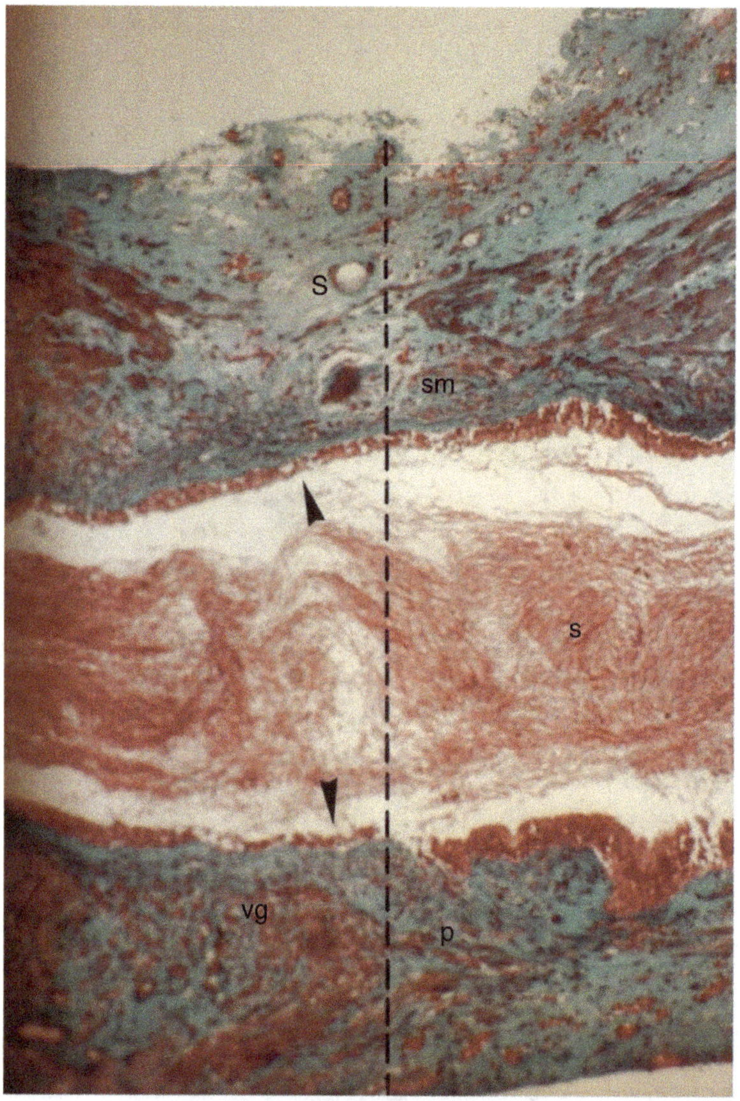

Figure 3 Longitudinal section through the proximal suture line of a vas autograft showing the patency of the anastomosis. The spermatozoa (s) filling the lumen, the suture (S), and the interrupted smooth muscle (sm) layers along the anastomosis site (dashed lines) are shown. Proximal vas (p), vas autograft (vg). Note the reduced length of the stereocilia (arrows) in the vas autograft 135x.

mature, male, unoperated, control rat was placed with the remaining nongravid females to eliminate the possibility of female infertility as a confounding factor.

Sperm motility studies

Sperm motility was assessed in all of the experimental animals after fertility assessments were completed. The right vas was cut 3 mm distal to the distal suture line, and spermatozoa were retrieved using a standard microaspiration technique [13]. The percentage of motile spermatozoa in each sample and their motility indices were calculated using the same routine visual analysis procedures recommended for human semen analysis. Sperm samples were also microaspirated from the convoluted vas at a level 3 mm proximal to the proximal suture line and analyzed as described above. Similar sample collection procedures and motility analyses were used to assess the motility of spermatozoa from the contralateral side. Similar sperm motility assessments were also performed on the ten unoperated control rats. Within-animal data were compared using Student's t-test, and sperm motility data from the same anatomical levels in experimental and control rats were compared using a one-way ANOVA (Minitab Statistical Software Inc., Pennsylvania, USA).

Autograft evaluation

After 90 days, fertility assessments were completed and each rat was sacrificed. The viability of the vas grafts evidenced by the presence of spermatozoa inside each autograft and in the adjacent vas above and below the graft were examined under low power magnification (9×) in all 15 experimental animals. The patency of the autografts

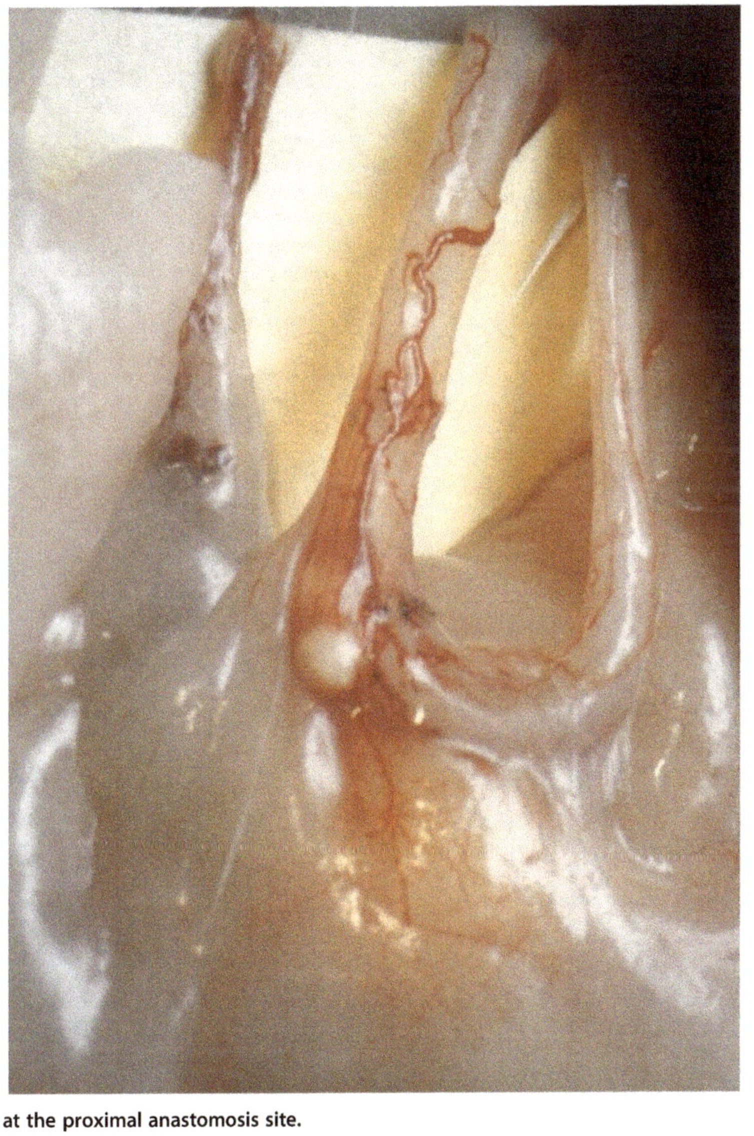

Figure 4 Minimal leakage at the proximal anastomosis site.

was evaluated under 9× magnification. The presence of a continuous white column of seminal fluid throughout the autograft and into the distal (abdominal) vas was indicative of graft patency. The presence of anastomotic leakage or granuloma was also documented. The autograft, including the proximal and distal anastomotic sites, was excised, preserved in Bouin's solution, and prepared for light microscopy. Longitudinal sections were cut through the anastomoses for further study of the operative sites. Four-micron-thick transverse sections were cut through the center of each autograft and from regions adjacent to the proximal and distal anastomosis sites to examine the vas autografts for any obvious histological changes. Sections stained with hematoxylin and eosin and Masson's trichrome were prepared from each paraffin block. Similar histological observations were made on vas samples obtained from similar regions in each of the ten unoperated control rats.

A grading system was devised to objectively assess the microscopic changes in autograft histology. The extent of smooth muscle degeneration was the basis for this system (see Figure 2 for a drawing of the vas grading system (0–3) with an appropriate description in the legend).

Results

Fertility assessment

Nine of the 15 (60%) rats established a pregnancy with at least one of the two females introduced into their cages following the twenty-day postoperative period of celibacy. Three pregnancies were achieved in rats with reversed polarity grafts and six in rats with normal polarity grafts. The fact that the same percentage (60%) was achieved in

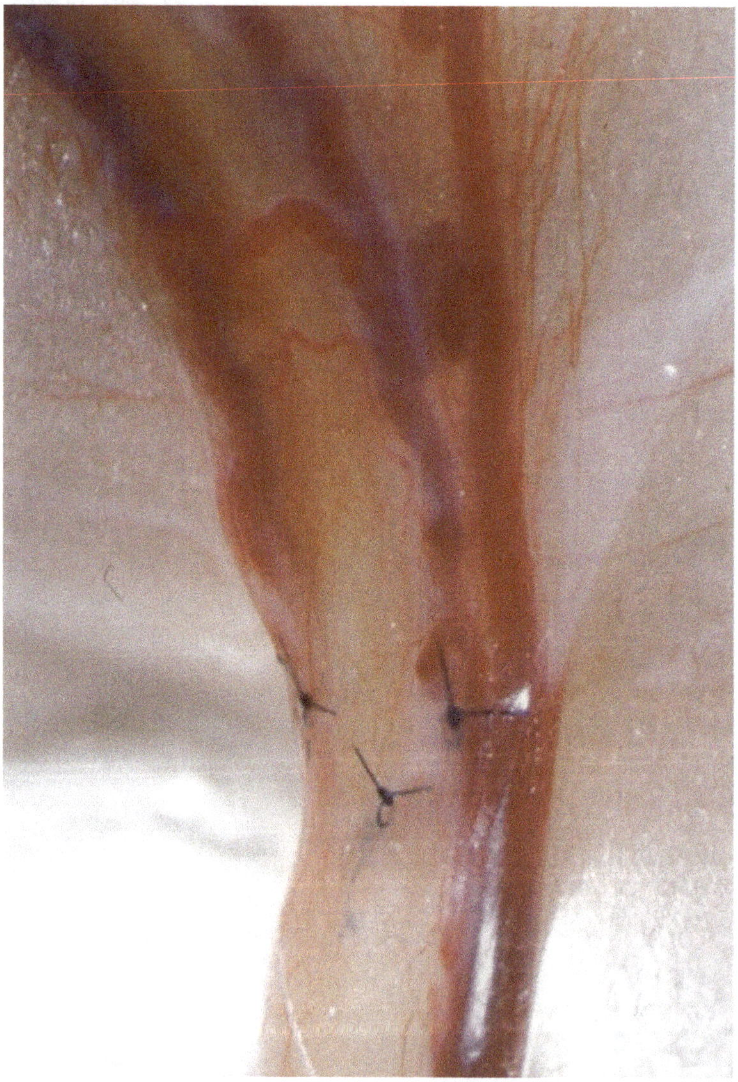

Figure 5 Prominent neovascularity.

both groups shows consistency. The fertility of all twelve (six pairs) of the female rats that failed to establish pregnancy during cohabitation with postoperative males was confirmed through breeding with control males.

Graft survival and patency of the anastomosis

Graft patency, tissue quality, and neovascularity were examined. Of the 30 vasautografts performed, 24 (80%) were patent and viable (Figure 3). Minimal unilateral fluid leakage was observed at six (20%) of the proximal anastomosis sites in those rats that had established pregnancies. No adverse effect of this leakage was observed on either graft patency or survival (Figure 4). Prominent neovascularity (Figure 5) was observed in all surviving autografts at 90 days. Large unilateral granulomata developed at the proximal anastomosis sites of the six (20%) autografts that ultimately failed. Histological degeneration was more profound in the vas graft segments immediately adjacent to these granulomata. The polarity of the autograft appeared to be inconsequential because 8 (80%) of reversed polarity grafts survived and the grafts that did not survive also had large unilateral granuloma at their proximal anastomosis sites.

Histological examinations

Grafts

All grafts showed some structural changes when compared with the controls (Figure 6). Light microscopic examination of tissue sections from the mid-portions of the viable autografts showed that they had all undergone some degeneration of the smooth muscle layers. The normal stellate configuration of the vas lumen was lost in all of the grafts. The lumina had become circular and smooth in appearance.

Two (6.6%) of the autografts demonstrated only grade 1 changes (i.e., loss of stellate lumen but maintenance of periluminal smooth muscle continuity) (Figure 7). Sixteen (53.3%) of the grafts showed grade 2 changes (Figure 8), and 12 (40%) showed grade 3 changes (Figure 9). In addition to fibrosis of the smooth muscle layers, we observed decreases in the luminal epithelial cell height and stereocilial length in all (100%) of autografts. Neovascularity was continuous with the adventitial blood supply of the proximal and distal native vas segments. Increased branching of the superficial vessels was observed as they traversed the anastomosis and supplied the autograft.

Observations of the spermatozoa

The presence of sperm distal to the patent grafts was confirmed by microaspiration. Motile spermatozoa were recovered from vas segments adjacent to the graft. No significant difference was observed in the percentage of motile spermatozoa, in the sperm motility index between samples collected from sites proximal and distal to the graft (Table 1), or between normal and reversed polarity patent grafts. Sperm motility parameters derived from the experimental rats did not differ significantly from those of sperm collected from comparable sites in the control rats (Table 1).

Discussion

The high graft survival and patency (80%) described in this study shows that vas grafts can be successfully autotransplanted in rats via microsurgical techniques. The

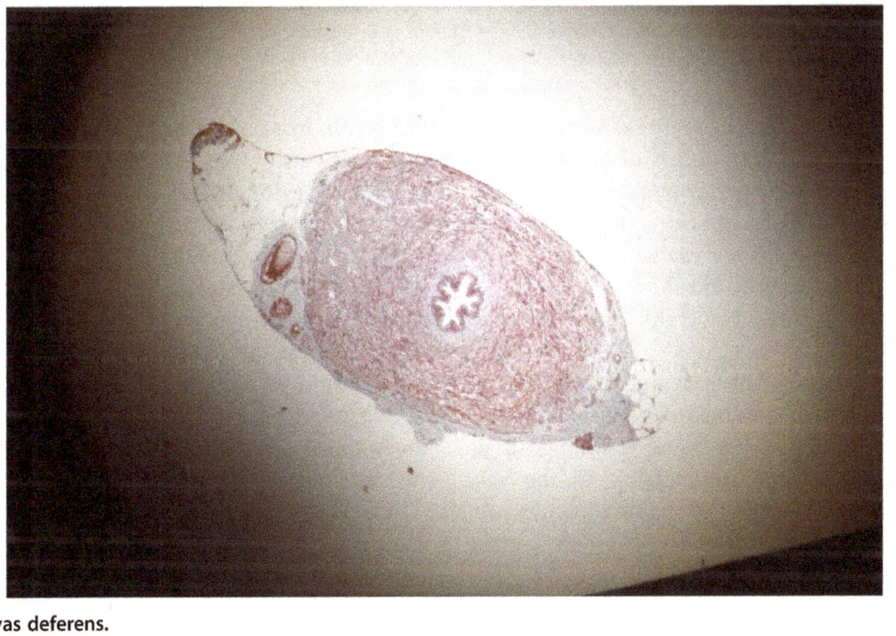

Figure 6 Normal vas deferens.

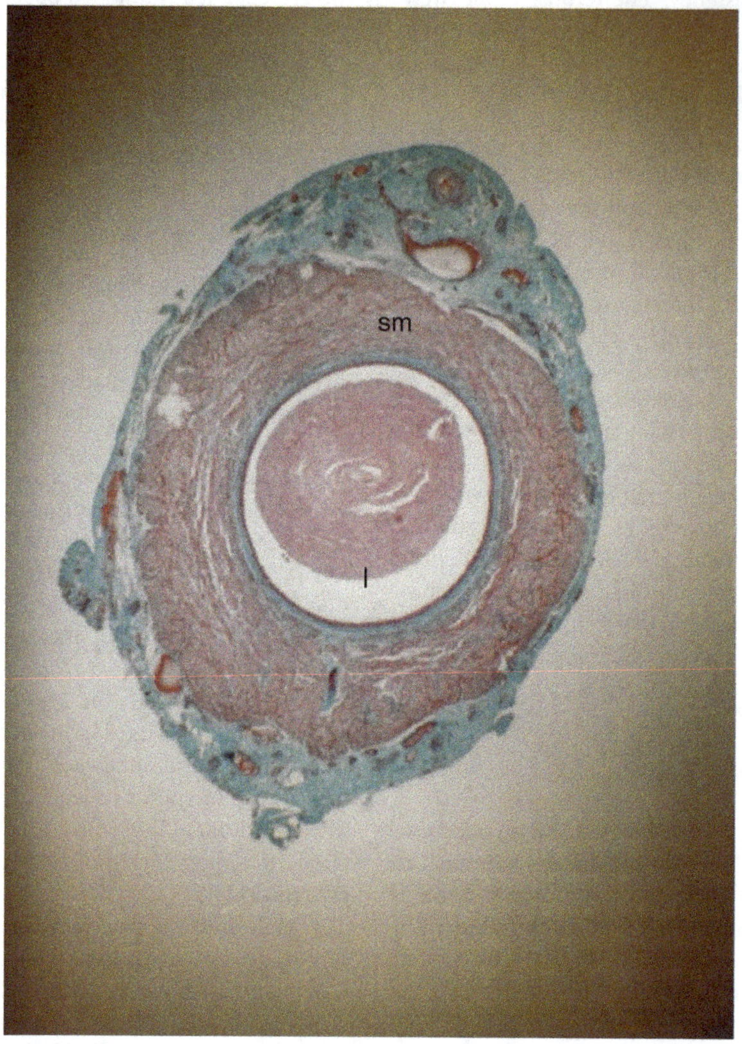

Figure 7 Transverse section through a vas autograft 1 month after surgery showing minimal changes. The slightly dilated lumen (l) has partially lost its stellate shape and contains few spermatozoa, and the smooth muscle (sm) layers have remained intact with thickened, revascularized adventitia (arrows). Note the presence of stereocilia on the epithelial cells as in controls 55x.

pregnancy data and post-mortem graft examination further substantiate the functional success of free vas autografts. A similar study was performed by Carringeret and associates using smaller vas segments or avascular grafts [14]. Although they did not evaluate pregnancy or the quality of spermatozoa, they did show that neovascularization of the transplanted vas grafts facilitated graft survival and patency.

Although extensive studies have demonstrated the superiority of a two-layer or modified one-layer microsurgical anastomosis in humans [6-8], only a simple, single layer anastomosis was technically feasible in the very thin, proximal rat vas. One of the major difficulties in using the rat model for developing a vas autograft is the predilection of the rat to develop granulomas [4,5]. The granulomata that were found adjacent to the proximal suture lines may have been caused by a pressure gradient forming in front of the hypoactive or inactive vas segment. It is noteworthy that the granulomata were found at the proximal anastomosis of each of the obstructed grafts. In men, granulomata formation at anastomotic sites plays a role in the postoperative results of vasectomy reversal [10]. Due to both the ability to perform a more watertight anastomosis and the lower incidence of granulomata, the use of the vas autografts in men would be less likely to suffer from obstruction. The low number of granulomata (3/30) found adjacent to the proximal anastomosis sites might have been due to the single layer anastomosis in rat vas autografts.

In contrast to the common development of convolutions in straight vas segments used in vasoepididymal anastomoses and vas-bridge procedures in rabbits [10], no convolutions developed in any of the rat vas autografts at one month after surgery.

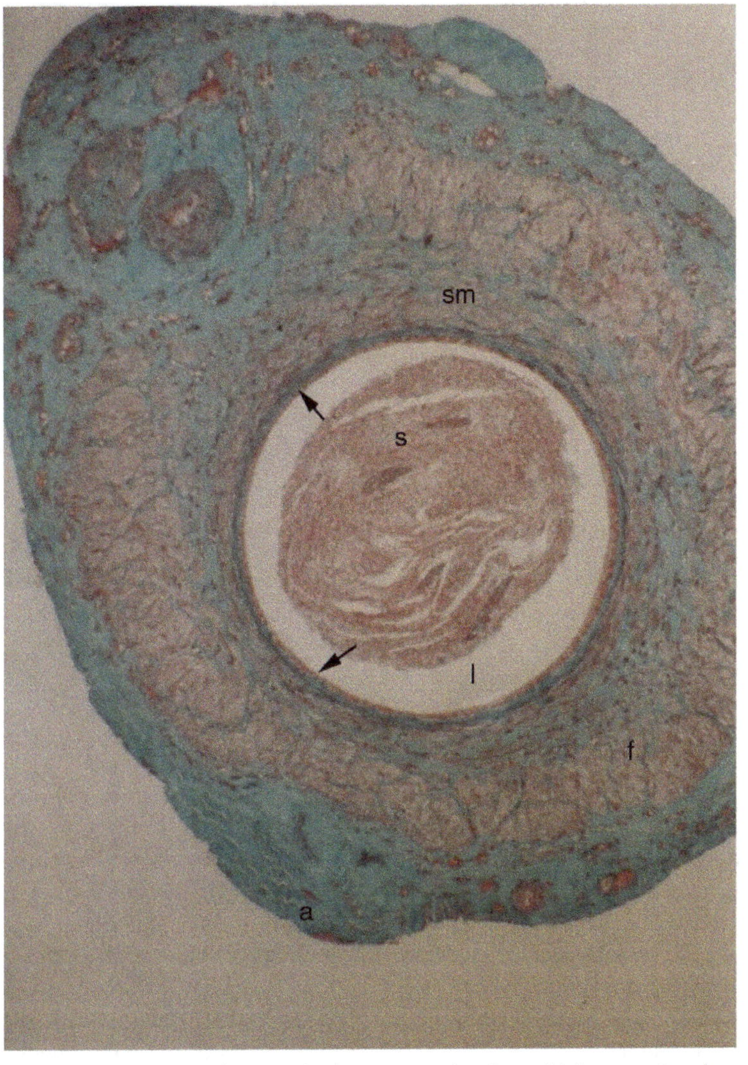

Figure 8 Transverse section through a vas autograft 1 month after surgery showing mild degenerative changes. The enlarged, rounded lumen (l) exhibits an increased presence of spermatozoa (s), and disrupted smooth muscle (sm) layers are partially replaced by fibrous tissue (f) surrounded by a revascularizing, thickened adventitia (arrows). Note the reduced epithelial height (arrow heads) and large perivasal pad of adipose tissue (a) 55x.

Despite the progressive nature of fibrotic changes in the smooth muscle layer of the grafts, the survival, revascularization, and early patency of these free autografts remain encouraging. The most obvious of these changes included the reduction in mass and progressive fibrosis of the layers of the longitudinal and circular smooth muscle and the associated changes in the luminal shape. In fact, there was an apparent relationship between the luminal shape and degeneration of the smooth muscle layers. In the grafts that were most severely affected, the lumen was round and packed with spermatozoa; in contrast, those in which the smooth muscle layers remained essentially unaffected exhibited a luminal shape more similar to the characteristic empty, stellate lumen of control vasa. This observation suggests that the change in luminal shape is caused by the loss of smooth muscle tone in the vas autografts. Two obvious factors may have led either separately or synergistically to the degenerative changes: 1) the temporary loss of the vascular supply and/or 2) the transection of nerves to the vas segment used as autografts. Similar degenerative changes have been reported in the smooth muscle layer of vascular grafts [15]. The structural changes occurring in all of the grafts suggested that transection of the nerve and blood supply altered the morphology of the vas without affecting its essential functions of sperm transport and maintenance of sperm viability. It is presumed that either sufficient smooth muscle activity to enable some transport was retained in the autograft segment or that backpressure

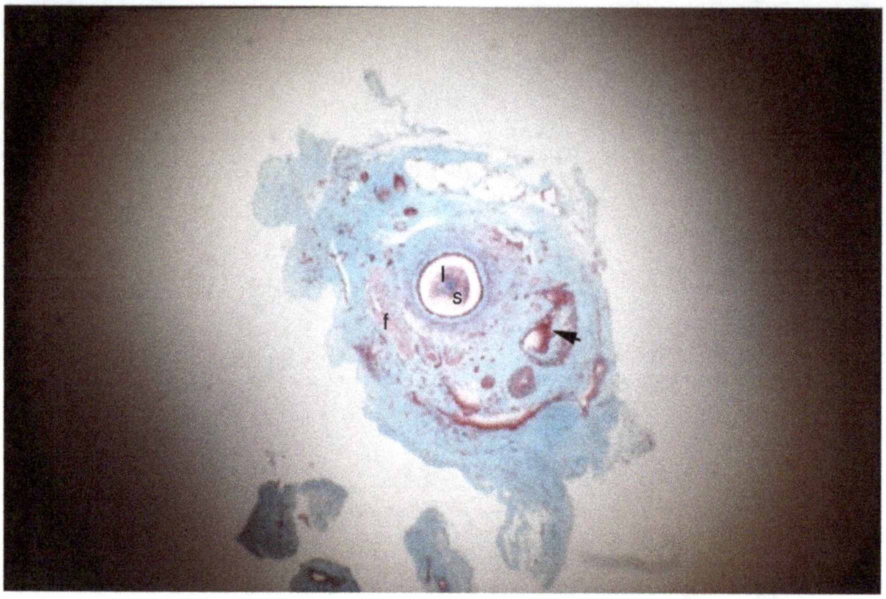

Figure 9 Transverse section through a vas autograft 1 month after surgery showing severe degenerative changes. The rounded lumen (l) exhibits an increased presence of spermatozoa (s), and smooth muscle (arrow heads) layers are largely replaced by fibrous tissue (f) surrounded by a revascularizing, thickened adventitia (arrows) 55x.

in the epididymis was sufficient to provide flow of luminal contents through the enlarged autograft lumen. The similarities in sperm motility of the samples taken above and below the graft, and the direct comparison of these with samples from equivalent regions in the control vasa, indicate that the histological changes observed in the epithelium of the autografts had no significant effect on sperm motility, sperm viability, or the autograft luminal environment.

None of the rats in this study were mated until at least twenty days postoperatively to ensure that no viable sperm remained in the distal vas deferens at the time of conception.

Table 1 Comparison of the percentage of motile spermatozoa and motility indices in sperm samples microaspirated from above and below the vas autografts (n = 15) and from identical vas sites in control animals (n = 5)

	Motility assessment		
	Control (n = 5)	Experimental (n = 15)	p
Proximal collection site			
% motile	59.1 + 24.6	51.1 + 12.3	0.34
Motility index	99.7 + 43.4	91.7 + 27.2	0.62
Distal collection site			
% motile	64.1 + 23.6	61.2 + 17.4	0.77
Motility index	109.8 + 47.1	102.2 + 28.9	0.66

No comparisons between the data using either Student's t-test (within animal data pair analysis) or one-way ANOVA (between animal data comparison) were found to be significantly different.

Kuwahara and Frick reported that more than 90% of the sperm remaining in the vas were decapitated, with motility falling to almost zero at six days following vas ligation [16]. Although sperm can survive for long periods in the epididymis, this study demonstrated that the vas was not conducive to long-term sperm survival.

Our previous work with pedicled vas bridges in rabbits suggested that the polarity of the graft might affect sperm survival and subsequent pregnancy as the sperm transit the graft. Unlike the pedicled bridges, which technically require a polarity change to complete the anastomoses, the polarity of the free vas autografts could be changed easily. In the present study, the graft survival, incidence of granulomata, and pregnancy rate were unaffected by graft polarity.

The clinical applications for successful vas autografts in men are potentially far-reaching. Insufficient vas length for performing tension-free vasovasostomy is a problem occasionally encountered by reproductive microsurgeons. Excessive scarring secondary to previous operative procedures and aggressive removal or extensive electrocautery of large vas segments during vasectomy are the most common causes of insufficient length for vasovasostomy. For patients presenting with the absence or atrophy of one testicle and insufficient vas length on the contralateral side, a vas autograft would be an ideal surgical option. Even in those men with two normal testes, using one vas as a free graft is attractive when both sides have long segments of scarred or absent vas deferens.

Conclusions

Translation of the autograft procedure from the rat model to a clinical procedure in men may improve the success of vasal microsurgery in cases where insufficient vas is available bilaterally to provide for tension-free vas anastomoses.

Competing interests

The authors declare that they have no competing interests.

Authors' contributions

TCK performed the operations, analysed and interpreted the data as well as preparing the manuscript. PDTS set up the scientific base for the concept for this study as well as previous similar animal experiments that led the path to this study and designed the study. GS tutored the microsurgical skills and perfected the microsurgical technique. All authors read and approved the final manuscript.

Author details

[1]Department of Urology, Istanbul School of Medicine, University of Istanbul, 34365 Istanbul, Turkey. [2]Department of Obstetrics and Gynaecology, Monash Medical Centre, Melbourne, Australia. [3]Melbourne Institute of Plastic Surgery, Melbourne, Victoria, Australia.

References

1. Koslov DS, Andersson KE: **Physiological and pharmacological aspects of the vas deferens-an update.** *Front Pharmacol* 2013, **4**:101.
2. Rajfer J, Bennett CJ: **Vasectomy.** *Urol Clin North Am* 1988, **15**:631.
3. Kelami A: **A new concept for macroscopic anastomosis of vas deferens; suture material and operative technique.** *Andrologia* 1980, **12**(3):245.
4. Bernie AM, Osterberg EC, Stahl PJ, Ramasamy R, Goldstein M: **Vasectomy reversal in humans.** *Spermatogenesis* 2012, **2**(4):273–278.
5. Parekattil SJ, Gudeloglu A: **Robotic assisted andrological surgery.** *Asian J Androl* 2013, **15**(1):67–74.
6. Kolettis PN: **Restructuring reconstructive techniques–advances in reconstructive techniques.** *Urol Clin North Am* 2008, **35**(2):229–234. viii-ix.
7. Southwick GJ, Temple-Smith PD: **Epididymal microsurgery: current techniques and new horizons.** *Microsurgery* 1988, **9**:266.
8. Monoski MA, Schiff J, Li PS, Chan PT, Goldstein M: **Innovative single-armed suture technique for microsurgical vasoepididymostomy.** *Urology* 2007, **69**(4):800–804.
9. Lee R, Li PS, Goldstein M, Tanrikut C, Schattman G, Schlegel PN: **A decision analysis of treatments for obstructive azoospermia.** *Hum Reprod* 2008, **23**(9):2043–2049. Epub 2008 Jun 13.
10. Temple-Smith PD, Southwick GJ, Herrera Castenada E, Hamer J, Mc Clatchey M: **Surgical manipulation of the epididymis: an experimental approach to sperm maturation.** In *Perspective in Andrology*, Volume 63. Edited by Serio M. New York: Raven Press, Serono Symposia Publications; 1989:281–290.
11. Wylie EJ: **Vascular replacement with arterial autografts.** *Surgery* 1965, **57**:14.
12. Leather RP, Shah DM, Buchbinder D, Annest SJ, Karmody AM: **Further experience with the saphenous vein used in situ for arterial bypass.** *Am J Surg* 1981, **142**(4):506.
13. Temple-Smith PD, Southwick GJ, Yates CA, Trounson AO, de Kretser DM: **Human pregnancy by in vitro fertilization (IVF) using sperm aspirated from the epididymis.** *J InVitro Fert Embryo Transf* 1985, **2**:119.
14. Carringer M, Pedersen J, Schnurer LB: **Experimental vas replacement by either vas or a vasculargraft.** *Scand J Urol Nephrol* 1995, **29**:97–102. Dept. Of UrologyandPathology, OrebroMedical Center, Orebro, Sweden.
15. Brook WH: **A histological review of the histology of patent autogenous vein grafts and vein patches.** *J Cardiovasc Surg* 1975, **16**:43.
16. Kuwahara M, Frick J: **The ligation of the male reproductive organs and the role of the spermatic cyst.** *Andrologia* 1975, **1**:1–14.

Men under the age of 55 years with screen detected prostate cancer do not have less significant disease compared to older men in a population of patients in Australia

Nandu D. Dantanarayana[1], Tania Hossack[2], Paul Cozzi[3], Andrew Brooks[1,2], Howard Lau[2], Warick Delprado[4] and Manish I. Patel[1,2*]

Abstract

Background: The American Urological Association (AUA) changed their Prostate-Specific Antigen (PSA) screening guidelines in 2013 to not recommend testing in men under 55 years of age without significant risk factors (such as a family history of prostate cancer or African ethnicity). The AUA argues that the rates of 'insignificant' prostate cancer (PC) in men under 55 are so high that the potential harms of PSA-testing in this population (over diagnosis and overtreatment) outweigh the benefits (early detection and treatment). Our study aims to identify and compare the rates of insignificant and high-risk PC in men diagnosed with PC ≤55 years and >55 years in two centres in Sydney, Australia.

Methods: Men with an abnormal screening PSA or DRE and diagnosed with PC by prostate biopsy were included in this study. A consecutive series of men were accrued from two major urology centres between the years 2006 and 2014. The analysis was divided into two parts, the first compared PC biopsy characteristics between men aged ≤55 years and those >55 years. The second analysis compared the prostatectomy pathological characteristics between the two groups. Differences were analysed by Chi squared and significance set at $p < 0.05$.

Results: A total of 598 prostate biopsies and 723 prostatectomy matched subjects were included. On prostate biopsies, 14.0 % of men ≤55 years and 11.9 % of men >55 years had insignificant PC ($X^2 = 0.32$, df = 1, $p = 0.57$), whilst 24.7 % of men ≤55 years and 25.1 % of men >55 years had high-risk PC ($X^2 = 0.007$, df = 1, $p = 0.93$). On prostatectomy specimens, 9.1 % of men ≤55 years and 6.5 % of men >55 years had insignificant PC ($X^2 = 1.25$, df = 1, $p = 0.26$), whilst 20.0 % of men ≤55 years and 24.0 % of men >55 years had high-risk PC ($X^2 = 0.83$, df = 1, $p = 0.36$).

Conclusion: We found no significant difference in the rates of insignificant and high-risk PC between men ≤55 years and >55 years, in either the prostate biopsies or prostatectomy specimens. Further trials need to be performed with comparable sample sizes and controlling of risk factors to assess the utility of PSA screening in younger men.

Keywords: Insignificant, Prostate Cancer, PSA testing, Prostatectomy, Biopsy

* Correspondence: mpatel@med.usyd.edu.au
[1]University of Sydney, Discipline of Surgery, Sydney, Australia
[2]Department of Urology, Westmead Hospital, Sydney, Australia
Full list of author information is available at the end of the article

Background

Prostate Specific Antigen (PSA) testing remains controversial with a diverse range of recommendations on whom to offer testing to amongst authorities worldwide [1]. In 2013, the American Urological Association (AUA) changed their PSA testing guidelines to not recommend testing in men under 55 years of age without significant risk factors (such as a family history of prostate cancer or African ethnicity) [2]. This is in contrast to the 2009 AUA guidelines that recommended PSA screening start at 40 years. The AUA argues that the rates of 'insignificant' prostate cancer in men under 55 are so high that the potential harms of PSA-testing in this population (over diagnosis and overtreatment) outweigh the benefits (early detection and treatment). The concept of insignificant prostate cancer is evolving but generally refers to a low grade, small volume, organ confined prostate cancer that is unlikely to manifest clinically in a patient's lifetime without treatment [3].

Furthermore, the AUA cites a lack of high-quality evidence to support PSA screening in men 40–55 years. Specifically, two recently performed large randomized clinical trials– the Prostate, Lung, Colorectal and Ovarian Cancer screening trial (PLCO) and European Randomised Study of Screening for Prostate Cancer (ERSPC) did not include men under 55 years and therefore do not inform the decision [4, 5].

In light of the AUA guideline changes, we aim to identify the rates of insignificant and high-risk prostate cancer in men diagnosed with prostate cancer in two centres in Sydney, Australia. In contrast to the AUA, we hypothesise that there is no significant difference between the rates of insignificant and high-risk cancer between men ≤55 years and >55 years.

Methods

Between January 2006 and February 2014 men with an abnormal screening PSA or DRE subsequently diagnosed with PC by prostate needle biopsy were included in this study. A consecutive series of patients were derived from three surgeons at Westmead hospital (Sydney, Australia) and one surgeon at St George hospital (Sydney, Australia). Patient data was de-identified and hence individual patient consent was not required for inclusion in the study. Data collected included patient age, pre-biopsy PSA score and clinical staging - obtained from audit databases maintained by each urologist in the study. Prostate biopsy data (age at biopsy, Gleason score, number of positive cores, tumour volume, PSA density) and radical prostatectomy data (age at prostatectomy, Gleason score, tumour volume, pathological staging) was obtained via histopathology reports stored on electronic databases at Douglass Hanley Moir (DHM) – a pathology company, all four surgeons use exclusively for reporting. African-American/Australian-African patients were excluded from the study since this is a known prostate cancer risk factor.

At DHM, radical prostatectomy specimens are fully processed but not whole mounted. They are embedded using standard cassettes, with each slide of the prostate fully embedded as quadrants in four separate cassettes. As such, all of the tissue is processed and examined. All of the tumour areas are drawn on a schematic and the diagram is used to calculate tumour volume, Gleason score and presence of extraprostatic extension.

The initial analysis compared PC biopsy characteristics between men ≤55 years and those >55 years at time of biopsy. From the prostate biopsy data, subjects were identified as having insignificant prostate cancer as per the Epstein criteria [6] (PSA density <0.15 ng/ml per gram, no Gleason pattern 4 / 5, <3 positives cores and <50 % involvement per core) or high-risk prostate cancer as per the D'Amico risk grouping [7] (at least one of Gleason score >7, PSA >20, Clinical stage > T2b). Whilst the Epstein biopsy criteria is controversial – with some advocating modifications such as including the presence of perineural invasion to increase criteria accuracy - it is still the most commonly used criteria for insignificant prostate cancer and hence included in this study [6].

The second analysis compared PC characteristics from prostatectomy specimens between men aged ≤55 years and those >55 years. This analysis is more robust in terms of actual pathological cancer differences but subject to selection bias as some men with low risk cancers may not have had curative treatment and older men may be more likely to have radiotherapy rather then surgery. Similarly, from the prostatectomy data subjects were identified as having insignificant prostate cancer as per the Stamey criteria [8] (tumour volume <0.5 cm^3, no Gleason pattern 4 or 5, and no extracapsular spread) or high-risk prostate cancer as per the D'Amico risk grouping.

The statistics package SPSS version 21 was used to perform Chi-square analyses for categorical and dichotomous data, and Student's t-tests for continuous data. Significance was set at $p < 0.05$. Ethics approval was sought and granted by the Western Sydney Local Health District Human Research Ethics Committee.

Results

There were 794 prostate biopsy subjects identified for the study, representing a consecutive series. Of these, the DHM electronic database had complete information for a total of 598 prostate biopsy and 723 prostatectomy subjects, which were matched. Missing data was attributed to procedures being performed prior to routine electronic uploading of histopathology reports. There were no stored hard copies of these missing reports and hence they were excluded from the study.

Table 1 shows the demographic and clinicopathologic characteristics of the 598 subjects that underwent prostate biopsy. As demonstrated, the minority of subjects (15.6 %) were ≤55 years whilst 84.4 % were >55 years ($p < 0.001$). The most frequent pre-biopsy PSA value range was 4.1–10 for both men ≤55 years (59.1 %) and men > 55 (67.7 %) ($p = 0.11$). A Gleason score of 3 + 4 was the most common for both age groups (41.9 % ≤55 years and 45.7 % >55 years) ($p = 0.50$) as was a clinical stage of T1c (69.9 % ≤55 years and 67.5 % >55 years) ($p = 0.65$).

Table 2 illustrates the prostate biopsy outcomes by age. 14.0 % of men ≤55 years and 11.9 % >55 years had insignificant prostate cancer as per the Epstein criteria, with no significant difference between the two age groups ($X^2 = 0.32$, df = 1, $p = 0.57$). Similarly, there was no significant difference between the two age groups in Gleason score >6 ($X^2 = 2.3$, $p = 0.13$), Gleason score >7 ($X^2 = 1.2$, $p = 0.27$), Gleason score as a continuous variable (t = −1.530, $p = 0.13$, mean difference = −0.195, 95 % CI of difference = −0.45 to 0.06), high-risk prostate cancer features ($X^2 = 0.007$, $p = 0.93$) or pre-biopsy PSA scores (t = 0.977, $p = 0.33$, mean difference = 1.45, 95 % CI of difference = −1.50 to 4.41).

The patient characteristics of the 723 subjects that underwent prostatectomy were similar in nature to the prostate biopsy patient characteristics (Table 3). There were less men ≤55 years (15.2 %) than >55 years (84.8 %) ($p < 0.001$), a common pre-biopsy PSA value of 4.1–10 in both men ≤55 years (56.4 %) and >55 years (65.6 %) ($p = 0.06$),and a common Gleason score 3 + 4

Table 1 Patient characteristics for prostate biopsy specimens for men ≤55 years compared to men >55 years

Characteristic	Age ≤55 years	Age >55 years	Total	Significance
Sample numbers	93 (15.6 %)	505 (84.4 %)	598 (100 %)	$X^2 = 283.9$, $p < 0.001$
Age (years)				
-Median	53	64	63	
-Range	41–55	56–79	41–79	
-Mean	51.9	64.3	62.4	
Clinical stage				
cT1c	65 (69.9 %)	341 (67.5 %)	406 (67.9 %)	$X^2 = 0.20$, $p = 0.65$
cT2a	10 (10.8 %)	64 (12.7 %)	74 (12.4 %)	$X^2 = 0.27$, $p = 0.61$
cT2b	2 (2.2 %)	25 (5.0 %)	27 (4.5 %)	$X^2 = 1.43$, $p = 0.23$
cT2c	14 (15.1 %)	73 (14.5 %)	87 (14.5 %)	$X^2 = 0.02$, $p = 0.88$
cT3a	0 (0 %)	0 (0 %)	0 (0 %)	-
cT3b	0 (0 %)	1 (0.2 %)	1 (0.2 %)	$X^2 = 0.18$, $p = 0.67$
Missing	2 (2.2 %)	1 (0.2 %)	3 (0.5 %)	$X^2 = 6.00$, $p = 0.01$
PSA score (ng/mL)				
<3	9 (9.7 %)	43 (8.5 %)	52 (8.7 %)	$X^2 = 0.134$, $p = 0.72$
3–4	12 (12.9 %)	41 (8.1 %)	53 (8.9 %)	$X^2 = 2.23$, $p = 0.14$
4.1–10	55 (59.1 %)	342 (67.7 %)	397 (66.4 %)	$X^2 = 2.59$, $p = 0.11$
10.1–20	14 (15.1 %)	73 (14.5 %)	87 (14.5 %)	$X^2 = 0.23$, $p = 0.88$
>20.1	3 (3.2 %)	6 (1.2 %)	9 (1.5 %)	$X^2 = 2.2$, $p = 0.14$
Gleason score				
3 + 3	32 (34.4 %)	135 (26.7 %)	167 (27.9 %)	$X^2 = 2.3$, $p = 0.13$
3 + 4	39 (41.9 %)	231 (45.7 %)	270 (45.2 %)	$X^2 = 0.46$, $p = 0.50$
4 + 3	13 (14.0 %)	69 (13.7 %)	82 (13.7 %)	$X^2 = 0.007$, $p = 0.94$
8	5 (5.4 %)	29 (5.7 %)	34 (5.7 %)	$X^2 = 0.02$, $p = 0.89$
9–10	4 (4.3 %)	41 (8.1 %)	45 (7.5 %)	$X^2 = 1.65$, $p = 0.20$
Biopsy				
No. cores mean	14.3	13.9	13.9	t = 1.17, $p = 0.24$, Mean difference = 0.48, 95 % CI of difference = −0.33 to 1.30
% of positive cores mean	31	34	34	t = −1.51, $p = 0.13$, Mean difference = −3.73, 95 % CI of difference = −8.58 to 1.11

Table 2 Prostate biopsy outcomes for men ≤55 years compared to men >55 years

Factor	Age ≤55 years	Age >55 years	Total	Significance
Insignificant prostate cancer (Epstein criteria)	13 (14.0 %)	60 (11.9 %)	73 (12.2 %)	$X^2 = 0.32$, $p = 0.57$
Total	93	505	598	
Gleason score				
>6	61 (65.6 %)	370 (73.3 %)	431 (72.1 %)	$X^2 = 2.3$, $p = 0.13$
>7	9 (9.7 %)	70 (13.9 %)	79 (13.2 %)	$X^2 = 1.2$, $p = 0.27$
Continuous variable	Mean = 2.03	Mean = 2.23		t = −1.53
	Std dev = 1.05	Std dev = 1.15		$p = 0.13$
				Mean difference = −0.20
				95 % CI of difference = −0.45 to 0.06
PSA comparison	Mean = 8.55	Mean = 7.10		t = 0.977
	Std dev = 14.26	Std dev = 3.98		$p = 0.33$
	Std error mean =1.48	Std error mean =0.18		Mean difference = 1.45
				95 % CI of difference = −1.50 to 4.41
High risk PC				
GS > 7	9 (12.5 %)	70 (13.9 %)	79 (13.2 %)	$X^2 = 1.2$, $p = 0.27$
PSA > 20	3 (3.2 %)	6 (1.2 %)	9 (1.5 %)	$X^2 = 2.2$, $p = 0.14$
Clinical stage > T2b	14 (15.1 %)	74 (14.7 %)	88 (14.7 %)	$X^2 = 0.03$, $p = 0.86$
At least one feature of high risk PC	23 (24.7 %)	127 (25.1 %)	150 (25.1 %)	$X^2 = 0.007$, $p = 0.93$

(51.8 % in men ≤55 years, 53.2 % in men >55 years) ($p = 0.79$). Additionally, the pathological stage was most frequently T2 in men ≤55 years (65.5 %) and men >55 years (59.5 %) ($p = 0.24$). Most often there was no seminal vesicle involvement (92.7 % in men ≤55 years, 92.3 % in men >55 years) ($p = 0.89$) and negative lymph nodes (62.7 % in men ≤55 years, 62.6 % in men >55 years) ($p = 0.99$). When comparing PSA as a continuous variable for the prostatectomy subjects there was no significant difference between men ≤55 and men >50 years (t = −0.365, $p = 0.72$, mean difference = −0.29, 95 % CI of difference = −1.86 to 1.28).

The prostatectomy outcomes paralleled the prostate biopsy outcomes, with similar rates of insignificant prostate cancer as per the Stamey criteria (9.1 % in men ≤55 years, 6.5 % in men >55 years) and no statistically significant difference ($X^2 = 1.25$, $p = 0.26$) (Table 3). Furthermore, there were similar mean tumour volumes (t = −1.63, df = 516, $p = 0.10$, 95 % CI = −1.01 to 0.95), Gleason score >6 ($X^2 = 4.23$, $p = 0.40$), Gleason score >7 ($X^2 = 0.95$, $p = 0.33$), Gleason score as a continuous variable (t = −2.000, $p = 0.05$, mean difference = −0.212, 95 % CI of difference = −0.42 to 0.00), margin positive status ($X^2 = 0.40$, $p = 0.84$) and high-risk prostate cancer ($X^2 = 0.83$, $p = 0.36$). As expected due to prostate hyperplasia with increasing age, the prostate weights in the men ≤55 years was significantly less than in men >55 years (t = −5.11, df = 191.8, $p < 0.001$, 95 % CI = −11.69 to −5.17). When pre-operative PSA levels are compared to prostatectomy tumour volumes, we find that PSA increases as tumour volume increases (t = 24.993, df = 515, $p < 0.001$). Also, men >55 years on average, have a higher PSA (6.83) and tumour volume (1.83) compared to men ≤55 years (mean PSA 6.22, mean tumour volume 1.37).

As described in Table 4, there were 27 men ≤50 years (4.5 %) and 571 men >50 years (95.5 %) who had prostate biopsies. Of these, 2 men ≤50 years (7.4 %) and 71 men >50 years (12.4 %) had insignificant prostate cancer (Epstein criteria), with no statistically significant difference between the two age groups ($X^2 = 0.55$, $p = 0.46$). Within the prostatectomy subjects there were 32 men ≤50 years (4.4 %) and 691 men >50 years (95.6 %). Of these, 2 men ≤50 years (1.8 %) and 48 men >50 years (7.8 %) had insignificant prostate cancer (Stamey criteria) with no significant difference between the younger and older men ($X^2 = 0.008$, $p = 0.93$) (Table 5).

When the group of men ≤55 years was subdivided into men ≤50 and 51–55 years, similar rates of insignificant prostate cancer were found in both prostate biopsy and prostatectomy specimens. From the prostate biopsies, 2 men ≤50 years and 11 men 51–55 years had insignificant prostate cancer ($X^2 = 1.238$, df = 1, $p = 0.27$). From the prostatectomy specimens, 2 men ≤50 years and 8 men 51–55 years had insignificant prostate cancer ($X^2 = 0.437$, df = 1, $p = 0.51$).

Discussion

Since the introduction of PSA testing, rates of prostate cancer diagnosis have dramatically increased whilst prostate cancer mortality has fallen [9]. Despite this, a large

Table 3 Prostatectomy patient characteristics and outcomes for men ≤55 years compared to men >55 years

Characteristic	Age ≤55 years	Age >55 years	Total	Significance
Sample numbers	110 (15.2 %)	613 (84.8 %)	723 (100 %)	$X^2 = 349.9$, $p < 0.001$
Age (years)				
-Median	53	64	63	
-Range	41–55	56–79	41–79	
-Mean	52.0	64.2	62.4	
PSA score (ng/mL)				
<3	11 (10.0 %)	67 (10.9 %)	78 (10.8 %)	$X^2 = 0.08$, $p = 0.77$
3–4	25 (22.7 %)	43 (7.0 %)	68 (9.4 %)	$X^2 = 27.02$, $p < 0.001$
4.1–10	62 (56.4 %)	402 (65.6 %)	464 (64.2 %)	$X^2 = 3.45$, $p = 0.06$
10.1–20	7 (6.4 %)	90 (14.7 %)	94 (13.4 %)	$X^2 = 5.56$, $p = 0.02$
>20.1	4 (3.6 %)	8 (1.3 %)	12 (1.7 %)	$X^2 = 3.11$, $p = 0.08$
Missing	1 (0.9 %)	3 (0.5 %)	4 (0.6 %)	$X^2 = 0.30$, $p = 0.59$
Continuous variable	110	613	723	(t = −0.365, $p = 0.72$, mean difference = −0.29, 95 % CI of difference = −1.86 to 1.28)
Gleason score				
3 + 3	26 (23.6 %)	96 (15.7 %)	122 (16.9 %)	$X^2 = 4.23$, $p = 0.40$
3 + 4	57 (51.8 %)	326 (53.2 %)	383 (53.0 %)	$X^2 = 0.70$, $p = 0.79$
4 + 3	19 (17.3 %)	128 (20.9 %)	147 (20.3 %)	$X^2 = 0.75$, $p = 0.39$
8	3 (2.7 %)	13 (2.1 %)	16 (2.2 %)	$X^2 = 0.16$, $p = 0.69$
9–10	5 (4.5 %)	50 (8.2 %)	55 (7.6 %)	$X^2 = 1.73$, $p = 0.19$
>6	84 (76.4 %)	517 (84.3 %)	601 (83.1 %)	$X^2 = 4.23$, $p = 0.40$
>7	8 (7.3 %)	63 (10.3 %)	71 (9.8 %)	$X^2 = 0.95$, $p = 0.33$
Continuous variable	mean = 2.13	mean = 2.34		t = −2.00
	Std dev = 0.96	Std dev = 1.04		$p = 0.05$
				Mean difference = −0.212
				95 % CI of difference = −0.42 to 0.00
Pathological stage				
pT2	72 (65.5 %)	365 (59.5 %)	437 (60.4 %)	$X^2 = 1.36$, $p = 0.24$
pT3a	24 (21.8 %)	167 (27.2 %)	191 (26.4 %)	$X^2 = 1.41$, $p = 0.24$
pT3b	14 (12.7 %)	80 (13.1 %)	94 (13.0 %)	$X^2 = 0.01$, $p = 0.93$
pT4	0 (0 %)	0 (0 %)	0 (0 %)	-
Missing	0 (0 %)	1 (0.2 %)	1 (0.1 %)	$X^2 = 0.18$, $p = 0.67$
Prostate weight	Mean = 46.40	Mean = 54.83		t = −5.11,
	Std dev = 14.86	Std dev = 20.72		df = 191.8,
				$p < 0.001$,
				95 % CI = −11.69 to −5.17
Tumour volume				
<0.5	21 (19.1 %)	109 (17.8 %)	130 (18.0 %)	$X^2 = 0.11$, $p = 0.74$
0.5-1	23 (20.9 %)	107 (17.5 %)	130 (18.0 %)	$X^2 = 0.75$, $p = 0.39$
1.1-2	17 (15.5 %)	106 (17.3 %)	123 (17.0 %)	$X^2 = 0.22$, $p = 0.64$
2.1+	13 (11.8 %)	123 (20.1 %)	136 (18.8 %)	$X^2 = 4.15$, $p = 0.04$
Missing	36 (32.7 %)	168 (27.4 %)	204 (28.2 %)	$X^2 = 1.30$, $p = 0.25$

Table 3 Prostatectomy patient characteristics and outcomes for men ≤55 years compared to men >55 years *(Continued)*

Mean tumour volume	Mean = 1.37 Std dev = 1.51	Mean = 1.82 Std dev = 2.34		t = −1.628, df = 516, $p = 0.104$, 95 % CI = −1.01 to 0.95
Seminal vesicle				
Negative	102 (92.7 %)	566 (92.3 %)	668 (92.4 %)	$X^2 = 0.02$, $p = 0.89$
Positive	8 (7.3 %)	47 (7.7 %)	55 (7.6 %)	
Lymph nodes				
Negative	69 (62.7 %)	384 (62.6 %)	453 (62.7 %)	$X^2 = 0.00$, $p = 0.99$
Positive	4 (3.6 %)	16 (2.2 %)	20 (2.8 %)	$X^2 = 0.37$, $p = 0.55$
Not taken	37 (33.6 %)	213 (29.5 %)	250 (34.6 %)	$X^2 = 0.05$, $p = 0.82$
Insignificant prostate cancer (Stamey criteria)	10 (9.1 %)	40 (6.5 %)	50 (6.9 %)	$X^2 = 1.25$, $p = 0.26$
Missing	10 (9.1 %)	29 (4.7 %)	39 (5.4 %)	
Total	110	613	723	
Clinical stage				
-Organ confined (pT2, N0NX)	72 (65.5 %)	363 (59.3 %)	435 (60.2 %)	$X^2 = 1.47$, $p = 0.23$
-Non-Organ confined (pT3/4, N0-1)	38 (34.5 %)	249 (40.7 %)	287 (39.8 %)	
Margin positive	27 (24.5 %)	156 (25.4 %)	183 (25.3 %)	$X^2 = 0.40$, $p = 0.84$
High risk PCa				
GS > 7	8 (7.3 %)	63 (10.3 %)	71 (9.8 %)	$X^2 = 0.95$, $p = 0.33$
PSA > 20	4 (3.6 %)	8 (1.3 %)	12 (1.7 %)	$X^2 = 3.11$, $p = 0.08$
Clinical stage > T2b	15 (13.6 %)	89 (14.5 %)	104 (14.4 %)	$X^2 = 0.06$, $p = 0.81$
At least one feature of high risk PCa	22 (20.0 %)	147 (24.0 %)	169 (23.4 %)	$X^2 = 0.83$, $p = 0.36$

proportion of those diagnosed with prostate cancer will have insignificant prostate cancer [10] – many of whom will have unnecessary treatment and subsequently experience morbidity and mortality. It is therefore important to define a population that would optimally benefit from PSA testing.

We chose to analyse differences in prostate cancer pathology on biopsy specimens between the age groups as this avoids selection bias to some extent. There would be some selection bias in who gets a prostate biopsy with an abnormal PSA, however we would expect the bias would favour older men having more significant cancer as these men would be more likely to avoid/not be recommended a biopsy at lower PSA levels [11]. We also studied the differences in prostatectomy specimen pathology between the age groups because Epstein criteria has inherent inaccuracies in detecting insignificant cancers [6]. Prostatectomy specimens allow more accurate determination of pathology but are subject to more selection bias. Again, we would expect the bias would be toward older men having more significant cancers, as younger men would elect to have surgery for less significant cancers and opt for active surveillance less readily then older men as a result of different life expectancies and co-morbidities [12]. In Australia, PSA screening is performed by the primary care physicians and patients

Table 4 Prostate biopsy characteristics and outcomes for men ≤50 years compared to men >50 years

Characteristic	Age ≤50 years	Age >50 years	Total	Significance
Sample numbers	27 (4.5 %)	571 (95.5 %)	598 (100 %)	
Age (years)				
-Median	49	63	63	
-Range	41–50	51–79	41–79	
-Mean	47.9	63.0	62.4	
Insignificant prostate cancer (Epstein criteria)	2 (7.4 %)	71 (12.4 %)	73 (12.2 %)	$X^2 = 0.55$, df = 1, $p = 0.46$
Total	27	571	598	

Table 5 Prostatectomy characteristics and outcomes for men ≤50 years compared to men >50 years

Characteristic	Age ≤50 years	Age >50 years	Total	Significance
Sample numbers	32 (4.4 %)	691 (95.6 %)	723 (100 %)	
Age (years)				
-Median				
-Range	41–50	51–79	41–79	
-Mean				
Insignificant prostate cancer (Stamey criteria)	2 (1.8 %)	48 (7.8 %)	50 (6.9 %)	$X^2 = 0.008$, df = 1, $p = 0.93$
Missing	3 (2.7 %)	36 (5.9 %)	39 (5.4 %)	
Total	110	613	723	

are generally referred to a urologist when the PSA is above the age specific reference range. We do not have data on the total number of men screened in each age group.

In our study population, there was no statistically significant difference in the rates of insignificant or high-risk prostate cancer between men ≤55 years and >55 years on either the prostate biopsy or prostatectomy specimens. Therefore, it would seem to follow that men ≤55 years would benefit from PSA testing by allowing early detection of significant prostate cancer in the same way as older men do. This in turn facilitates early treatment and prevents presentation with advanced disease. Early diagnosis of significant prostate cancer may be particularly important in men <55 years as high grade and locally advanced prostate cancer in this younger group may paradoxically have worse outcomes compared to their older counterparts - potentially reflecting differing prostate cancer biology in this population [13].

There is currently contradictory evidence in the literature about the benefit of prostate cancer screening in terms of reducing prostate cancer-specific mortality. The PLCO and ERSPC trials are often quoted as the most rigorous of the available studies, though these give conflicting results. PLCO concluded that there was no significant prostate cancer-specific mortality benefit (RR 1.15, 95 % CI 0.86 to 1.54) from screening, whilst ERSPC showed a significant benefit (RR 0.84, 95 % CI 0.73 to 0.95) [1]. Unfortunately, neither study included men <55 years, therefore do not reliably contribute to the discussion of PSA screening in this age group.

Of the trials that included men <55 years, the Goteborg population-based randomised trial showed a reduction in metastatic disease and prostate cancer-specific mortality when screening started at 50 years [14]. The Quebec trial included men as young as 45 years though has demonstrated no benefit in prostate-specific mortality with PSA testing when using an intention-to-treat analysis [15]. A Cochrane review exploring the prostate cancer-specific mortality according to the age of participants at screening identified no significant difference in prostate cancer-specific mortality regardless of whether the men were screened from age 45 years (RR 1.01; 95 % CI 0.76–1.33), 50 years (RR 0.93; 95 % CI 0.69–1.27) or 55 years (RR 1.12; 95 % CI 0.92–1.37) [1].

In a retrospective study, Twiss et al. (2005) found that men under 50 years had similar rates of significant prostate cancer as men over 50 years when analysing radical retropubic prostatectomy specimens - implying that there would be utility in PSA testing both populations [16]. In contrast, Howard et al. (2009) found that prostate cancer screening beginning at 40 years compared to 50 years would prevent less than 1 prostate cancer death per 1000 men screened [17]. This is due to the fact that the rate of prostate cancer detection in the younger age group is lower than older men. Our study has shown however that when a cancer is detected in this younger age group, it is no less aggressive.

The role of a baseline PSA test in younger men for predicting future risk of prostate cancer is also controversial. There is evidence that PSA testing in men in their 40's can stratify risk of developing prostate cancer in the future, particularly if the baseline PSA is in the highest centiles above the median [18, 19]. This strategy would allow men with a high-risk PSA to undergo close monitoring, whilst sparing men with a low-risk PSA from regular PSA testing.

This raises the question of at which age PSA testing should actually be implemented. It may be when below a certain age there is a statistically significant difference in the rates of insignificant prostate cancer. In our data set, when the rates of insignificant prostate cancer in men ≤50 years were compared to those >50 years in both the prostate biopsy and prostatectomy specimens - there remained no difference, suggesting that screening may still be appropriate at this age.

We acknowledge that the definition of insignificant cancer has not been well defined clinically and validated and as such is controversial. Factors such as age and family history and life-expectancy will have to be included in any real pathological definition of insignificant cancer. In the absence of a well-established definition of insignificant cancer, we chose the Epstein criteria for needle biopsy and Stamey definition for prostatectomy specimens, as these are the most commonly reported.

Larger studies need to be designed to assess whether our findings remain consistent, particularly amongst different geographical/ethnic populations. Future trails should include men >40 years to more thoroughly assess prostate cancer screening benefits in terms of prostate cancer-specific mortality. Ideally, there would be exclusion of subjects with a family history of prostate cancer- as this is a known prostate cancer risk factor that alters PSA screening choice. Nevertheless, it is estimated that only 5–10 % of prostate cancer is related to a positive family history [20] and this would not explain the similarities in rates of high-risk prostate cancer in men ≤55 and >55 years in our study.

Limitations of this study include reliance on a third-party for availability of recorded and collected data. There were cases of missing subject data that resulted in the exclusion of some participants. Ideally, there would be an equal sample size of men ≤55 and >55 years in the study, however if consecutive subjects are chosen this is challenging to accomplish as more men >55 years have PSA testing and prostate biopsies. Screening calculators such as the Prostate Cancer Prevention Trial (PCPT) screening calculator may be used for an individualised assessment of prostate cancer risk.

Conclusions

PSA testing remains controversial and guidelines will continue to evolve in the coming years. We found no significant difference in the rates of insignificant and high-risk prostate cancer between men ≤55 years and >55 years, in either the prostate biopsies or prostatectomy specimens. The optimal age to begin PSA testing is yet unclear, however, our findings suggest that it should be less than 55 years. Further trials need to be performed with comparable sample sizes and controlling of risk factors to assess the utility of PSA screening in younger men.

Abbreviations

PC: Prostate cancer; PSA: Prostate specific antigen; AUA: American Urological Association; DRE: Digital rectal examination.

Competing interests

Manish I. Patel is supported by a NSW Cancer Institute Fellowship (10/ECF/2-29). There are no disclosures relevant to this research from any of the authors.

Authors' contributions

ND – Involved in data collection, manuscript drafting. TH – Conceived study, involved in manuscript drafting. PC – Involved in data collection of own patients. AB – Involved in data collection of own patients. HL – Involved in data collection of own patients. WD – Assisted in data collection and data retrieval organisation. MP – Conceived study, involved in data collection of own patients and manuscript drafting. All authors read and approved the final manuscript.

Acknowledgements

We would like to acknowledge Douglas Hanley Moir, the pathology company, for their invaluable contribution in data retrieval of the prostate biopsy and prostatectomy specimen histopathology.

Author details

[1]University of Sydney, Discipline of Surgery, Sydney, Australia. [2]Department of Urology, Westmead Hospital, Sydney, Australia. [3]St George Hospital, Sydney, Australia. [4]Douglass Hanley Moir Pathology, Sydney, Australia.

References

1. Ilic D, Neuberger MM, Djulbegovic M, Dahm P. Screening for prostate cancer. Cochrane Database Syst Rev. 2013;1:CD004720.
2. Carter HB, Albertsen PC, Barry MJ, et al. Early detection of prostate cancer: AUA Guideline. J Urol. 2013;190:419–26.
3. Ploussard G, Epstein JI, Montironi R, et al. The contemporary concept of significant versus insignificant prostate cancer. Eur Urol. 2011;60:291–303.
4. Schroder FH, Hugosson J, Roobol MJ, et al. Screening and prostate cancer mortality: results of the European Randomised Study of Screening for Prostate Cancer (ERSPC) at 13 years of follow-up. Lancet. 2014;384:2027–35.
5. Andriole GL, Crawford ED, Grubb 3rd RL, et al. Prostate cancer screening in the randomized Prostate, Lung, Colorectal, and Ovarian Cancer Screening Trial: mortality results after 13 years of follow-up. J Natl Cancer Inst. 2012;104:125–32.
6. Oon SF, Watson RW, O'Leary JJ, Fitzpatrick JM. Epstein criteria for insignificant prostate cancer. BJU Int. 2011;108:518–25.
7. Hernandez DJ, Nielsen ME, Han M, Partin AW. Contemporary evaluation of the D'amico risk classification of prostate cancer. Urology. 2007;70:931–5.
8. Stamey TA, Freiha FS, McNeal JE, Redwine EA, Whittemore AS, Schmid HP. Localized prostate cancer. Relationship of tumor volume to clinical significance for treatment of prostate cancer. Cancer. 1993;71:933–8.
9. Oliver SE, May MT, Gunnell D. International trends in prostate-cancer mortality in the "PSA ERA". Int J Cancer. 2001;92:893–8.
10. Haas GP, Delongchamps N, Brawley OW, Wang CY, de la Roza G. The worldwide epidemiology of prostate cancer: perspectives from autopsy studies. Can J Urol. 2008;15:3866–71.
11. Oesterling JE, Jacobsen SJ, Chute CG, et al. Serum prostate-specific antigen in a community-based population of healthy men. Establishment of age-specific reference ranges. JAMA. 1993;270:860–4.
12. Stangelberger A, Waldert M, Djavan B. Prostate cancer in elderly men. Rev Urol. 2008;10:111–9.
13. Lin DW, Porter M, Montgomery B. Treatment and survival outcomes in young men diagnosed with prostate cancer: a Population-based Cohort Study. Cancer. 2009;115:2863–71.
14. Hugosson J, Carlsson S, Aus G, et al. Mortality results from the Goteborg randomised population-based prostate-cancer screening trial. Lancet Oncol. 2010;11:725–32.
15. Labrie F, Candas B, Cusan L, et al. Screening decreases prostate cancer mortality: 11-year follow-up of the 1988 Quebec prospective randomized controlled trial. Prostate. 2004;59:311–8.
16. Twiss C, Slova D, Lepor H. Outcomes for men younger than 50 years undergoing radical prostatectomy. Urology. 2005;66:141–6.
17. Howard K, Barratt A, Mann GJ, Patel MI. A model of prostate-specific antigen screening outcomes for low- to high-risk men: information to support informed choices. Arch Intern Med. 2009;169:1603–10.
18. Vickers AJ, Ulmert D, Sjoberg DD, et al. Strategy for detection of prostate cancer based on relation between prostate specific antigen at age 40–55 and long term risk of metastasis: case-control study. BMJ. 2013;346:f2023.
19. Lilja H, Cronin AM, Dahlin A, et al. Prediction of significant prostate cancer diagnosed 20 to 30 years later with a single measure of prostate-specific antigen at or before age 50. Cancer. 2011;117:1210–9.
20. Hemminki K, Czene K. Age specific and attributable risks of familial prostate carcinoma from the family-cancer database. Cancer. 2002;95:1346–53.

18

Extranodal nasal-type natural killer/T-cell lymphoma with penile involvement

Xiaotian Wang[1], Zimu Gong[2], Shawn Xiang Li[2,3], Wei Yan[2] and Yongsheng Song[1*]

Abstract

Background: Extranodal natural killer/T-cell lymphoma (ENKTL) usually presents as a localized disease in the nasal cavity; extension to the male genitourinary system is very rare and has been characterized only recently. Most cases present with predominantly extranodal involvement, advanced stage disease, highly aggressive course, and strong association with Epstein-Barr virus (EBV). While metastasis is common in ENKTLs, the penis is rarely involved in both nasal and non-nasal ENKTLs and only one report was published to date.

Case presentation: One patient with NK/T-cell lymphoma, presented initially with a penile mass, is reported. The 58-year-old man who presented with progressive painless penile swelling underwent penectomy for penile tumor. Histologically, the glans and foreskin revealed neoplastic infiltration of medium-sized lymphoma cells expressing CD56, CD3, granzyme-B, and labeled for EBV-encoded RNA in situ hybridization. Findings were consistent with NK/T-cell lymphoma. By detailed history, we learned that the patient had nasal obstruction for more than 10 years. Nasopharyngeal involvement was screened with PET-CT; ENKTL was diagnosed after a nasopharyngeal biopsy. The final diagnosis was primary nasal NK/T-cell lymphoma, with metastasis to the penis. Additional sites of disease appeared soon afterward (adrenal gland, liver, spleen and lymph nodes). The patient died within 4 months.

Conclusion: This study suggested that penile NK/T-cell lymphoma tends to disseminate early and pursues an aggressive course. It is imperative to distinguish nasal NK/T lymphoma from other types of tumors, because the prognosis and treatment differ significantly for secondary metastases.

Keywords: NK/T lymphoma, Penile malignancy

Background

Extranodal natural killer/T-cell lymphoma (ENKTL) is a distinct entity of non-Hodgkin lymphoma with unique characteristics in both biological features and clinical behavior. ENKTL is most commonly seen in young to middle-aged patients, with a male preponderance of 2–4:1. Despite its rarity in the Caucasian population, ENKTL had a significantly higher incidence in East Asia and Latin America [1].

The common and primary sites which ENKTL arises from include the nasal cavity, upper aerodigestive tract, and other midline facial structures [2]. Invasion to adjacent tissues and metastasis to distant organs are also common [3, 4]. Overall, ENKTL is associated with an aggressive disease course and poor clinical outcome, especially with metastatic disease beyond the nasal cavity, in which the complete remission rate is only about 30%, and median survival is 4.3 months [5].

Since the primary lesion is often occult without causing significant symptoms, ENKTL is often diagnosed in relatively advanced stages when metastatic lesions occur. The most commonly involved metastatic sites include skin, gastrointestinal tract, testis, kidney, and breast. The morphological characteristics of metastatic lesions are often less typical than that of the primary lesion, and extensive necrosis further compromises the accuracy of histopathological diagnosis. Therefore, it is crucial to investigate potential nasal lesion when metastatic ENKTL is suspected.

* Correspondence: songyongsheng123@hotmail.com
[1]Department of Urology, Shengjing Hospital of China Medical University, 36 Saohao Road, Shenyang, Liaoning, China
Full list of author information is available at the end of the article

We herein report a case of penile metastatic NK/T cell lymphoma in which the diagnosis was established first at the metastatic site, and the primary lesion in the nasal cavity was uncovered later.

Case presentation

Clinical history

A 58-year-old male was admitted to our hospital with diffuse swelling of the penis, followed by sclerosis and ischemic changes in the glans and anterior segment of the penis, without bloody or purulent discharge. On review of systems, he denied fever, night sweat, and weight loss. Past medical and family history are not contributory. On admission, his vital signs were within normal limits. On physical examination, his face was thin and worn. No lymphadenopathy was palpated in the neck and supraclavicular region; visual examination of the genitals manifested a diffused enlargement of the penis with local ulcer and necrotic tissue in the glans penis.

Laboratory findings showed the white blood cell count as 8100/mm^3, hemoglobin as 12.5 g/dL, and a platelet count of 276,000/mm^3, and liver function, kidney function, and the serum lactate dehydrogenase (LDH) levels were within normal limits. The EBV IgG was positive in the serum, the EBV DNA determination was negative in the blood, and CRP was 22.9 mg/mL.

Pelvic enhanced MRI showed space-occupying lesions in the forward part of the penis, urethral orifice stenosis, and cavernosal swelling (Fig. 1a-c). No lesion in the bladder was identified upon cystoscopy. CT scans of chest and abdomen did not detect enlarged lymph nodes. The liver and spleen were of normal size and shape. Bone marrow biopsy showed lymphoma cell infiltration up to 3.2%.

Pathologic finding and treatment

Microscopic findings of the penile mass showed infiltration of medium-sized cells with irregular nuclei, inconspicuous nucleoli, and many apoptotic bodies. The lymphoma cells exhibited a notable angioinfiltrative growth pattern, with homocentric arrangement around small arteries, and coagulative necrosis was also observed (Fig. 2a and b). On immunohistochemical staining, the atypical cells were positive for CD3, CD56, vimentin, LCA, TIA-1, and granzyme B, but negative for cytokeratin, CD20, bcl-2, bcl-6, and ALK (Fig. 2c-e). In the case of in situ hybridization for EBV encoded RNA (EBER), most atypical cells were also labeled (Fig. 2f). These findings were consistent with NK/T-cell lymphoma.

By detailed history, we learned that the patient had nasal obstruction for more than 10 years. PET-CT found a high-FDG metabolic mass in the nasal cavity and the nasopharyngeal cavity. Space-occupying lesion in the nasal cavity was observed and biopsied with sinoscopy. Histological examination showed diffuse infiltration of small to medium-sized lymphoid cells with angiodestructive growth pattern, and apoptotic bodies were present (Fig. 3a). The tumor cells were positive for CD3, CD56, EBER; they were negative for CD20 and granzyme B (Fig. 3. b-d). Based on the endoscopic and immunophenotypical findings, the diagnosis of penile metastasis from extranodal nasal-type NK/T-cell lymphoma was established.

Twenty days after neoplasm resection, the patient consented to chemotherapy treatment followed by radiotherapy and autologous stem cell transplantation. CHOP-L regimen (cyclophosphamide, doxorubicin, vincristine, prednisone, and L-asparaginase) was planned to be given every 3 weeks, with six cycles in total. However, the third cycle of chemotherapy was delayed due to ascites, fever, and grade 4 myelosuppression. Subsequently, he developed tachypnea, abdominal pain, fever, and diarrhea. According to the CT results, His lymphoma was refractory to chemotherapy and metastases developed in the adrenal gland, liver, spleen and lymph

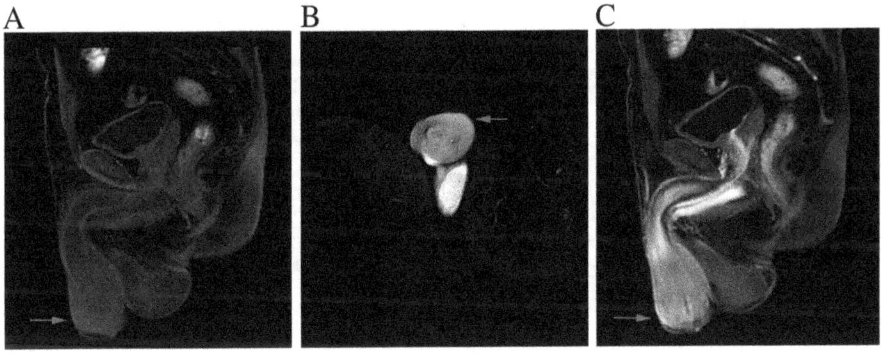

Fig. 1 **a** Sagittal T1-weighted magnetic resonance imaging scan showing mass around the corpus cavernosum (arrow); **b** Axial T2-weight magnetic resonance imaging scan showing ill-defined mass around the corpus cavernosum (arrow); **c** Sagittal T1-weighted fat suppression contrast-enhanced magnetic resonance imaging scan showing enhanced mass around the corpus cavernosum (arrow)

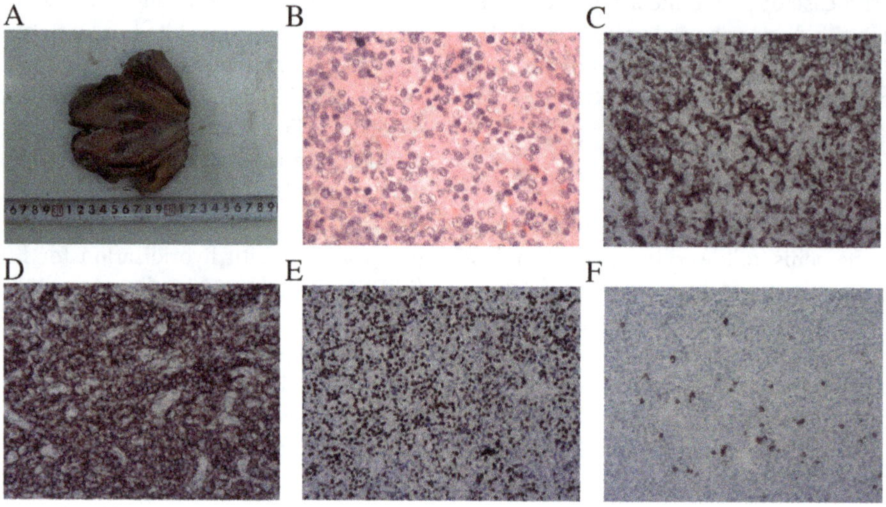

Fig. 2 Pathologic gross (**a**) and microscopic features of thespecimen. **b** Histological examinations stained with hematoxylin and eosin revealed infiltration of medium-sized cells with irregular nuclei, inconspicuous nucleoli, and many apoptotic bodies(H&E stains × 100). **c** Immunohistochemical staining showed positive reactivity for CD3(×100). **d** Immunohistochemical staining showed positive CD56(×100). **e** In situ hybridization for Epstein-Barr virus-encoded RNA showed positive reaction in atypical cells(×100). **f** Immunohistochemical staining showed negative CD20(×100)

nodes. The patient died of disease 1 month later, which is approximately 4 months after the diagnosis was made.

Informed consent was obtained from the patient for publication of this case report and any accompanying image.

Discussion

Lymphoma of the NK cell phenotype is rare. International T-cell Lymphoma Project reported that 10.4% of T cell lymphoma was of the NK/T-cell type [6]. WHO recognized entities include extranodal NK/T-cell

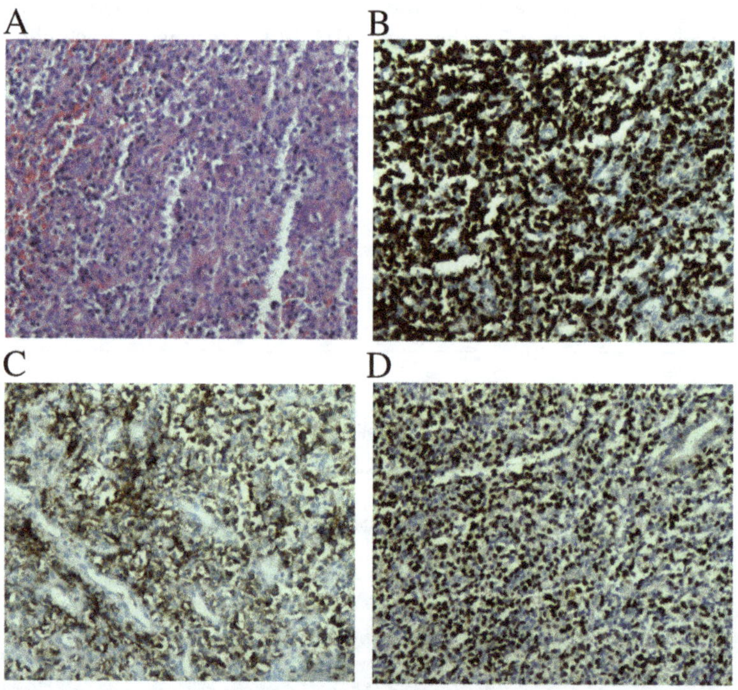

Fig. 3 **a** Pathological features of sinoscopical biopsy showed diffuse infiltration of small to medium-sized lymphoid cells with angiodestructive growth pattern, and apoptotic bodies were present (H&E stains ×100). **b** Immunohistochemical staining showed positive reactivity for CD3(×100). **c** Immunohistochemical staining showed positive CD56(×100). **d** In situ hybridization for Epstein-Barr virus-encoded RNA showed positive reaction in atypical cells(×100)

lymphoma, nasal type, aggressive NK cell leukemia, and chronic lymphoproliferative disorders of NK cells [7]. Among these entities, the last one is indolent but the other two exhibit an aggressive course and short survival. Diagnosis of NK cell lymphoma may be challenging. The characteristic immunophenotype of NK/T-cell lymphoma is CD56+, CD2+, surface CD3-, LCA+. Also, CD56 is a useful marker [8]. EBER is a diagnostic requisite of NK/T-cell lymphoma and is especially useful in metastatic sites where the CD56 expression might be lost [9].

NK/T-cell lymphoma often occurs in the nasal cavity and the upper aerodigestive tract, and it is associated with a poor prognosis. Bone marrow involvement occurs in <10% of patients. Distant metastasis of NK/T-cell lymphoma is sporadically reported, with the most commonly involved site including skin, testis, gastrointestinal tract, eyes, lungs, adrenal glands, breast, and brain [10, 11]. ENKTL with penis involvement is very rare, with only one case reported. We reviewed these ENKTL cases with involvement of male genitourinary system, whose clinical characteristics are summarized in Table 1 [12–27].

Lymphoma of the penis can present as a solitary nodule, non-healing ulcer, or diffuse penile swelling [28]. Upon reviewing the literature, most reported cases of penile lymphoma were classified as diffuse large B-cell lymphoma (DLBCL) [29]. Primary penile NK/T-cell lymphoma is never reported. In combination with clinical history and pathological results, the final diagnosis of penile metastasis secondary to extranodal nasal-type NK/T-cell lymphoma was established in our case. The diagnosis of the rare diseases has always been a challenging process. The final diagnosis of lymphoma of the penis was made on the histopathological examination of tissue biopsy. Histological analyses must include comprehensive immunohistochemistry tests to differentiate lymphoma from undifferentiated sarcomas or carcinoma and to distinguish between different types of lymphomas.

Nasal type NK/T cell lymphoma is associated with poor prognosis and often follows a rapidly progressive course. Age, symptoms, local tumor invasion, clinical stage, treatment response, NK/T cell IPI, LDH, and EBV infection were reported to be prognostic in ENKTL [30]. Although lacking statistical data, some literature reported distant metastasis and bone marrow involvement, with a very poor prognosis [31]. Our patient had unfavorable prognostic factors (EBV infection, distant metastasis, and bone marrow involvement), and the available data on optimal treatment strategies are limited. Systemic chemotherapy and involved field radiotherapy is the current standard of care for nasal-type NK/T-cell lymphoma, and CHOP is a very commonly used regimen.

Table 1 Clinical features of ENKTL cases with involvement of male genitourinaty system

Location	Age	Presentation	Treatment	Outcome	Ref
Kidney	72	Left flank pain	RT	DOD	[12]
Kidney	35	Urinary symptoms	CT	DOD	[13]
Prostate	59	Fever and dysuria	CT	DOD	[14]
Testis	38	Nasal granuloma	Orchiectomy RT,CT	DOD	[15]
Testis	61	Right testicular swelling	Orchiectomy, CT	AWR	[16]
Testis	68	Left testicular swelling	Orchiectomy, CT	NA	[16]
Testis	40	Left testicular swelling with B symptom	Orchiectomy, CT	DOD	[16]
Testis	44	Bilateral testicular swelling with B symptom	Orchiectomy, CT	DOD	[16]
Testis	45	Left testicular swelling	Orchiectomy, CT	NA	[16]
Testis	13	Right testicular swelling with B symptom	Orchiectomy, CT	NA	[16]
Testis	22	Right testicular swelling with B symptom	Orchiectomy, CT	AWD	[16]
Testis	0.67	Enlarged scrotum	CT, CBSCT	AWD	[17]
Testis	28	Painful testicular mass	CT	DOD	[18]
Testis	76	Left painless testicular enlargement	Orchiectomy, CT	AWD	[19]
Testis	36	Left testicular swelling fatigue weight-loss night sweat	CT, RT, allo-SCT	AWR	[20]
Testis	81	Right thigh soft tissue mass	Bilateral orchiectomy	DOD	[21]
Testis	30	Bilateral scrotal swelling and fever	RT, CT	DOD	[22]
Testis	52	Right testicle swelling	Chemo/RT	DOD	[23]
Testis	66	Painless enlargement of right testis	Orchiectomy	AWD	[24]
Testis	35	Right testicular swelling	Orchiectomy, CT	NA	[25]
Testis	47	Left scrotal swelling, weight loss	RT, CT	DOD	[26]
Testis	71	Nontender left testicular mass	Orchiectomy	DOD	[26]
Testis	55	Left scrotal swelling, fever and weight loss	Orchiectomy and CT	DOD	[26]
Penis	48	A painful mass in the penile shaft	CT	AWR	[27]

Abbreviations: *ENKTL* extranodal natural killer/T-cell lymphoma, *CT* chemotherapy, *RT* radiotherapy, *allo-SCT* allogeneic stem cell transplantation, *CBSCT* cord blood stem cell transplantation, *AWR* alive with relapse, *DOD* died of disease, *AWD* alive with disease, *NA* not available

The introduction of L-asparaginase-containing regimens led to further improvement in outcome, as most studies using L-asparaginase-containing regimens in a relapsed or refractory setting reported response rates of around 50% [32]. Therefore, the use of L-asparaginase-containing regimens may be superior to the use of CHOP regimen alone. The prognosis of ENKTL involving male genitourinary system is poor: most reported that patients died due to complications of the disease or of the treatment. Patients need chemotherapy combined with other effective treatments. A recent study showed that autologous stem cell transplantation is a feasible and effective therapy for high-risk nasal-type NK/T-cell lymphoma. We reviewed these trials, whose clinical outcomes are summarized in Table 2 [33–38]. The patient was also recommended to undergo autologous stem cell transplantation. However, unfortunately, he rapidly died due to disease progression, before that could be possible.

There are certain strengths and a major limitation to this study. An obvious strength is that this is a case report of a very rare case that can illuminate future treatment of similar cases. The treatment plans may be of value to future clinical guidelines. The primary limitation is self-evident. This is a case report of a single case; single-case reports are inherently limited. Our treatment regimen did not work effectively. With the hindsight of this case, more effective treatments may be developed in the future.

Table 2 Clinical outcomes of autologous stem cell transplantation in patients with ENKTL

Author	Cases	Median age	Male: female	Median follow-up(M)	Outcome	Ref
Fox	28	47	17:11	33	1-year NRM:11%, 2-year PFS:41%	[33]
Yhim	62	45.5	43:19	43.3	CR:61.3%; PR:38.7%	[34]
					3-year PFS:52.4%, 3-year OS:60%	
Wang	31	43	22:9	70	ORR:90.3%,1-year ORR:96.8%	[35]
Lee	47	42	34:13	116.5	5-year OS:56%	[36]
					In people who were in CR: disease-specific 5-year OS:87.3%	
Cui	22	38	38:19	24	5-year OS:79.3%	[37]
					5-year-PFS:36.4%	
Kim	16	36	5:3	22.4	2-year OS:71.3%, RFS:25.8%	[38]

Abbreviations: *NRM* non-relapse mortality, *PFS* progression-free survival, *ORR* overall response rate, *OS* overall survival, *CR* complete response, *PR* partial response, *RFS* relapse free survival

Conclusion

In conclusion, we present a case with primary NK/T-cell lymphoma with metastasis to the penis. The incidence of such condition is extremely low but has significant clinical value. This case broadened the spectrum of differential diagnosis of penile tumors and exhibited the value of detailed history taking and comprehensive workup. After all, patients with suspected metastasized ENKTL should undergo appropriate workup to investigate possible nasal lesions, and early biopsy should be done for suspected lesions to avoid delay in diagnosis. Due to the rapid progress and poor prognosis of this malignant disease, doctors need to make joint efforts to develop more effective therapeutic regimens.

Abbreviations

CHOP-L: Cyclophosphamide, doxorubicin, vincristine, prednisone, L-asparaginase; DLBCL: Diffuse large B-cell lymphoma; EBER: EBV encoded RNA; EBV: Epstein-Barr virus; ENKTL: Extranodal NK/T-cell lymphoma; LDH: Lactose dehydrogenase

Acknowledgements

None.

Funding

None.

Authors' contributions

XW discovered the case and treated patient. ZG, SL, WY carried out literature research, participated in design, and all participated in drafting of the case, YS participated in drafting case, provided guidance, and is the corresponding author. All authors actively contributed to the case on an intellectual level. All authors read and approved the final manuscript.

Competing interests

The authors declare that they have no competing interests.

Author details

[1]Department of Urology, Shengjing Hospital of China Medical University, 36 Saohao Road, Shenyang, Liaoning, China. [2]Department of Hematology, Shengjing Hospital of China Medical University, Shenyang, China. [3]International College, China Medical University, Shenyang, China.

References

1. Gill H, Liang RH, Tse E. Extranodal natural-killer/T-cell lymphoma, nasal type. Adv Hematol. 2010;2010:627401.
2. Kwong YL. The diagnosis and management of extranodal NK/T cell lymphoma, nasal-type and aggressive NK-cell leukemia. J Clin Exp Hematop. 2011;51:21–8.
3. Lim ST, Hee SW, Quek R, et al. Comparative analysis of extranodal NK/T-cell lymphoma and peripheral T-cell lymphoma: significant differences in clinical characteristics and prognosis. Eur J Haematol. 2008;80:55–60.

4. Li S, Feng X, Li T, et al. Extranodal NK/T-cell lymphoma, nasal type: a report of 73 cases at MD Anderson Cancer Center. Am J Surg Pathol. 2013;37:14–23.
5. Au WY, Weisenburger DD, Intragumtomchai T, et al. Clinical differences between nasal and extranasal natural killer/T-cell lymphoma: a study of 136 cases from the international peripheral T-cell lymphoma project. Blood. 2009;113:3931–7.
6. Savage NM, Johnson RC, Natkunam Y, et al. The spectrum of lymphoblastic, nodal and extranodal T-cell lymphomas: characteristic features and diagnostic dilemmas. Hum Pathol. 2013;44:451–7.
7. Chan JKC, Quintanilla-Martinez L, Ferry JA, et al. Extranodal NK/T-cell lymphoma, nasal type. In: Swerdlow SH, Campo E, Harris NK, et al., editors. World Health Organization classification of Tumours of Haematopoietic and lymphoid tissues. Lyon: IARC Press; 2008. p. 285–8.
8. Chan JK, Sin VC, Wong KF, et al. Nonnasal lymphoma expressing the natural killer cell marker CD56: a clinicopathologic study of 49 cases of an uncommon aggressive neoplasm. Blood. 1997;89:45014–4513.
9. Au WY, Pang A, Choy C, et al. Quantification of circulating Epstein-Barr virus(EBV) DNA in the diagnosis and monitoring of natural killer cell and EBV-positive lymphomas in immunocompetent patients. Blood. 2004;104: 243–9.
10. Baykal C, Polat Ekinci A, Öztürk Sarı S, et al. Annular erythematous patches as the presenting sign of extranodal natural killer/T-cell lymphoma. Yurk J Hematol. 2016;33:355–70.
11. Tse E, Kwong YL. Nasal NK/T-cell lymphoma: RT, CT, or both. Blood. 2015; 126:1400–1.
12. Sem Liew M, Chan AM, Galloway S, et al. Extra-nasal NK/T cell lymphoma masquerading as renal infarction. Leuk Lymphoma. 2010;51:1139–41.
13. Thompson MA, Habra MA, Routbort MJ, et al. Primary adrenal natural killer/ T-cell nasal type lymphoma: first case report in adults. Am J Hematol. 2007; 82:299–303.
14. Jiang Q, Liu S, Peng J, et al. An extraordinary T/NK lymphoma, nasal type, occurring primarily in the prostate gland with unusual CD30 positivity case report and review of the literature. Diagn Pathol. 2013;8:94.
15. Naboush A, Farhat F, Nasser SM, et al. Bifocal presentation of primary testicular extranodal NK/T-cell lymphoma: a case report and review of the literature. Case Rep Oncol Med. 2013;2013:267389.
16. Liang DN, Yang ZR, Wang WY, et al. Extranodal nasal type natural killer/T-cell lymphoma of testis: report of seven cases with review of literature. Leuk Lymphoma. 2012;53:1117–23.
17. Yagasaki H, Ohashi H, Ito M, et al. A novel mechanism of transplacental cancer transmission: natural killer/T-cell lymphoma in the paratesticular region is of maternal origin. Blood. 2011;117:6046–7.
18. Ayadi L, Makni S, Toumi N, et al. Aggressive nasal-type natural killer/T-cell lymphoma associated with Ebstein Barr virus presenting as testicular tumor. Tunis Med. 2010;88:196–8.
19. Mastuda M, Iwanaga T, Hashimoto S, et al. Primary Epstein-Barr virus-negative nasal-type natural killer/T-cell lymphoma of the testis. Leuk Res. 2009;33:e119–20.
20. Ornstein DL, Bifulco CB, Braddock DT, et al. Histopathologic and molecular aspects of CD56+ natural killer/T-cell lymphoma of the testis. Int J Surg Pathol. 2008;16:291–300.
21. Morelli L, Pisctoli I, Licci S, et al. T/natural killer cell lymphoma of the testis with cutaneous and subcutaneous doft tissue involvement: a management problem. Ann Hematol. 2007;6:469–70.
22. Ballereau C, Leroy X, Morschhauser F, et al. Testicular natural killer T-cell lymphoma. Int J Urol. 2005;12:223–4.
23. Kim YB, Chang SK, Yang WI, et al. Primary NK/T cell lymphoma of the testis. A case report and review of the literature. Acta Haematol. 2003;109:95–100.
24. Totonchi KF, Engel G, Weisenberg E, et al. Testicular natural killer/T-cell lymphoma, nasal type, of the natural killer-cell origin. Arch Pathol Lab Med. 2002;126:1527–9.
25. Guler G, Altinok G, Uner A, et al. CD56+ lymphoma presenting as a testicular tumor. Leuk Lymphoma. 1999;36:207–11.
26. Chan JK, Tsang WY, Lau WH, et al. Aggressive T/natural killer cell lymphoma presenting as testicular tumor. Cancer. 1996;77:1198–205.
27. Lan SK, Lin CW, Ho HC, et al. Penile metastasis secondary to nasal NK/T-cell lymphoma. Urology. 2008;72:1014–5.
28. Chu L, Mao W, Vikramsingh KC, et al. Primary malignant lymphoma of glans penis: a rare case report and review of the literature. Asian J Androl. 2013; 15:571–2.
29. Gallardo F, Pujol RM, Barranco C, et al. Progressive painless swelling of glans penis uncommon clinical manifestation of systemic non Hodgkin's lymphoma. Urology. 2009;73:929. e3-5
30. Suzuki R, Takeuchi K, Ohshima K, Nakamura S. Extranodal NK/T-cell lymphoma: diagnosis and treatment cues. Hematol Oncol. 2008;26:66–72.
31. Mo ZY, Wang P, Yang HW, et al. Esophageal metastasis secondary to extranodal nasal-type natural killer/T-cell lymphoma: a case report. Mol Clin Oncol. 2016;5:207–9.
32. Obama K, Tara M, Niina K. L-asparaginase-based induction therapy for advanced extranodal NK/T-cell lymphoma. Int J Hematol. 2003;78:248–50.
33. Fox CP, Boumendil A, Schmitz N, et al. High-dose therapy and autologous stem cell transplantation for extra-nodal NK/T lymphoma in patients from the western hemisphere: a study from the European Society for Blood and Marrow Transplantation. Leuk Lymphoma. 2015;56:3295–300.
34. Yhim HY, Kim JS, Mun YC, et al. Clinical outcomes and prognostic factors of up-front autologous stem cell transplantation in patients with extranodal natural killer/T cell lymphoma. Bio Blood Marrow Transplantation. 2015;21: 1597–604.
35. Wang CB, Bai H, Xi R, et al. Curative efficacy for nasal type extranodal NK/T-cell lymphoma by autologous peripheral blood stem cell transplantation after sequencing chemotherapy and radiotherapy. Zhongguo Shi Yan Xue Ye Xue Za Zhi. 2013;21:1477–81.
36. Lee J, Au WY, Park MJ, et al. Autologous hematopoietic stem cell transplantation in extranodal natural killer/T cell lymphoma: a multinational, multicenter, matched controlled study. Biol Blood Marrow Transplant. 2008; 14:1356–64.
37. Cui XZ, Wang HQ, Liu XM, et al. Treatment outcome and prognosis of autologous hematopoietic stem cell transplantation combined with high dose radiotherapy/chemotherapy in 22 patients with nasal NK/T cell lymphoma. Zhonghua Xue Ye Xue Za Zhi. 2007;28:609–11.
38. Kim HJ, Bang SM, Lee J, et al. High-dose chemotherapy with autologous stem cell transplantation in extranodal NK/T-cell lymphoma: a retrospective comparison with non-transplantation cases. Bone Marrow Transplant. 2006; 37:819–24.

19

TMPRSS2:ERG gene aberrations may provide insight into pT stage in prostate cancer

Zoran Krstanoski[1*], Nadja Kokalj Vokac[2], Andreja Zagorac[2], Boris Pospihalj[3], Miha Munda[4], Saso Dzeroski[5] and Rastko Golouh[6]

Abstract

Background: *TMPRSS2:ERG* gene aberration may be a novel marker that improves risk stratification of prostate cancer before definitive cancer therapy, but studies have been inconclusive.

Methods: The study cohort consisted of 202 operable prostate cancer Slovenian patients who underwent laparoscopic radical prostatectomy. We retrospectively constructed tissue microarrays of their prostatic specimens for fluorescence in situ hybridization, with appropriate signals obtained in 148 patients for subsequent statistical analyses.

Results: The following genetic aberrations were found: *TMPRSS2:ERG* fusion, *TMPRSS2* split (a non-*ERG* translocation) and *ERG* split (an *ERG* translocation without involvement of *TMPRSS2*). *TMPRSS2:ERG* gene fusion happened in 63 patients (42 %), *TMPRSS2* split in 12 patients and *ERG* split in 8 patients. Association was tested between *TMPRSS2:ERG* gene fusion and several clinicopathological variables, i.e., pT stage, extended lymph node dissection status, and Gleason score, correcting for multiple comparisons. Only the association with pT stage was significant at $p = 0.05$: Of 62 patients with pT3 stage, 34 (55 %) had *TMPRSS2:ERG* gene fusion. In pT3 stage patients, stronger (but not significant) association between eLND status and *TMPRSS2:ERG* gene fusion was detected. We detected *TMPRSS2:ERG* gene fusion in 64 % of the pT3 stage patients where we did not perform an extended lymph node dissection.

Conclusions: Our results indicate that it is possible to predict pT3 stage at final histology from *TMPRSS2:ERG* gene fusion at initial core needle biopsy. FISH determination of *TMPRSS2:ERG* gene fusion may be particularly useful for patients scheduled to undergo a radical prostatectomy in order to improve oncological and functional results.

Keywords: FISH, Predicting pT stage, Radical prostatectomy, Prostate cancer, *TMPRSS2:ERG* fusion

Background

Prostate cancer (PCa) is the most common cancer in males and one of the major leading causes of morbidity and mortality. The incidence is higher in Western Europe (>200 per 100,000) than in Eastern Europe [1]. With the widespread use of serum prostatic specific antigen (PSA) screening, almost 90 % of PCa cases can be diagnosed. On the other hand, screening is associated with overdiagnosis and overtreatment with an impact on the patient's quality of life [2, 3]. Whether underestimated clinically localized cancers should be treated, and if treated, how aggressively they should be treated, remains an important management dilemma. The clinical stage, Gleason grade and the serum PSA levels are used for prognosis and treatment stratification at the time of diagnosis. However, these indicators do not always accurately predict a clinical outcome on an individual patient basis [4]. Thus, more specific diagnostic modalities, prognostic indicators of progression and a better understanding of PCa biology are high priorities in PCa research [5].

The identification of the common *TMPRSS2:ERG* gene fusion in PCa could enable us to detect the disease in an earlier stage and also make it possible to design the proper therapy for each patient. With that we could predict disease outcomes [5, 6], more easily. In this study we examined potential associations between *TMPRSS2:ERG*

* Correspondence: zkrst@yahoo.com; zoran.krstanoski@sb-sg.si
[1]Department of Urology, General Hospital Slovenj Gradec, Gosposvetska 1, 2380 Slovenj Gradec, Slovenia
Full list of author information is available at the end of the article

gene fusion and clinicopathological characteristics with the aim of helping predict the cancer outcome.

Methods

Study population

The study cohort consisted of 202 operable PCa patients who underwent laparoscopic radical prostatectomy at the General Hospital Slovenj Gradec in Slovenia, but only 148 patients yielded appropriate signals for futher analysis. Patients were operated in the period between January 2010 and July 2011. Conventional clinicopathological data were evaluated. The mean age of the patients at the time of diagnosis was 64 years (range 47–78) years. The mean value of PSA before operation (Op) was 8.7 ng/ml (range 0.1–110). Extended lymph node dissection (eLND) was performed in 26 patients (13 %), 8 of which had positive lymph nodes (N1) and 18 had no tumor metastasis (N0). The median follow-up time of patients was 36 months. Fifteen patients experienced a biochemical recurrence and underwent hormonal therapy. Up until July 2015, none of these patients had died.

Generation of tissue microarrays (TMA)

The original haematoxylin and eosin (H&E) slides and paraffin-embedded tumour tissues were retrieved from the archives of the Department of Pathology, General Hospital Slovenj Gradec. H&Estained slides of tumour tissue were reviewed by two pathologists to identify representative tumour regions without necrosis or prostatic intraepithelial neoplasia. Three tissue cylinders with a diameter of 0.6 mm were obtained for each corresponding tumour block and arrayed into a recipient new paraffin block using the tissue chip microarrayer (Beecher Instruments, Silver Spring, MD). Thirty-nine recipient tissue blocks were constructed. The blocks were subsequently cut into 2_3 μm sections and fixed on silanized glass slides (Knittel Glaeser, Germany) to support adhesion of the tissue samples for subsequent fluorescence in situ hybridization (FISH) analysis.

Interphase

Interphase FISH was performed using the ZytoLight® SPEC *ERG/TMPRSS2* TriChech™ DNA Probe (ZytoVision GmbH, Bremerhaven, Germany), designed to detect deletions between the *ERG* and *TMPRSS2* genes at 21q22 and other translocations affecting either of these genes. FISH was performed on pretreated slides (that had undergone dewaxing, proteolysis, and post-fixation) using the Vysis Paraffin Pretreatment Reagent Kit (Abbott Molecular Inc., Des Plaines, IL, USA), following the manufacturer's instructions. Slides were denatured in 70 % formamide for 10 min at 73 °C, and the probe was denatured for 10 min at 75 °C. The probe was applied to each slide and the slide was covered by a 2–22 mm plastic coverslip and hybridized overnight in a moist chamber at 37 °C. After 16 h, the coverslips were gently removed, and slides were washed in 0.4 × saline sodium citrate (SSC) 0.05 % Tween for 2 min at 73 °C and 2 × SSC 0.05 % Tween for 2–60 s at RT. The cells were counterstained with 4',6-diamidino-2-phenylindole (DAPI) and embedded in an antifade solution. Images were acquired using a Zeiss Axioplan 2 microscope (Goettingen, Germany) equipped with Chroma optical filters (Chroma Technologies, Brattleboro, VT). The FISH results were evaluated by two independent screeners using a 63× objective. In normal interphase nuclei, two red/green/blue fusion signals were expected, representing two normal (non-rearranged) 21q22.13-q22.3 loci.

Statistical analysis

We tested significance of the association between several nominal clinicopathological variables (i.e., pT stage, eNLD status, Gleason score) and *TMPRSS2:ERG* fusion. For this purpose, we used Fisher's exact test for two-by-two contingency tables, as well as its Freeman-Halton extension for two-rows by three-columns contingency tables, as appropriate. The significance level was set at 0.05. To correct for the multiple tests, we used Bonferroni correction: Since we test a total of 4 hypotheses (the association of eNLD and *TMPRSS2:ERG* fusion on the subpopulation of pT3 stage patients), the corrected significance level for the individual hypotheses is set to 0.0125. For a significance level of 0.1, the corrected significance level for the individual hypotheses would be 0.025.

Results

We performed FISH analyses on 202 operable PCa patients. The sample was classified as aberrant if a staining pattern other than two red/green/blue fusion signals was detected in at least 20 cells in the tumor. *TMPRSS2:ERG* fusion, in wich the 21q22 locus is affected by a 21q22.2 deletion, was indicated as one red/blue fusion signal and the loss of one green signal (Fig. 1a). An *ERG* split without involvement of *TMPRSS2* was indicated by a separated red signal and green/blue fusion signal (Fig. 1b). A *TMPRRS2* split was indicated by a separated blue signal and red/green fusion signal (Fig. 1c). Tumor samples with very weak signals or lack of signals were considered to provide insufficient results and were not considered for further analysis. A resulting 148 patients were considered appropriate for subsequent statistical analysis.

The following genetic aberrations were found in the samples of the 148 patients: *TMPRSS2:ERG* fusion, *TMPRSS2 split* (a non-*ERG* translocation) and *ERG* split (an *ERG* translocation without involvement of *TMPRSS2*). Samples from 79 patients (53 %) had gene aberrations, while no aberrations were detected in 69 patients (47 %).

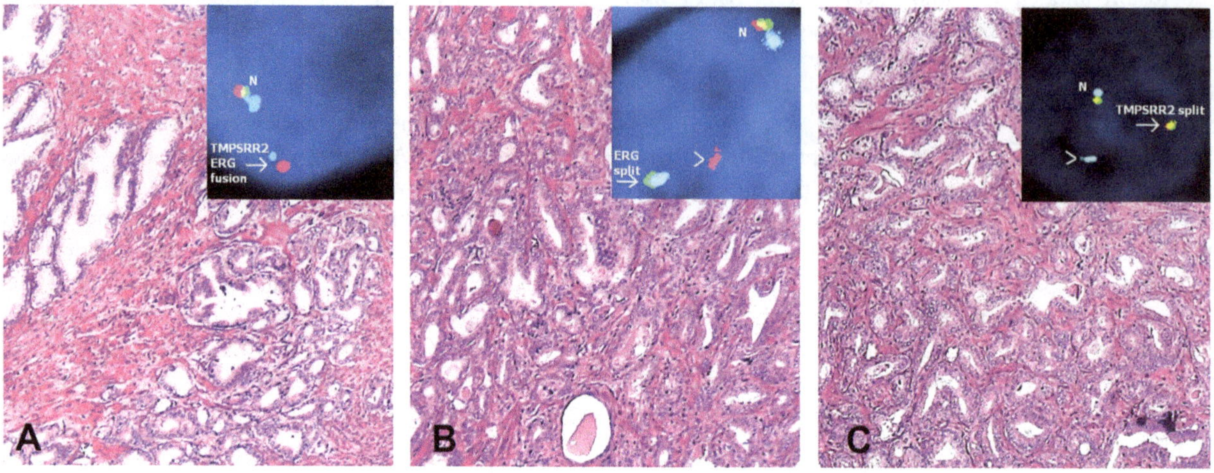

Fig. 1 Three cases of invasive adenocarcinoma of the prostate (H&E, 20×) with corresponding FISH staining. Arrow heads show gene aberration (split and fusion) and N shows normal signal. **a** One normal red/green/blue fusion signal and *TMPRSS2:ERG* fusion as indicated by one red/blue fusion signal with loss of one green signal. **b** One normal red/green/blue fusion signal and an *ERG* split as indicated by one green/blue fusion signal with the separated red signal. **c** One normal red/green/blue fusion signal and a *TMPRSS2* split as indicated by one red/green fusion signal with separated blue signal

We found *TMPRSS2:ERG* gene fusion in 63 patients (42 %), *TMPRSS2* split in 12 patients and *ERG* split in 8 patients. One patient had both *TMPRSS2:ERG* gene fusion and a *TMPRSS2* split. In three patients, *TMRRSS2:ERG* gene fusion and an *ERG* split were detected.

Table 1 summarizes the clinicopathological characteristics of the 148 patients included in the study. Averages (and counts) are given for all patients, as well as for the groups with/without aberrations and with/without *TMPRSS2:ERG* gene fusion. We tested for significant differences between *TMPRSS2:ERG* gene fusion positive and fusion negative cases in terms of pT stage, N stage and GS before a surgery (Tables 2, 3, and 4).

The association between *TMPRSS2:ERG* fusion and pT stage (with values divided into two groups, pT2 and pT3) was significant. The exact p-value obtained by Fisher's exact test was 0.01, which after the Bonferroni correction still makes the association significant at the 0.05 level. From 62 patients with pT3 stage, *TMPRSS2:ERG* gene fusion was detected in 34 (55 %) (Table 2).

The association between *TMPRSS2:ERG* fusion and Gleason score before operation was not significant. The exact p-value was 0.19. The contingency table is given in Table 3. This was obtained by the Freeman-Halton extension of Fisher's exact test.

The association between *TMPRSS2:ERG* fusion and N stage (eLND status) was examined next, considering the subgroups of eLND, pN0 and pN1 patients. In the entire population of 148 patients, the association was very weak and thus not significant. The exact p-value was 0.66 (Table 4). Again, the p-value was obtained by the Freeman-Halton extension of Fisher's exact test.

For further statistical analysis, we considered only the patients with pT3 stage. We re-examined the association between *TMPRSS2:ERG* fusion and N stage in this subpopulation. Here, the association was much stronger (exact p-value of 0.02), but not significant at the 0.05 level due to the Bonferroni correction. It is only significant at the weaker 0.1 level. In the group of patients on which we did not perform eLND, we detected *TMPRSS2:ERG* gene fusion in 25 patients (64 %).

Discussion

Many new biomarkers have been recently tested to enhance the accuracy of diagnosis, prediction of stage, estimation of metastatic potential and biochemical recurrence of PCa. So far, only a few have shown positive results and promising practical use in everyday practice. One of the most promising biomarkers is *TMPRSS2:ERG* gene fusion. This fusion is important not only for its high prevalence (or combining with other biomarkers), sensitivity and specificity in early diagnosis of PCa [7, 8], but also in predicting the stage [9–11], aggressiveness [9, 12] and metastatic potential of the tumor [11, 13].

In our study of 148 patients, we observed a prevalence of gene fusion in 42 %, which is similar to published data reporting prevalence ranges of 44–50 % [14–16]. Futhermore, we found no differences between fusion positive and negative cases in relation to age, PSA and GS. This is in concordance with the study by Magi-Galluzzi et al. that included 42 Caucasians, 64 African-Americans, and 44 Japanese patients who underwent radical prostatectomy [17]. *TMPRSS2:ERG* gene fusion correlated with ethnicity ($p = 0.03$) and marginally correlated with pathologic stage ($p = 0.06$), but did not correlate

Table 1 A summary of the clinico-pathological data of the 148 patients: Overall, with and without gene aberrations and with/without *TMPRSS2:ERG* fusion

	All Patients	Patients without gene aberrations	Patients with gene aberrations	Patients with fusion *TMPRSS2:ERG*	Patients with no fusion *TMPRSS2:ERG*
	148	69	79	63	85
pT stage					
pT2a	9	5	4	3	6
pT2b	12	7	5	4	8
pT2c	65	34	31	22	43
pT3a	49	20	29	26	23
pT3b	13	3	10	8	5
AGE (years)	64.37 (47–78)	64.50 (47–78)	64.24 (49–76)	64.27 (49–76)	64.44 (47–78)
N stage					
eLND	122	57	65	53	69
pN0	18	8	10	6	12
pN1	8	4	4	4	4
PSA before OP (ng/ml)	8.95 (0.1–110)	9.39 (0.1–110)	8.56 (0.71–43.2)	8.37 (0.71–43.2)	9.38 (0.1–110)
GS before OP (N°)					
6	62	35	27	21	41
7	78	32	46	38	40
≥8	8	2	6	4	4
PSA 1 month after OP ng/ml	0.26 (0.0–20)	0.42 (0.0–20)	0.11 (0.00–2.8)	0.14 (0.00–2.8)	0.35 (0.001–20)
GS after OP (N°)					
6	47	28	19	15	32
7	88	36	52	42	46
≥8	13	5	8	6	7

with other clinicopathologic parameters, such as age, preoperative PSA levels, and GS. Pettersson et al. [18] did not find any statistical significance between TMPRSS2:ERG gene fusion and GS (either low grade or high grade). Their cohort study includes 1180 patients after radical prostatectomy. with 694 patients showing GS ≤ 7 and 355 with positive gene rearrangement; a total of 486 patients had poorly differentiated prostate carcinoma GS ≥8 and 229 patients had gene fusion ($p = 0.58$). Similarly, Perner et al. [11] did not observe any significant associations between GS and *TMPRSS2:ERG* status in their study of 118 patients.

Table 2 Association of pT (stage) with gene fusion: Contingency table. The *p*-value obtained by the Fisher's exact test for two-by-two contingency tables is 0.01. After Bonferroni correction for testing 4 hypotheses, this is still significant at the 0.05 level

	TMPRSS2-ERG	No fusion	Total
pT2	29	57	86
pT3	34	28	62
Total	63	85	148

Gopalan et al. [19] reported different results. The authors found a statistically significant correlation between gene fusion and low GS ($p = 0.02$). Gene fusion was found in 71 patients (32 %) with GS < 7, 118 patients (54 %) with GS = 7 and 16 patients (7 %) with GS > 7. Seventy-four patients (24 %) showed GS < 7, while 182 patients (60 %) with GS = 7 and 40 patients (13 %) with GS > 7 had no gene fusion.

In the study of Darnel et al. [20] of 196 patients, the authors found a statistically significant correlation between *TMPRSS2:ERG* gene fusion and lower primary

Table 3 Association of Gleason score (before operation) with gene fusion: Contingency table. The *p*-value obtained by the Freeman-Halton extension of Fisher's exact test for two-by-three contingency tables is 0.19. After Bonferroni correction for testing 4 hypotheses, this is not significant at the 0.05 level

Gleason score	*TMPRSS2-ERG*	No fusion	Total
6	21	41	62
7	38	40	78
≥8	4	4	8
Total	63	85	148

Table 4 Association of N stage (eLND status) with gene fusion: Contingency table. The *p*-value obtained by the Freeman-Halton extension of Fisher's exact test for two-by-three contingency tables is 0.66. After Bonferroni correction for testing 4 hypotheses, this is not significant at the 0.05 level

	TMPRSS2-ERG	No fusion	Total
eLND	53	69	122
pN0	6	12	18
pN1	4	4	8
Total	63	85	148

Gleason pattern. Gene fusion was detected in 42 % of patients with primary Gleason pattern 3 and 27 % in primary Gleason pattern 4 ($p = 0.014$).

Demichelis et al. [12] showed a statistical significance between *TMPRSS2:ERG* gene fusion and higher GS ($p = 0.01$). Similar connections between gene fusion and GS ≥ 8 were shown in study by Font-Tello et al. [21].

The results of our study show a significant association between *TMPRSS2:ERG* gene fusion and pT stage. Perner S. et al. [11] reported high percentage of *TMPRSS2:ERG* rearrangements in patients with pT3 stage, i.e., 50/91 patients (55 %) and $p = 0.03$. Mehra et al. [10] reported similar findings for pT2b, but in the other direction. The authors found a statistically significant association between *TMPRSS2* gene rearrangement and the presence of advanced pathologic tumour stage ($p = 0.04$), defining advanced stage as pT2b. In their study, a total of 24 out of 37 (65 %) patients with positive *TMPRSS2* rearrangements had pathologic tumour stage ≤ pT2b. Font-Tello et al. [21] analyzed the mRNA levels of *TMPRSS2-ERG, ERG, PTEN,* and AR ($n = 83$), as well as *ERG* immunostaining ($n = 78$) in a series of prostate tumors. They found *TMPRSS2:ERG* gene fusion in 57 patients and it was associated with stage T3-T4 tumors. Saramäki et al. [22] did not find correlation between gene fusion and T3 stage ($p = 1.0$).

In our study *TMPRSS2:ERG* gene fusion was twice as frequent in the group of pT3 patients who did not undergo eLND compared with the group of pT3 patients who did undergo eLND. This finding indicates that we probably underestimate the group of patients with classical prognostic factors that characterise these patients as low or intermediate risk of PCa.

As we only had five patients with *ERG* split alone and three patients with both *ERG* split and *TMPRSS2:ERG* gene fusion, which was only 10 % of all gene rearrangements, the number of this subgroup was too small for statistical analyis.

Methodological differences in the patient cohorts could lead to these discrepancies. Some recent studies have shown that genetics diferences in prostate cancer among interracial groups can also be a reason for these discrepancies [23].

This study had several limitations. The study is retrospective in nature and prone to selection and collection bias. In addition, the sample size was fairly low, limiting subgroup data analyses. Therefore, all data should be confirmed in large possible prospective cohorts.

If confirmed in larger studies gene rearrangements on biopsies or postoperative specimens could be useful adjunct to clinical routine markers. In addition, it may be possible to detect these rearrangements in urine samples, eliminating the need for invasive specimen collection.

Conclusions

Based on our results, we expect that more than half of the patients with *TMPRSS2:ERG* gene fusion at their initial core needle biopsy will have a pT3 stage at their final histology in more than one half of the cases. This is especially important for patients with preoperative PSA and GS values indicating a low or intermediate risk of PCa. For one half of them, their preoperative clinical stage is probably underestimated. If, in these patients, we expect a pT3 stage (at their final histology), this could help us to achieve a lower percentage of positive section margins, as published (33.5–66 %) [24]. Namely, in patients with a clinical pT3 stage, we expect higher prevalence of positive lymph nodes (7.9–49 %) [24]. Following the results of our present study, we have to indicate eLND in patients with confirmed gene fusion, even if they have "false" low risk PCa (as indicated by their preoperative PSA and GS values). To conclude, *TMPRSS2:ERG* gene fusion at the initial core needle biopsy may be associated with pT3 stage and may therefore represent a biomarker for clinical routine. FISH determination of *TMPRSS2:ERG* gene fusion may be particularly useful for patients scheduled to undergo a nerve-sparing procedure in order to improve oncological and functional results. However, it is difficult to support the theory that patients with gene fusion will have worse prognosis.

Abbreviations

eLND, extended lymph node dissection; FISH, fluorescence in situ hybridization; GS, Gleason score; N0, negative lymph node; N1, positive lymph node; Op, operation; PCa, prostate cancer; PSA, prostatic specific antigen; TMA, tissue microarrays

Acknowledgements

There were no particular people or institutions to be acknowledged during this study.

Funding

We have no sources of funding.

Authors' contributions
ZK and RG conceived and designed the study. Data acquisition was conducted by ZK and MM. Analyses and interpretation of data were performed by NKV, AZ, BP and RG. ZK and RG drafted and wrote the manuscript, and RG and NKV provided critical review. Statistical analyses were performed by SD. All authors read and approved the final manuscript.

Competing interests
The authors declare that they have no competing interests.

Author details
[1]Department of Urology, General Hospital Slovenj Gradec, Gosposvetska 1, 2380 Slovenj Gradec, Slovenia. [2]Laboratory of Medical Genetics, University Medical Centre Maribor, Maribor, Slovenia. [3]Division of Gynecology, Department of Gynecological Pathology and Cytology, University Medical Center Ljubljana, Ljubljana, Slovenia. [4]Institute for Anatomy, Histology and Embryology, Medical Faculty, University of Maribor, Maribor, Slovenia. [5]Jozef Stefan Institute, Ljubljana, Slovenia. [6]Institute of Pathology, Medical Faculty University of Maribor, Maribor, Slovenia.

References

1. Arnold M, Karim-Kos HE, Coebergh JW, et al. Recent trends in incidence of five common cancers in 26 European countries since 1988: Analysis of the European Cancer Observatory. Eur J Cancer. 2013;51(9):1164–87.
2. Vasarainen H, Malmi H, Määttänen L, et al. Effects of prostate cancer screening on health-related quality of life: Results of the Finnish arm of the European randomized screening trial (ERSPC). Acta Oncol. 2013;52:1615–21.
3. Heijnsdijk EA, Wever EM, Auvinen A, et al. Quality-of-life effects of prostate-specific antigen screening. N Engl J Med. 2012;367:595–605.
4. Holmberg L, Bill-Axelson A, Helgesen F, et al. A randomized trial comparing radical prostatectomy with watchful waiting in early prostate cancer. N Engl J Med. 2002;347:781–9.
5. Kumar SH, Tomlin SA, Chinnaiyan AM. Recurrent gene fusions in prostate cancer. Nat Rev Cancer. 2008;8:497–511.
6. Choudhury A, Eeles R, Freedland S, et al. The role of genetic markers in the management in prostate cancer. Eur Urol. 2012;62:577–87.
7. Salami SS, Schmidt F, Laxman B, et al. Combining urinary detection of TMPRSS2:ERG and PCA3 with serum PSA to predict diagnosis of prostate cancer. Urol Oncol. 2013;31:566–71.
8. Robert G, Jannink S, Smit F, et al. Rational basis for the combination of PCA3 and TMPRSS2:ERG gene fusion for prostate cancer diagnosis. Prostate. 2013;73:113–20.
9. Rostad K, Hellwinkel OJ, Haukaas SA, et al. TMPRSS2:ERG fusion transcripatients in urine from prostate cancer patients correlate with a less favorable prognosis. APMIS. 2009;117:575–82.
10. Mehra R, Tomlins RS, Shen R, et al. Comprehensive assessment of TMPRSS2 and ETS family gene aberrations in clinically localized prostate cancer. Modern Pathol. 2007;20:538–44.
11. Perner S, Demichelis F, Beroukhim R, et al. TMPRSS2:ERG fusion-associated deletions provide insight into the heterogeneity of prostate cancer. Cancer Res. 2006;66:8337–41.
12. Demichelis F, Fall K, Perner S, et al. TMPRSS2:ERG gene fusion associated with lethal prostate cancer in a watchful waiting cohort. Oncogene. 2007;26:4596–9.
13. Attard G, Clark J, Ambroisine L, et al. Duplication of the fusion of TMPRSS2 to ERG sequences identifies fatal human prostate cancer. Oncogene. 2008;27:253–63.
14. Tomlins SA, Bjartell A, Chinnaiyan AM, et al. ETS gene fusions in prostate cancer: from discovery to daily clinical practice. Eur Urol. 2009;56:275–86.
15. Jiangling JT, Rohan S, Kao J, et al. Gene fusions between TMPRSS2 and ETS family genes in prostate cancer: Frequency and transcript variant analysis by RT-PCR and FISH on paraffin-embedded tissues. Modern Pathol. 2007;20:921–8.
16. Mosquera JM, Mehra R, Regan MM, et al. Prevalence of TMPRSS2-ERG fusion prostate cancer among men undergoing prostate biopsy in the United States. Clin Cancer Res. 2009;15:4706–11.
17. Magi-Galluzzi C, Tsusuki T, Elson P, et al. TMPRSS2-ERG gene fusion prevalence and class are significantly different in prostate cancer of Caucasian, African-American and Japanese patients. Prostate. 2011;71:489–97.
18. Pettersson A, Graff RE, Bauer SR, et al. The TMPRSS2:ERG rearrangement, ERG expression, and prostate cancer outcomes: a cohort study and meta-analysis. Cancer Epidemiol Biomarkers Prev. 2012;21(9):1497–509.
19. Gopalan A, Leversha MA, Satagopan JM, et al. TMPRSS2-ERG gene fusion is not associated with outcome in patients treated by prostatectomy. Cancer Res. 2009;69(4):1400–6.
20. Darnel AD, Lafargue CJ, Vollmer RT, et al. TMPRSS2-ERG fusion is frequently observed in Gleason pattern 3 prostate cancer in a Canadian cohort. Cancer Biol Ther. 2009;8(2):125–30.
21. Font-Tello A, Juanpere N, de Muga S. Association of ERG and TMPRSS2-ERG with grade, stage, and prognosis of prostate cancer is dependent on their expression levels. Prostate. 2015;75(11):1216–26.
22. Saramäki OR, Harjula AE, Martikainen PM, et al. TMPRSS2:ERG fusion identifies a subgroup of prostate cancers with a favorable prognosis. Clin Cancer Res. 2008;14(11):3395–400.
23. Zhau HE, Li Q, Chung LW. Interracial differences in prostate cancer progression among patients from the United States, China and Japan. Asian J Androl. 2013;15:705–7.
24. Joniau S, Hsu CY, Lerut E, et al. A pretreatment table for the prediction of final histopathology after radical prostatectomy in clinical unilateral T3a prostate cancer. Eur Urol. 2007;51:388–96.

20

Cancer-specific and overall survival in patients with recurrent prostate cancer who underwent salvage extended pelvic lymph node dissection

Daniar K. Osmonov, Alexey V. Aksenov*, David Trick, Carsten M. Naumann, Moritz F. Hamann, Amr Abou Faddan and Klaus-Peter Jünemann

Abstract

Background: The aim was to evaluate cancer-specific survival (CSS) and overall survival (OS) in patients with prostate cancer (PCa) recurrence who underwent salvage extended pelvic lymph node dissection (ePLND), taking into consideration pre- and postoperative androgen deprivation therapy (ADT).

Methods: Salvage ePLND was performed in a cohort of 54 patients with PCa recurrence, and data from 45 patients were analyzed. The indications for salvage ePLND were biochemical recurrence (BCR) of PCa and suspect findings on ^{11}C-choline PET/CT. PSA-level, biochemical response (BR), duration of biochemical recurrence freedom (BCRF), number of metastases, OS and CSS were analyzed retrospectively.

Results: The average follow-up was 42.7 ± 20.8 months. Thirty-three patients (73.3 %, 95 % CI: 60.5–83.6 %) achieved BCRF during follow-up. The mean BCRF-period was 31.4 ± 19.7 months. CSS and OS were both 91.7 % ± 4.8 % (3-year survival) and 80.6 ± 8.6 % (5-year survival). Twenty-four patients (53.3 %, 95 % CI: 40.0–66.3 %) with castration-resistant PCa (CRPC) responded again to ADT after salvage ePLND.

Conclusions: Salvage ePLND for selected patients with BCR and clinically recurrent nodal disease can achieve an immediate complete PSA response (i. e. BCRF) in nearly half of the patients. Patients with CRPC responded again to ADT after ePLND. Multicenter prospective studies with a control group are needed.

Keywords: Recurrent prostate cancer, Biochemical relapse, Salvage therapy, Lymph node dissection, Cancer-specific survival

Abbreviations: ADT, Androgen deprivation therapy; BCR, Biochemical recurrence; BCRF, Biochemical recurrence free(dom); BR, Biochemical response; CRPC, Castration-resistant prostate cancer; CSS, Cancer specific survival; ePLND, Extended pelvic lymph node dissection; Ga-PSMA, ^{68}Gallium- Prostate-specific membrane antigen; GS, Gleason score; iPSA, Initial PSA level; LHRH, Luteinising hormone-releasing hormone; LN(s), Lymph node(s); LND, Lymph node dissection; OS, Overall survival; PCa, Prostate cancer; RP, Radical prostatectomy; RT, Radiotherapy; SD, Standard deviation

* Correspondence: Alexey.Aksenov@uksh.de
Department of Urology and Pediatric Urology, University Hospital Schleswig-Holstein, Campus Kiel, Arnold-Heller Strasse 3, Haus 18, D-24105 Kiel, Germany

Background

The standard treatment options for patients with prostate cancer (PCa) recurrence after radical prostatectomy (RP) are radiotherapy (RT) and/or androgen deprivation therapy (ADT) [1, 2]. Salvage extended pelvic lymph node dissection (ePLND) is neither mentioned in the European Association of Urology (EAU) guidelines, nor in the German S-3 and the US guidelines. However, it might be an alternative treatment approach in a selected group of the patients. Moreover, our data show that patients who had ceased to respond to ADT (i. e. CRPC patients) responded again to ADT after salvage ePLND.

RT is the most common option in cases of pelvic PCa recurrence. Salvage RT should be offered to patients with biochemical recurrence (BCR) or local recurrence after RP if there is no evidence of distant metastatic disease [3]. Briganti et al. performed a multicenter retrospective analysis of 472 node-negative patients who experienced BCR after RP and received salvage RT. The rate of 5-year BCR-free survival after early salvage RT was 73.4 %. The authors have developed the first nomogram to predict the outcome after salvage RT [4].

ADT is a standard method in node-positive patients with BCR after primary RP and RT [5]. Intermittent androgen deprivation results in non-inferior oncological efficacy when compared with continuous ADT in well-selected populations [2].

Sciarra et al. showed that 29.7 % of the patients with BCR after RP who received intermittent ADT developed castration-resistant prostate cancer (CRPC) and 14.2 % of the cases showed clinical progression, with a mean duration of 88.4 ± 14.3 months and 106.5 ± 20.6 months, respectively [6]. Prolonged ADT exposure increases the risk of cardiovascular disease and diabetes in men aged >75 years with PCa [7].

New substances such as abiraterone and enzalutamide represent new therapeutic options. Their mechanism of action regarding renewed ADT response is not clear, especially in consideration of insufficient control possibilities. In one-third of patients receiving abiraterone, the PSA level showed no tendency to decrease [8].

An alternative treatment option for patients with recurrent PCa, especially in CRPC, is salvage ePLND. The effect of the salvage surgery on the response to ADT after surgery is not clear. In the past 5 years there has been an increase in publications on the outcomes of salvage PLND. There is a partial or even a complete PSA response to salvage LND in patients with nodal recurrence of PCa. Despite the relatively small patient numbers and the lack of a long-term follow-up, the available data mark a preliminary success and demonstrate this technique to be a promising new approach [9–11].

The data presented in these and other similar studies were collected and analyzed in different centers and published independently of each other, but the outcome of all these studies was surprisingly similar. Salvage ePLND can take a more significant place in the treatment of patients with BCR. Some authors point out that a more extended type of PLND at the time of primary RP is to be favored. A high percentage of patients with pelvic LN recurrence responded with reduced PSA after salvage surgery, and thus, they might have already benefited from more extensive PLND during primary surgery [9, 10, 12].

In this single center retrospective study, we analyzed CSS and overall survival (OS) data, as well as the influence of salvage surgery on the response to ADT in patients with previous CRPC. This evaluation provides us with sufficient preliminary evidence to initiate a further study or to join a similar study with prospective randomized design.

Methods

We analyzed a cohort of 54 patients with PCa recurrence. Most of the patients visited our clinic on their own initiative. They had expressed a wish to be treated in an alternative surgical way. All patients were informed about the absence of prospective multicenter data and about the fact that salvage ePLND is not mentioned in US, European or S3 guidelines.

All patients gave signed informed consent. Thirteen patients [28.9 %, 95 % confidence interval (CI): 18.2–41.9 %] were aged >70 years at the time of salvage ePLND. Recurrence was defined as an increase of PSA >0.5 ng/ml. We introduced salvage ePLND in Kiel in November 2003. We could eventually only evaluate the data from 45 of 54 patients, as the other patients continued follow-up treatment at their local urologist and we were unable to collect their data. The mean follow-up period was 42.7 ± 20.8 months.

Preoperatively, all patients underwent positron emission tomography (PET)/computed tomography (CT) imaging. ADT was aborted at least 4 weeks prior to PET/CT examination. There was no bone metastasis prior to salvage ePLND. The indications for salvage ePLND were BCR and/or positive PET/CT scan. Salvage ePLND was done in thirteen patients (37.1 %), who had undergone primary RP without LND; some of these had a negative PET/CT scan result, but all had a proven BCR.

We used the D'Amico risk classification to describe a primary tumor (Table 1). We defined an initial PSA level (iPSA) as a PSA level prior to primary treatment. Ten of 45 patients (22.2 %) had RT as primary treatment and underwent RP during salvage ePLND as well. Thirteen patients (28.9 %) had primary RP without any LND. In 22 patients (48.9 %) with primary LND, the mean number of removed LNs was 13.3 (range: 3–26) and LN metastases were found in five of those patients. R1 stage

Table 1 Summary of results of initial treatment ($n = 35$ with initial RP and $n = 10$ with initial RT, summary $n = 45$)

Total number of evaluated patients	45	100 %
Initial RT (%)	10	22.2 %
Initial RP without LND (%)	13	28.9 %
Initial RP with LND (%)	22	48.9 %
Average number of removed LN´s ($n = 22$)	13.3	3-26
Average number of N1 (%)	5	22.7 %
Mean iPSA, ng/ml (SD)	6.7	±1.6
Risk classification[a]		
Low (%)	1	2.2 %
Intermediate (%)	21	46.7 %
High (%)	21	46.7 %
T stage after RP		
T2 (%)	15	33.3 %
T3 (%)	27	60.0 %
T3a (%)	12	26.7 %
T3b (%)	15	33.3 %
Tx (%)	3	6.7 %
Gleason Score after RPGS 6 (%)		
GS 7 (%)	4	8.9 %
GS 8 (%)	17	37.8 %
GS 9 (%)	10	22.2 %
GS 10 (%)	10	22.2 %
GSx (non detectable) (%)	2	4.4 %
	2	4.4 %
R1 after initial PR (out of 35 patients) (%)	12	34.3 %

[a]In two patients, the initial risk group was unknown

after primary prostatectomy were diagnosed in 12 (34.3 %) out of 35 patients. Gleason score (GS) subgroups were as follows: four (8.9 %) patients had GS 6; 17 (37.8 %) had GS 7; 10 (22.2 %) had GS 8; 10 (22.2 %) had GS 9; and two (4.4 %) had GS 10; and two (4.4 %) patients had a non-detectable GS (Table 1). Most patients had undergone primary RP ex domo.

We performed salvage ePLND according to the surgical template developed at our department [13]. The surgical regions of the Kiel template are defined as follows: (1) para-aortic LNs; (2) LNs along the common iliac artery; (3) LNs along the external iliac artery; (4) LNs along the internal iliac artery; (5) LNs in the Marcille's triangle; (6) obturator LNs; and (7) presacral LNs. The Kiel principles of salvage ePLND are: (1) exclusively transperitoneal access; (2) definition of landmarks such as the iliac vessels prior to LND; and (3) careful separation of the ureter from the surrounding tissue. Subsequent to these measures, LND is systematically performed from the top downwards. Small or medium clips are used to avoid extensive ligation. Moreover, we used a harmonic scalpel to seal the lymph vessels and shorten the operation time [14]. The operation was performed no later than 4 months after PET/CT. None of the patients had bone metastases at the time of the intervention. The removed LNs were cut into 4-mm slices and examined further at our Pathology Institute.

PSA measurements were performed 40 days after surgery and thereafter every 3–6 months. In case of biochemical progression, PET/CT and bone scintigraphy were performed to exclude clinical progression. The data on the occurrence of bone metastases have been presented in our paper. There was no standard protocol for postoperative imaging diagnostics.

BR was defined as PSA regression immediately after salvage surgery, measured 40 days after surgery, regardless of whether the level was above or under BCR criteria. Some patients received ADT directly after salvage ePLND, prescribed by the local urologist. The patients who were followed up in our department received ADT on occurrence of renewed BCR after salvage ePLND. These patients have continuously received complete androgen blockage.

We analyzed the number of removed LNs, number of positive LNs, changes in PSA level, CSS and OS. Key points in the clinical outcome of salvage ePLND were BCR-free survival and its duration, as well as CSS and OS, taking into consideration the administration of ADT and the occurrence of bone metastases during follow-up. On analyzing the data, we found out that 80 % of the patients who underwent salvage ePLND had shown castration resistance (CRPC) prior to surgery, although CRPC was not a primary indication criterion for salvage surgery. We analysed the influence (whether negative or positive) of salvage ePLND + ADT on PSA recurrence after salvage ePLND in these particular patients.

95 % CIs for frequencies were determined based on the binomial distribution, with $p = 0.05$. Statistically significant differences of frequencies were determined by the exact variant of criterion χ^2. Risk factors affecting survival were determined using Cox regression. CSS and OS were determined using Kaplan-Meier analysis.

The research was performed with the approval of the appropriate ethics committee (Ethics Commission, Faculty of Medicine, CAU Kiel University, reference number – D474/15).

Results

The patient data are listed in Table 2 and Figs. 1, 2, 3 and 4. The PSA was measured ca. 40 days after salvage ePLND. At this point, 22 patients (48.9 %, 95 % CI: 35.8–62.1 %) were BCR-free. 16 of 22 patients (72.7 %) with immediate complete BR after salvage ePLND were treated with ADT prior to surgery. During follow-up, 33 patients (73.3 %, 95 % CI: 60.5–83.6 %) achieved

Table 2 Summary of results of salvage treatment ($n = 45$)

Follow-up (months), mean (SD)	42.7	(±20.8)
Median PSA-nadir after salvage ePLND, ng/ml (SD)	4.4	± 1.5
N-stage after salvage ePLND		
N0 (%)	19	(42.2 %)
N1 (%)	26	(58.7 %)
No. of LNs removed (range)	971	(4–76)
Mean no. of LNs removed per patient (SD)	21.6	(±9)
No. of positive LNs (range)	183	(1–42)
No. of positive LNs per patient (range)	4,1	(1–42)
No. of deaths (%)	7	(15.6 %)
Time to death (months), mean (range)	48.8	5–105
BR after salvage ePLND n (% patients)	31	(68.9 %)
BCRF immediately after salvage ePLND (complete BR) n (% patients)	22	(48.9 %)
BCRF during follow-up n (% patients)	33	(73.3 %)
Mean BCRF duration (months) (SD)	31.4	(±19.7)
ADT before salvage ePLND No. (%) patients	36	(80.0 %)
ADT after salvage ePLND No. (%) patients	40	(88.9 %)
Bone metastases in follow-up after salvage ePLND No. (%) patients	10	(22.2 %)

BCR-freedom (BCRF), including those who received and responded to ADT again (Fig. 1) The mean follow-up in these 33 patients is 46.7 ± 25.0 months (median follow-up 47 months). In 10 patients (22.2 %, 95 % CI: 12.9–34.6 %), bone metastases appeared during follow-up. The mean duration until diagnosis of bone metastases was 25.9 ± 18.4 (median 21.5 months). Seven patients (15.6 %, 95 % CI: 8.0–26.8 %) died and six of these had bone metastases. In these patients, the average follow-up between salvage ePLND and occurrence of bone metastases was 34.2 ± 9.5 months [in this and similar cases, the data are represented as mean ± standard deviation (SD)]. BCR-free survival in patients with and without bone metastases was dramatically different (Fig. 2).

It is notable that the mean iPSA in patients without bone metastases was 5.5 ng/ml compared with 29.1 ng/ml in those with postoperatively diagnosed bone metastases. The mean PSA nadir after salvage ePLND was 4.7 ng/ml. We used an interval of 40 days for PSA nadir.

CSS and OS were equal at 91.7 ± 4.8 % (3-year CSS and OS) and 80.6 ± 8.6 % (5-year CSS and OS) (Figs. 3 and 4).

A total of 971 LNs were removed during 45 salvage ePLNDs, with a mean of 21.6 LNs (median 20, SD 9) per operation. Metastases were found in 183 (18.8 %) of 971 removed LNs. The mean number of positive LNs per patient was 4.1 (Table 2). In 22 patients (48.9 %, 95 % CI: 35.8–62.1 %) >20 LNs were removed per operation. In 26 patients (57.8 %, 95 % CI: 44.3–70.4 %), N1 stage was histologically confirmed. In four patients (8.9 %, 95 % CI: 3.7–18.3 %), just one LN was positive; in two patients (4.4 %, 95 % CI: 1.4–11.8 %) two LNs were positive; in 12 patients (26.7 %, 95 % CI: 16.4–39.5 %) 3–5 LNs were positive; in three patients (6.7 %, 95 % CI: 2.5–15.1 %) 6–10 LNs were positive; and in five patients (11.1 %, 95 % CI: 5.1–21.2 %) >10 LNs were positive (Table 3).

We have divided the patients into subgroups differentiating between pre- and postoperative ADT receivers and non-receivers and their post-operative ADT-response in Table 4.

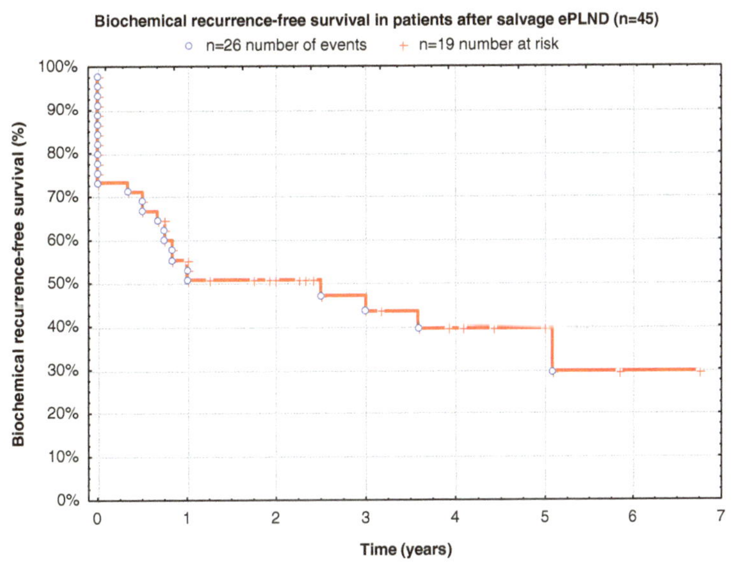

Fig. 1 Biochemical recurrence-free survival in patients after salvage ePLND ($n = 45$)

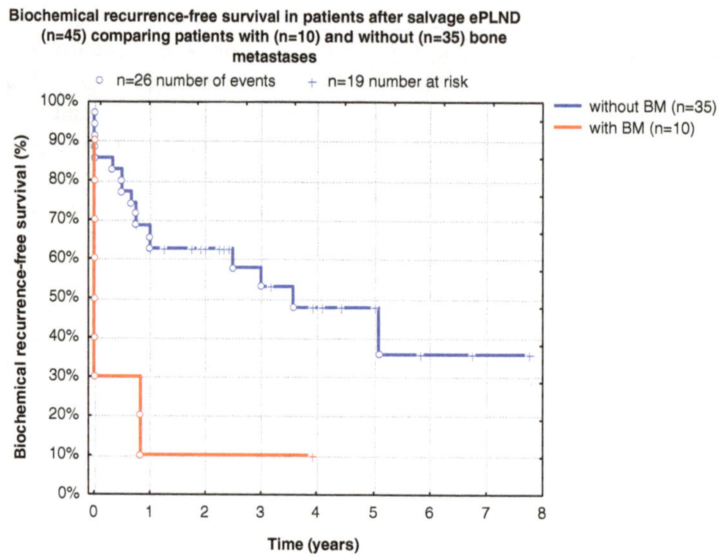

Fig. 2 Biochemical recurrence-free survival in patients after salvage ePLND ($n = 45$) comparing patients with ($n = 10$) and without ($n = 35$) bone metastases

The following complications were observed in seven patients (15.6 %, 95 % CI: 8.0–26.8 %); all related to Grade IIIb Clavien–Dindo complications: two patients (4.4 %, 95 % CI: 1.4–11.8 %) with postoperative relevant bleeding: two (4.4 %, 95 % CI: 1.4–11.8 %) with ureteral stricture; one with rectovesical fistula (2.2 %, 95 % CI: 0.5–7.9 %), and two (4.4 %, 95 % CI: 1.4–11.8 %) with lymphocele.

We analyzed the risk factors for cancer-specific mortality. Only the occurrence of bone metastases during follow-up after salvage ePLND was shown to be a significant risk factor (Table 5).

Discussion

According to our results, we cannot postulate any benefit of salvage ePLND because of the limitation of the study, in particular its' small retrospective character and heavily selected cohort of patients. Despite of that, the results have showed, that in the majority of patients BCRF were achieved, even in those with no histologically

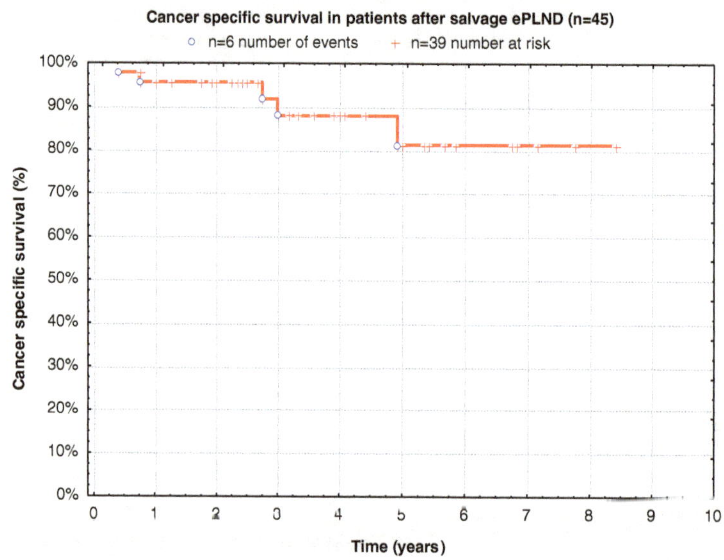

Fig. 3 Cancer specific survival in patients after salvage ePLND ($n = 45$)

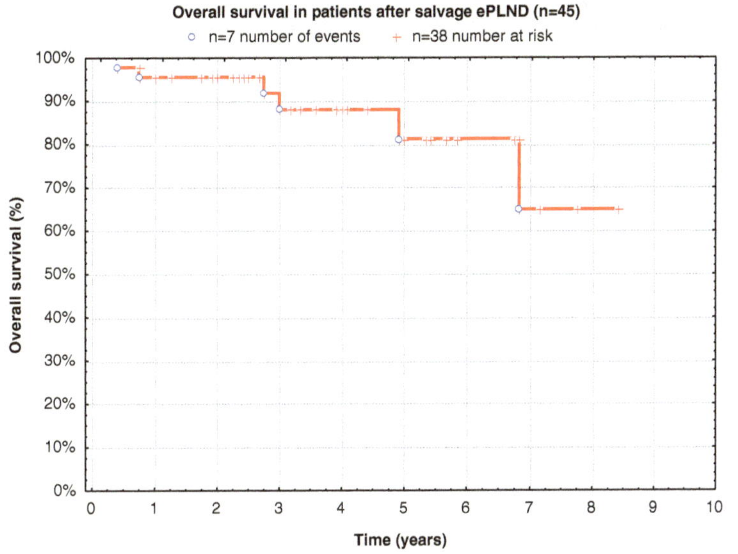

Fig. 4 Overall survival in patients after salvage ePLND ($n = 45$)

proven LN metastases. Moreover, CSS and OS data compared with acceptable complications rate makes this procedure feasible for selected patients. Similar results were found in previous studies on salvage ePLND. Thus, the data collected in different centers demonstrate comparable results [15] The most important two parameters are (1) complete biochemical response within 40 d after surgery (range: 46 %; 48.9 % up to 56.9 %) and (2) achievement of BCR-freedom after salvage ePLND with rates of up to 71.8 %. The role of ADT after salvage surgery remains a critical and unresolved issue, however.

The retrospective character of the study does not provide us with the opportunity to divide the patients into different groups with and without ADT. Moreover, the concept of recurrent PCa salvage treatment makes it impossible to split salvage ePLND and ADT; both treatments can and should be used in a combined approach. This approach has allowed us and other centers to achieve similarly high rates of CSS ranging between 75 % and 80.6 % [15].

We believe that the aim of any further research is to demonstrate that patients benefit from salvage ePLND. The selection of patients, taking into consideration the above-shown absence of reliable LN recurrence imaging tools, remains a matter of dispute.

Table 3 Number of positive LNs per patient

No. of patients	Positive LNs per patient
19 (42.2 %)	Node-negative (N0)
4 (8.9 %)	1 LN+
2 (4.4 %)	2 LNs+
12 (26.7 %)	3-5 LNs+
3 (6.7 %)	6-10 LNs+
5 (11.1 %)	>10 LNs+
Summary: 45 patients	Mean LN+ pro patient 4.1 (range 1–42)

13 (68.4 %) of 19 node-negative patients showed a BR immediately after salvage ePLND. 16 (84.2 %) reached BCRF during postoperative follow-up with a mean duration of 33 ± 22 months, median 28.5 (min 6 – max 81) months. However, 17 (89.5 %) undergone ADT after salvage ePLND in follow-up.

Again, 84.2 % patients with stage N0 after salvage surgery were BCR free. We discussed possible explanations for this with our pathologist and during various international meetings. For a better understanding, we also need to consider the method of pathological examination.

Pathological examination of removed LNs may miss micrometastases, which are defined in different ways depending on the cancer entity. In malignant melanoma, for example, one isolated tumor cell is already considered a micrometastasis according to the American Joint Committee on Cancer, although it can only be detected by means of immunohistochemistry. In breast cancer, micrometastases are defined as >200 µm (and/or >200 tumor cells) and <2 mm in diameter. Such micrometastases can be detected by light microscopy. In penile cancer, a micrometastasis is defined as being <2 mm [16].

There is no clear definition of micrometastasis with respect to PCa or cancer of other parenchymal organs. The International Society of Urological Pathology has no consensus on the definition of micrometastasis in PCa [17]. The problem is that something that is not clearly defined cannot be found.

However, we believe that we did remove LNs carrying micrometastases or even true metastases that were

Table 4 BCRF-survival in subgroups of patients according to pre- and postoperative ADT receivers and non-receivers and their postoperative ADT-response

ADT post-op / ADT pre-op		*Without* ADT after surgery	*With* ADT after surgery
Patients *without* preoperative ADT, $n = 9$ (20 %)	Total *without / with* ADT	3 (33.3 %)	6 (66.7 %)
	Of the above: BCRF-survival after salvage ePLND, n (%)	2 of 3 (66.7 %)	5 of 6 (83.3 %)
	Duration of BCRF-survival after salvage ePLND (months): 1. mean duration ± SD	18 ± 3	33.4 ± 15.8
	2. median duration	18	36
	3. min-max duration	15–21	6–53
Patients *with* preoperative ADT $n = 36$ (80 %)	Total *without / with* ADT	2 (5.6 %)	34 (94.4 %)
	Of the above: BCRF-survival after salvage ePLND, n (%)	2 of 2 (100 %)	24 of 34 (70.6 %)
	Duration of BCRF-survival after salvage ePLND (months): 1. mean duration ± SD	54.5 ± 5.5	30.1 ± 25.2
	2. median duration	51.75	23.5
	3. min-max duration	49–60	4–93

missed using the applied pathological method. We systematically removed all potentially positive LNs from various areas following the Kiel surgical template of salvage ePLND [14]. Most of the positive LNs were found in the area of the common iliac artery (37.5 %), paraaortal area (20 %), sacral area (12.5 %), and in the area of the triangle of Marcille (5 %). This is an important argument in favor of template-oriented surgery rather than selective or limited LN removal.

The small number of studies [15] shows the outcome of salvage ePLND, but it is more difficult to assess the difference in survival of patients after salvage ePLND alone versus patients after salvage ePLND and adjuvant ADT. In addition, it is difficult to assess the independent impact of these two therapeutic measures on progression-free survival. We observed an interesting phenomenon: in patients with CRPC and BCR, ADT can be effective again after salvage ePLND. We reported this side effect of salvage surgery at the 2014 meetings of the German Society of Urology, EAU and American Urological Association. This effect was detected after analysing all data and is a largely unexpected result of our study. We describe this effect with caution and as a preliminary statement. Moreover, we still lack an adequate explanation for this effect. However, we believe that this finding will have a major impact on the role of salvage ePLND if our data are confirmed by other study groups, ideally in a prospective setup with larger patient cohorts and in multicenter trials.

Table 5 Risk factors of cancer-specific mortality (univariate analysis)

Risk factor (CSS)	p (significance)
Decrease of PSA level after salvage ePLND	0.268
Immediate BCRF after salvage ePLND	0.062
BCR	0.026
R-stage	0.253
T-stage	0.032
N-stage	0.299
Number of LNs	0.296
No. of LNs removed	0.42
Risk-group (D'Amico)	0.619
Bone metastases at follow-up	<0.001
Age at moment of salvage ePLND	0.249
Surgical complications	0.745

Our hypothesis so far is based on the tumor biology of PCa. The PCa tumor architecture is heterogeneous and probably depends on the different c-types and their mutation characteristics. There are a few theories about this heterogeneity, which can have an impact on the aggressiveness and speed of metastatic spread. In breast cancer, for example, the BRCA-1 and BRCA-2 genes indicate a strong dependency between BRCA-gene types and lymphatic and hematogeneous metastatic spread [18]. These two genes are found in LN or organ metastases of PCa. However, we believe that heterogeneity in PCa metastasis is even more complex. Based on the described facts, we see the potential reason for the renewed ADT response as the removal of aggressive tumor cells, which are probably chiefly responsible for metastatic spread of the tumor.

The interest in lesion-targeted salvage therapies has increased recently [19]. The outcome of salvage surgery and other diagnostic methods for positive LN detection compared to pathological examination needs to be evaluated further. Moreover, salvage surgery needs to be included in PCa guidelines. Lesion-targeted or selective salvage PLND can only be enhanced with development of new diagnostic imaging. Some recent studies have shown promising results with Ga-PSMA (^{68}Gallium- Prostate-specific membrane antigen) PET/magnetic resonance imaging (MRI) and Ga-PSMA PET/CT [20, 21].

Most of the studies describing the clinical outcome of salvage ePLND are based on the findings of ^{18}F choline PET/CT findings. Application of the tracer ^{18}F-2-fluoro-2-deoxyglucose in PET/CT is successfully used in many tumor types. However, a benefit in PCa diagnosis has been questioned by several authors [22, 23].

There have been divergent results on choline-PET/CT regarding PCa recurrence. In several studies the detection rates were analyzed in relation to the PSA level. These studies have shown the sensitivity of choline-PET/CT for detection of LN metastases to be as low as 41.1 % [24]. Therefore, extensive salvage treatment is needed to maximize the chance of cure [19]. However, these results are insufficient to standardize the indications for salvage ePLND.

Data from our own department show a low specificity of 18.2 % with a relatively satisfactory sensitivity of 85.2 %. Most importantly, the positive predictive value and negative predictive value were 56.1 % and 50.0 %, respectively [25]. Therefore, we conclude that the reliability of PET/CT imaging for detection of LN metastases is limited by a high false-positive rate, and the findings in patients with low PSA values were associated with a high ratio of errors. In this situation, there is still no alternative to the template-based salvage ePLND to remove all LNs and thus to detect all metastatic LNs, including those that were false negative by PET/CT.

Here, as well as in the validation of the method mentioned above, a prospective study design should be set up for a full analysis of false-positive and false-negative results regarding LN metastasis. This will only be possible if histological verification is done after template-based ePLND.

Looking at the largest studies in this field, the CSS results in patients who underwent salvage ePLND seem to be similar despite the different cohorts analyzed by different workgroups. Thus, Jilg et al. reported 5-years CSS of 77.7 %, Rigatti et.al – 75 %, and our current data show 80.6 % [9, 10].

In the absence of evidence-based guidelines regarding salvage ePLND, our study and the publications listed in Table 1 allow us to conclude that salvage ePLND is effective and useful in selected patients. The only statistically significant finding in this study is that bone metastasis is associated with more rapid mortality. This is an important point which can help us define the indication criteria for salvage ePLND, but it should not be used to question the clinical significance of salvage surgery.

The requirements placed on the surgeon are high, however. The current situation remains unsatisfactory due to the lack of prospective multicenter randomized studies. We concede that our study was only a retrospective analysis. However, there are two good reasons for publishing these data. First, we needed to evaluate our own patient data in order to decide whether we can go further with salvage ePLND as a treatment option. Second, this analysis will serve as a basis for a prospective trial, for example, by joining in the SALPRO study of our colleagues from Freiburg, Germany. Finally, the low rate of complications that we found justifies further pursuit of this strategy.

Conclusion

Salvage ePLND resulted in an immediate complete PSA response in nearly 50 % of the patients and in a BR in more than two-thirds. CSS and OS were equal at 91.7 ± 4.8 % (3-year CSS and OS) and 80.6 ± 8.6 % (5-year CSS and OS). In addition, one of the most important results of our study was the fact that 53.3 % of previous CRPC patients respond to ADT again after salvage ePLND. Bone metastasis is a poor prognostic surveillance factor after salvage ePLND. We do not wish to suggest that salvage surgery should be performed in patients with bone metastases, but we believe that salvage ePLND should find a place in the guidelines for selected groups of patients, especially as an additional option for CRPC patients. Multicenter prospective studies with control groups are needed to achieve a reliable output.

Acknowledgements

We would like to thank Ms. Kalz for her kind editing of the English text. We would like to thank Prof. Andrey N. Gerasimov from the I.M. Sechenov First Moscow State Medical University for his professional help with the statistical analysis of our data.

Funding

Not applicable.

Authors' contributions

DO made substantial contributions to study conception, data interpretation, and manuscript revision. AA made substantial contributions to study conception and design, and analysis and interpretation of data, created the figures, tables and manuscript text, drafted and submitted the manuscript. DT was involved in revising the manuscript and gave some suggestions on the pathological sections. CN and MH were involved in conception of manuscript as well as revision. AF was involved in drafting of the manuscript. K-PJ made substantial contributions to study conception and design, and was involved in revision of the manuscript. All authors read and approved the final version of the manuscript.

Authors' information

All the authors are employees of the University Hospital Schleswig-Holstein, Campus Kiel (Germany). Further information regarding the position, clinical focus and contact data of the authors can be found on www.urologie-kiel.de.

Competing interests

The authors declare that they have no competing interests.

References

1. Wirth M, et al. S3-Guidelines prostate cancer (Germany) Version 3.1, Oktober 2014. AWMF-Register-Number 043/022OL; http://leitlinienprogramm-onkologie.de.
2. Heidenreich A, Bastian PJ, Bellmunt J, Bolla M, Joniau S, van der Kwast T, et al. EAU guidelines on prostate cancer. Part II: treatment of advanced, relapsing, and castration-resistant prostate cancer. Eur Urol. 2014;65:467–79.
3. Thompson IM, Valicenti RK, Albertsen P, Davis BJ, Goldenberg SL, Hahn C, et al. Adjuvant and salvage radiotherapy after prostatectomy: AUA/ASTRO Guideline. J Urol. 2013;190:441–9.
4. Briganti A, Karnes RJ, Joniau S, Boorjian SA, Cozzarini C, Gandaglia G. Prediction of outcome following early salvage radiotherapy among patients with biochemical recurrence after radical prostatectomy. Eur Urol. 2014;66:479–86.
5. Mottet N, Bellmunt J, Bolla M, Joniau S, Mason M, Matveev V, et al. EAU guidelines on prostate cancer. Part II: treatment of advanced, relapsing, and castration-resistant prostate cancer. Eur Urol. 2011;59:572–83.
6. Sciarra A, Cattarino S, Gentilucci A, Alfarone A, Innocenzi M, Gentile V, et al. Predictors for response to intermittent androgen deprivation (IAD) in prostate cancer cases with biochemical progression after surgery. Urol Oncol. 2013;31:607–14.
7. Morgans AK, Fan KH, Koyama T, Albertsen PC, Goodman M, Hamilton AS, et al. Influence of age on incident diabetes and cardiovascular disease in prostate cancer survivors receiving androgen deprivation therapy. J Urol. 2015;193(4):1226–31.
8. Giacinti S, Bassanelli M, Aschelter AM, Milano A, Roberto M, Marchetti P. Resistance to abiraterone in castration-resistant prostate cancer: a review of the literature. Anticancer Res. 2014;34:6265–9.
9. Jilg CA, Rischke HC, Reske SN, Henne K, Grosu AL, Weber W, Drendel V, et al. Salvage lymph node dissection with adjuvant radiotherapy for nodal recurrence of prostate cancer. J Urol. 2012;188:2190–7.
10. Rigatti P, Suardi N, Briganti A, Da Pozzo LF, Tutolo M, Villa L, et al. Pelvic/retroperitoneal salvage lymph node dissection for patients treated with radical prostatectomy with biochemical recurrence and nodal recurrence detected by [11C] choline positron emission tomography/computed tomography. Eur Urol. 2011;60:935–43.
11. Suardi N, Briganti A, Salonia A, Rigatti P. Salvage lymphadenectomy in postprostatectomy patients with prostate-specific antigen recurrence. Curr Opin Urol. 2011;21:237–40.
12. Stenzl A. Salvage lymph node dissection in recurrent prostate cancer patients. Eur Urol. 2011;60:944–5.
13. Osmonov DK, Aksenov AV, Boller A, Kalz A, Heimann D, Janssen I, et al. Extended salvage pelvic lymph node dissection in patients with recurrent prostate cancer. Adv Urol. 2014;2014:321619. doi:10.1155/2014/321619.
14. Osmonov DK, Aksenov AV, Naumann CM, Hamann MF, Jünemann K-P. Kiel template of salvage extended pelvic lymph node dissection in patients with prostate cancer recurrence. Eur Urol Suppl. 2015;14/2:e449.
15. DK Osmonov, AV Aksenov, CA Jilg, W Schultze-Seeman, CM Naumann, MF Hamann, K Bothe, KP Jünemann. Salvage lymphadenectomy in patients with prostate cancer recurrence: A review. Urologe A. 2015 Dec 19. [Epub ahead of print] German.
16. Naumann CM, Macquarrie A, Van Der Horst C, Hamann MF, Al-Najar A, Kaufmann S, et al. Histological detection of minimal metastatic disease in inguinal non-sentinel lymph nodes in penile cancer. Anticancer Res. 2010;30:467–71.
17. Berney DM, Wheeler TM, Grignon DJ, Epstein JI, Griffiths DF, Humphrey PA, et al. ISUP Prostate Cancer Group. International Society of Urological Pathology (ISUP) Consensus Conference on Handling and Staging of Radical Prostatectomy Specimens. Working group 4: seminal vesicles and lymph nodes. Mod Pathol. 2011;24:39–47.
18. Castro E, Goh C, Olmos D, Saunders E, Leongamornlert D, Tymrakiewicz M, et al. Germline BRCA mutations are associated with higher risk of nodal involvement, distant metastasis, and poor survival outcomes in prostate cancer. J Clin Oncol. 2013;31:1748–57.
19. Passoni NM, Suardi N, Abdollah F, Picchio M, Giovacchini G, Messa C, et al. Utility of [(11)C]choline PET/CT in guiding lesion-targeted salvage therapies in patients with prostate cancer recurrence localized to a single lymph node at imaging: results from a pathologically validated series. Urol Oncol. 2014;32:38. e9-38.e16.
20. Afshar-Oromieh A, Haberkorn U, Schlemmer HP, Fenchel M, Eder M, Eisenhut M, et al. Comparison of PET/CT and PET/MRI hybrid systems using a 68Ga-labelled PSMA ligand for the diagnosis of recurrent prostate cancer: initial experience. Eur J Nucl Med Mol Imaging. 2014;41:887–97.
21. Afshar-Oromieh A, Zechmann CM, Malcher A, Eder M, Eisenhut M, Linhart HG, et al. Comparison of PET imaging with a (68)Ga-labelled PSMA ligand and (18)F-choline-based PET/CT for the diagnosis of recurrent prostate cancer. Eur J Nucl Med Mol Imaging. 2014;41:11–20.
22. Sanz G, Robles JE, Giménez M, Arocena J, Sánchez D, Rodriguez-Rubio F, et al. Positron emission tomography with 18fluorine-labelled deoxyglucose: utility in localized and advanced prostate cancer. BJU Int. 1999;84:1028–31.
23. Liu IJ, Zafar MB, Lai YH, Segall GM, Terris MK. Fluorodeoxyglucose positron emission tomography studies in diagnosis and staging of clinically organ-confined prostate cancer. Urology. 2001;57:108–11.
24. Scattoni V, Picchio M, Suardi N, Messa C, Freschi M, Roscigno M, et al. Detection of lymph-node metastases with integrated [11C]choline PET/CT in patients with PSA failure after radical retropubic prostatectomy: results confirmed by open pelvic-retroperitoneal lymphadenectomy. Eur Urol. 2007; 52:423–9.
25. Osmonov DK, Heimann D, Janßen I, Aksenov A, Kalz A, Juenemann KP. Sensitivity and specificity of PET/CT regarding the detection of lymph node metastases in prostate cancer recurrence. Springerplus. 2014;3:340.

21

The prostate cancer detection rates of CEUS-targeted versus MRI-targeted versus systematic TRUS-guided biopsies in biopsy-naïve men

A. W. Postema[1*], M. J. V. Scheltema[1], C. K. Mannaerts[1], R. J. G. Van Sloun[2], T. Idzenga[1], M. Mischi[2], M. R. E. Engelbrecht[3], J. J. M. C. H. De la Rosette[1] and H. Wijkstra[1,2]

Abstract

Background: The current standard for Prostate Cancer (PCa) detection in biopsy-naïve men consists of 10–12 systematic biopsies under ultrasound guidance. This approach leads to underdiagnosis and undergrading of significant PCa while insignificant PCa may be overdiagnosed. The recent developments in MRI and Contrast Enhanced Ultrasound (CEUS) imaging have sparked an increasing interest in PCa imaging with the ultimate goal of replacing these "blind" systematic biopsies with reliable imaging-based targeted biopsies.

Methods/design: In this trial, we evaluate and compare the PCa detection rates of multiparametric (mp)MRI-targeted biopsies, CEUS-targeted biopsies and systematic biopsies under ultrasound guidance in the same patients. After informed consent, 299 biopsy-naïve men will undergo mpMRI scanning and CEUS imaging 1 week prior to the prostate biopsy procedure. During the biopsy procedure, a systematic transrectal 12-core biopsy will be performed by one operator blinded for the imaging results and targeted biopsy procedure. Subsequently a maximum of 4 CEUS-targeted biopsies and/or 4 mpMRI-targeted biopsies of predefined locations determined by an expert CEUS reader using quantification techniques and an expert radiologist, respectively, will be taken by a second operator using an MRI-US fusion device. The primary outcome is the detection rate of PCa (all grades) and clinically significant PCa (defined as Gleason score ≥7) compared between the three biopsy protocols.

Discussion: This trial compares the detection rate of (clinically significant) PCa, between both traditional systematic biopsies and targeted biopsies based on predefined regions of interest identified by two promising imaging technologies. It follows published recommendations on study design for the evaluation of imaging guided prostate biopsy techniques, minimizing bias and allowing data pooling. It is the first trial to combine mpMRI imaging and advanced CEUS imaging with quantification.

Keywords: Prostate cancer, Prostate cancer imaging, mpMRI, CEUS, Contrast enhanced ultrasound, Targeted prostate biopsies

* Correspondence: a.w.postema@amc.nl
[1]Department of Urology, AMC University Hospital, Amsterdam, The Netherlands
Full list of author information is available at the end of the article

Background

The incidence of PCa has increased in the 1990's, due to increased awareness and prolific Prostate Specific Antigen (PSA) screening. Although in the United States this trend has partly reversed, PCa is still the most common cancer in men representing 21% of cancer cases and it is estimated that 180,890 men will be diagnosed with PCa in United States in 2016 [1]. In Europe the incidence has increased, with 417,00 new PCa diagnoses in 2012 [2]. According to current standards, patients with a clinical suspicion of PCa based on elevated serum PSA and/or digital rectal examination should undergo 10–12 systematic transrectal ultrasound (TRUS)-guided prostate biopsies to confirm the diagnosis [3]. These systematic "blind" prostate biopsies lead to a considerable rate of overdiagnosis of clinically insignificant PCa as well as underdiagnosis and undergrading of significant PCa [4]. Image - guided targeted biopsy approaches have been proposed to address these problems [5]. Prostate cancer imaging has thus far developed on two platforms: MRI and Ultrasound. On the MRI platform, multiparametric MRI(mpMRI) in which diffusion - weighted MRI and dynamic contrast- enhanced MRI sequences are added to anatomical T2-weighted imaging has become the standard for PCa imaging [6]. A 2015 systematic review on the accuracy of mpMRI for the detection of prostate cancer found 12 studies and reported a negative predictive value for the detection of clinically significant prostate cancer between 63 and 98% and positive predictive values of 34–68% [7]. However, these results should be interpreted with caution since several used biopsy pathology as the reference standard to calculate sensitivity and specificity. Several meta-analyses have addressed the value of mpMRI - targeted biopsy cores and these show an improved per-core detection rate and a beneficial increased per-patient detection rate in patients with a persistent clinical suspicion after prior negative biopsies [5, 8]. The 2016 update of the EAU (European Association of Urology) guidelines on PCa now recommends performing mpMRI in these patients. However, at this point, the value of using mpMRI and MRI-targeted biopsies at initial biopsy in biopsy-naïve patient is debated [3]. Even though high negative predictive values for detecting significant prostate cancer have been reported, significant disease can still be missed by MRI - targeted biopsy. Furthermore, considerable heterogeneity and risk of selection bias of published results exists. [8, 9]. The EAU guidelines therefore recommend combining systematic and targeted biopsies [3]. The review by Van Hove et al. shows a 1–43% absolute and 2–430% relative increase in per-patient detection rate can be achieved by adding mpMRI - targeted cores to systematic cores [9]. Several methods of using the information obtained by mpMRI to target the region of interest with prostate biopsies exist: in cognitive targeting, the operator makes a visual estimation of where the MRI lesion is located during a TRUS-guided biopsy procedure. Taking in-bore biopsies during MRI scanning reduces the risk of targeting error but due to its magnet time consuming and therefore costly nature, it is not used often. Fusion devices have been developed that register the MRI images and US together, guiding the observer towards the MRI lesion during the TRUS procedure [10, 11].

Prostate cancer may be visible on standard B-mode TRUS. However, the sensitivity is generally reported to be around 11–35% and the positive predictive value is often cited to be between 17 and 57%, although some studies have shown slightly better numbers [12, 13]. Hence, B-mode ultrasound is widely regarded as insufficiently accurate for tumor detection making systematic ultrasound-guided biopsies necessary. A conclusion that is supported by the guidelines [3, 14]. Contrast - Enhanced Ultrasound (CEUS) has been proposed to improve the accuracy of TRUS to detect Prostate Cancer. In CEUS, an intravascular Ultrasound Contrast Agent (UCA) is used to visualize the changes in vascularity that are typical for significant PCa, particularly angiogenesis. It has been demonstrated that angiogenesis is essential for prostate tumors to progress from small indolent lesions below 2 mm in size to clinically significant disease [15]. The UCA's consist of gas-filled micro bubbles of 1–10 μm with a lipid or protein shell that have an intravascular lifespan of several minutes. A systematic review on CEUS demonstrated a sensitivity and specificity of 70 and 74% or PCa detection. It must be noted that this meta-analysis contains a mixture of biopsy - controlled studies and prostatectomy - controlled studies as well as different variants of CEUS. Of particular interest is the analysis by van Hove et al. that shows a 2–8% absolute or 7–35% relative increase in per-patient detection rate was attained by adding CEUS - targeted cores to systematic biopsy protocols [9]. This analysis indicates improved per-patient detection rates can be achieved with adding CEUS-targeted cores, however CEUS-targeted biopsy at this point cannot replace systematic biopsy. Traditional drawbacks of CEUS are its user-dependency, the limited number of planes that can be visualized in one setting, and the fact that the cues that signify a suspicious focus are subtle and present in the image studies in a matter of seconds. To overcome these drawbacks, computer-aided quantification, a relatively new method to analyze CEUS recordings, is used to assist in the CEUS interpretation [16]. In the present trial, we will use the Contrast Ultrasound Dispersion Imaging (CUDI) method with computer-aided quantification developed at the Eindhoven University of Technology [17]. In short, this method entails constructing per-pixel Time-Intensity-Curves (TICs) during the

UCA inflow phase of CEUS recordings. Several parameters calculated from the spatiotemporal distribution of these TICs have shown very promising results in predicting PCa presence with Area Under the Curve (AUC) values reaching up to 0.88–0.89 [17, 18]. These results were obtained by estimating how well CUDI could predict whether pixels belonged to a benign or malignant region of interest using radical prostatectomy specimens as the reference standard. In the present study we will evaluate the value of targeted biopsy procedures with mpMRI and CEUS + CUDI quantitative imaging by performing both procedures with systematic biopsies in the same patients scheduled for initial prostate biopsies. This way we will be able to determine how successful these tools can be used for targeting biopsies and how these targeting procedures compare to each other and to systematic biopsies. Additionally, we will analyze to what extent the imaging tools overlap in the tumors they detect or miss, and therefore to what extent they can be used complementary to each other.

Methods/design

Study objectives

Primary

- To compare the per-patient (significant) prostate cancer detection rate for mpMRI-US fusion - targeted biopsies and CEUS + CUDI-targeted biopsies with 12-core systematic biopsies.

Secondary

- To evaluate the value of using both mpMRI and CEUS + CUDI for targeted prostate biopsies.

Expected outcomes

Based on previous studies that used a fusion device to take 2–4 mpMRI - targeted biopsy cores in biopsy naïve patients, we expect a per-patient cancer detection rate (CDR) between 40–54% for the mpMRI - targeted biopsies. With the targeted cores, CDRs were achieved that were between 1% absolute higher and 13% absolute lower than the CDRs of systematic biopsies in the same series. Of note is that the biggest series used 3 different methods of targeting the mpMRI cores: cognitive targeting, rigid fusion and elastic fusion. Their best result with targeted cores relative to the systematic cores was achieved with the elastic fusion method (33% CDR for systematic cores and 47% for targeted cores). The Artemis (Eigen, Grass Valley, USA) fusion system that will be used in our trials uses elastic registration. The majority of series have performed a similar analysis in patients with previous negative systematic biopsies or mixed patient cohorts which tend to show a better performance of targeted cores relative to systematic cores [19]. In our biopsy naïve cohort we expect to find a per-patient CDR for all PCa grades that is in the same range as the systematic biopsies. In contrast, we expect the per-patient CDR for clinically significant (Gleason >3 + 4) disease of the mpMRI - targeted biopsies to be relatively higher compared to systematic biopsies.

Limited data is available for the value of CEUS-targeted cores. Van Hove et al. reviewed 6 studies that compared the CDRs for CEUS-targeted biopsies and systematic biopsies [9]. They report that targeted biopsy cores achieved CDRs between 13% absolute lower and 4% absolute higher than systematic cores in these heterogeneous studies with mixed patient groups and various CEUS variants used. None of the studies in this review have included the use of quantitative techniques. A previous study done in our own institution, that retrospectively correlated CEUS imaging with and without quantification with systematic biopsy results, showed improved significant PCa detection with the use of quantification. In 82 patients, 5.6% of biopsy locations that were classified benign on imaging showed clinically significant disease when quantification software was used, compared to 8.5% for CEUS without quantification [20]. Unfortunately, no targeted biopsies were taken in this retrospective analysis. We hypothesize that the use of CUDI quantification software in our current study will result in a CDR for significant disease up to the level of systematic biopsies or better. To our knowledge, there are no published data on the complementarity of mpMRI and CEUS in prostate cancer detection and biopsy targeting. Based on the available data on the separate techniques, we expect that the combination will result in a CDR higher than that of systematic biopsies, especially for the detection of clinically significant disease.

Study design

This study is a prospective in-vivo study in humans in which we perform MRI imaging and CEUS imaging in biopsy-naïve patients scheduled for prostate biopsies. Targeted prostate biopsies based on these images will be taken besides current standard of care systematic biopsies. Since both imaging modalities and targeted biopsies will be performed in the same patients, every patient effectively serves as his own control. Patients will undergo mpMRI imaging and CEUS imaging approximately 1 week before the scheduled biopsy appointment. During this week, MRI reading will be performed by a specialized uroradiologist with approximately 10 years of prostate mpMRI experience using the European Society of Urogenital Radiology (ESUR) Prostate Imaging Reporting and Data System standardised scoring system, version 2 (PIRADS v2) [21]. The radiologist is blinded to CEUS and CUDI results. The CEUS recordings will be analysed using the CUDI quantification technique. An observer experienced in CEUS of the prostate will read the CEUS recordings and CUDI-maps, while blinded to the MRI results. Before the biopsy procedure, the MRI - based biopsy targets and CEUS + CUDI - based biopsy targets are therefore predetermined independently from each other. During the biopsy session, approximately 1 week after the imaging is recorded, a physician who is blinded to all imaging results and the targeted biopsy procedure will first perform the standard 12-core systematic biopsy to prevent potential bias by post-biopsy haemorrhage seen on ultrasound after targeted biopsies. Then a separate observer, using an MRI-US fusion device, takes a maximum of 4 targeted biopsies from the MRI lesions delineated by the radiologist followed by a maximum of 4 targeted cores from the CEUS + CUDI lesions identified by the CEUS expert. Per-patient CDRs and tumor differentiation grades are compared between each of the biopsy regimens: MRI - targeted biopsies, CEUS + CUDI - targeted biopsies and systematic biopsies.

Population

Two hundred ninety-nine biopsy-naïve men above the age of 18 years that are scheduled for initial prostate biopsies on the basis of a suspicious DRE and/or elevated serum PSA (above 3 ng/ml) will be included in the study. Patients will be recruited at the AMC University Hospital and all study procedures will be performed at that institution. Exclusion criteria are mostly related to the MRI, the UCA used for CEUS imaging and biopsy procedures(Table 1). Patients will be informed about study procedures, risks and benefits, and are only included after written informed consent has been obtained.

Study procedures

Multiparametric magnetic resonance imaging

Prior to the mpMRI acquisition, a rectal preparation with a laxative suppository (Bisacodyl) will be performed and just before mpMRI scanning an anti-Peristaltic Drug (Buscopan or Glucagon) will be given. mpMRI will be performed in supine position on a 1.5 Tesla AVANTO® MRI scanner (Siemens Healthcare, Erlangen, Germany) or on a 3 Tesla INGENIA® without endorectal coil (Philips Medical Systems, Best, The Netherlands). The scanning protocol starts with T2-weighted sequences which will be performed in sagittal, coronal and axial planes covering the prostate and seminal vesicles. Then, a single-shot-echo planar diffusion-weighted sequence with fat suppression pulse is acquired and ADC maps are calculated. Finally, dynamic contrast-enhanced images using 0.1 mmol of gadopentetate dimeglumine (Gadolinium DTPA, Gadovist) per kg of body weight, are obtained. More details on the mpMRI conduct can be found in Table 2. mpMRI will be evaluated by a specialized uroradiologist (blinded for CEUS results) on prostate volume and area's suspicious for PCa. Scoring of suspicion will be performed using PIRADS v2 [21]. All lesions will be marked and delineated for MRI-TRUS fusion using the ProFuse (Eigen, Grass Valley, USA) software package that accompanies the Artemis fusion device.

Contrast-enhanced ultrasound and quantification

Contrast Ultrasound scanning will be performed in the left-lateral decubitus position using a Philips IU22 ultrasound scanner with a C10–3V endocavity probe (Philips Healthcare, Bothell, USA) with power modulation at 3.5 MHz and a mechanical index (MI) of 0.06. A total of four CEUS recordings will be made: from the base, mid-base, mid apical and apical planes. The locations of these planes within the prostate are stored using the Artemis fusion device, for future targeting of suspicious lesions. Each of the 2 min recordings will be started following the administration of a 2.4 mL bolus of the contrast agent SonoVue® (Bracco, Geneva, Switzerland) through an intravenous cannula. After each recording a pause of 3 min is observed to allow sufficient UCA breakdown to assess the inflow of the next UCA bolus. The CEUS recordings are anonymized and transferred through a secure connection to the Eindhoven University of Technology for CUDI quantitative analysis. The CUDI maps are

Table 1 Inclusion and exclusion criteria

Inclusion Criteria	Exclusion Criteria
1. Age ≥ 18 years	1. Is incapable of understanding the language in which the information for the patient is given
2. Signed informed consent	2. Has undergone previous prostate biopsies
3. Referred for prostate mpMRI and prostate biopsies	3. Active (urinary tract) infection or prostatitis
	4. History of any clinically evidence of cardiac right-to-left shunts
	5. Receives treatment that includes dobutamine
	6. Severe pulmonary hypertension (pulmonary artery pressure >90 mmHg) or uncontrolled systemic hypertension or respiratory distress syndrome
	7. Any medical condition or other circumstances which would significantly decrease the chances of obtaining reliable data, achieving study objectives, or completing the study
	8. Any (further) contraindication to undergo mpMRI or CEUS imaging

mpMRI multiparamteric Magentic Resonance Imaging, *CEUS* Contrast - Enhanced Ultrasound

Table 2 MRI conduct

mpMRI Conduct		
Unit	Philips 3 Tesla INGENIA®	Siemens 1.5 Tesla AVANTO®
Slice Thickness		
T2-Weighted	3 mm	3 mm
DW-MRI	4 mm	5 mm
DCE-MRI	2 mm	4 mm
T2-weighted planes	axial, coronal and sagittal	axial, coronal and sagittal
DCE-MRI		
Temporal resolution	5.00 s	3.06 s
Post-processing model	Tofts model using Dynacad (In Vivo, Best, The Netherlands)	Tofts model using Dynacad (In Vivo, Best, The Netherlands)
DW-MRI,		
B-values,	B0, B100, B1000	B50, B800
Imaging sets	ADC, calculated B1500	ADC
Quantitative analysis	primarily qualitative, quantitative in unclear cases	primarily qualitative, quantitative in unclear cases

mpMRI multiparamteric Magentic Resonance Imaging, *DW-MRI* Diffusion - Weighted Magnetic Resonance Imaging, *DCE-MRI* Dynamic Contrast- Enhanced Magnetic Resonance Imaging

transferred back to the physicians to aid in the CEUS interpretation and selection of the biopsy targets. This is done by a CEUS expert, who is blinded to MRI results.

Biopsy procedure

Patients are prepared for the biopsy procedure with a 2 day course of fluoroquinolone prophylaxis. The biopsy procedure is performed in the left-lateral decubitus position using the same ultrasound device and probe as used for the CEUS imaging. A first operator blinded to the targeted biopsy procedure planning and imaging results will take a standard 12-core systematic biopsy that includes 2 medial and 4 laterally directed cores of the peripheral zone of the prostate on each side. Then a second physician, using the Artemis fusion device for guidance, takes a maximum of 4 biopsies from targets designated by the radiologist and a maximum of 4 biopsies from the targets designated by the CEUS expert. The needle biopsy cores will be analysed for tumour presence and grading by our institution's specialized uropathologist in accordance with current pathology guidelines.

Sample size and statistical analysis

Statistical analysis

The per-patient PCa detection rates of both targeted biopsy regimens will be tested separately for non-inferiority against current standard 12-core systematic biopsies using a one sided non-inferiority test for correlated proportions [22, 23]. To evaluate if image- targeted biopsies can be used complementarily, we will also perform the same comparative analysis for the targeted biopsy results combined, compared to the systematic biopsies. Moreover, the per-patient CDR's of all three biopsy protocols will be directly compared using McNemars test for correlated proportions. The same analyses will be performed including all tumors and including clinically significant tumors only, defined as PCa with a Gleason score $\geq 3 + 4 = 7$.

Sample size calculation

The sample size calculation is based on the non-inferiority test between the targeted biopsy procedures and the systematic biopsies. For this test we performed a power analysis, with the detection rate for systematic biopsies set at 45% [24], a power of 80% and the significance level (alpha) of 5%. The maximum allowable difference in detection rate for the targeted biopsies to be considered non-inferior to systematic biopsies was set at 1%. We expect a maximum proportion of discordant pairs of 15% and a detection rate difference of 5%. The required sample size according to these specifications is 260 patients. Based on the estimation that 15% of the patients that are scheduled for biopsies will not receive targeted biopsies due to the absence of PCa suspected lesions on imaging; a total number of 299 patients will be enrolled in the study.

Literature shows that of all positive biopsies about 25% is Gleason >6 [25–27]. Results from our institution differ from literature as only 40% of all the patients with PCa at biopsy have a Gleason score 6 PCa, while 60% of them have a Gleason score >6 PCa. Thus, numbers of positive biopsies and Gleason score > 6 are higher than reported in literature. Based on our historical data we expect that by including 299 patients in the study we will find ~65 cases with a Gleason score = 6 and ~100 cases with a Gleason score > 6. For differentiation between Gleason score we hypothesize that we need at least 40 people in both Gleason grade groups.

Quality and patient safety

The quality of the data obtained and patient safety will be continuously monitored by the investigators. Periodical (yearly) reporting of study progression and patient safety will be performed to the reviewing Institutional Review Board (IRB). In accordance to section 10, subsection 4, of the Wet Medisch-Wetenschappelijk Onderzoek met Mensen (Medical Research Involving Human Subjects Act), the investigators will suspend the study if there is sufficient ground that continuation of the study will jeopardise subject health or safety. The investigators will notify the accredited IRB without undue delay of a temporary halt including the reason for such an action. The study will be suspended pending a further positive decision by the accredited IRB. The investigator will take care that all subjects are kept informed.

Risks and benefits

The mpMRI and TRUS - guided prostate biopsies are already performed routinely in our institution. The extra targeted prostate biopsies are considered to convey minimal additional risk over the systematic biopsy cores that were already planned. When contraindications for mpMRI and necessary preparations for prostate biopsies (proper antibiotic prophylaxis and management of anticoagulant medications) are followed, these investigations are considered safe [3]. After use in thousands of patients, adverse events related to micro bubble UCA's appear to be transient, mild and rare [28–30]. The most frequent minor side-effects are a transient alteration of taste, local pain at the injection site and facial or general flush (1–5%) [31]. Serious adverse events, which consists of hypersensitivity allergic reactions, are rare (<0.01%) [32]. In a study with SonoVue® in patients with chronic obstructive pulmonary disease, CEUS appeared to be as safe and well tolerated as in a healthy control group [28]. The Committee for Medicinal Products for Human Use has granted SonoVue® a marketing authorization, but it should not be used together with the medicine dobutamine and in pregnant or breastfeeding women (http://www.ema.europa.eu). Although patients are informed about the experimental nature of CEUS imaging, a potential benefit of participation is the real possibility of finding (significant) PCa in one of the targeted biopsies that would otherwise have remained undetected.

Discussion

Improvement of the PCa diagnostic pathway is necessary, and will likely depend on the advances in PCa imaging. Multiparametric MRI has a recognized value before a second biopsy in case of a persistent clinical suspicion for PCa. The value in biopsy - naïve patients and the possibility to omit systematic biopsies is debated [3]. Contrast -enhanced ultrasound has shown promising results, but should currently be viewed as experimental. This trial will provide data on both these techniques, allowing comparison and assessment of complementarity. The study design chosen is in line with recommendations formulated by the Standards of reporting for MRI-targeted biopsy studies (START) Working Group [33] and by van Hove et al [9]. To validate imaging - targeted prostate biopsy protocols van Hove et al. recommend using either one of two study designs: randomize patients to undergo either systematic biopsies alone or systematic biopsies and targeted biopsies. In the other option every patient undergoes both targeted biopsies and systematic biopsies by separate blinded observers. In our study design all patients undergo both imaging procedures and both targeted and systematic biopsies. The targeted biopsies and systematic biopsies are performed by separate observers. The targeted biopsy locations are predetermined by blinded readers and targeted through a fusion device. To prevent potential bias by post-biopsy haemorrhage seen on ultrasound the targeted biopsies are performed after the systematic biopsies. This way we prevent information gathered from one imaging technique to influence biopsy targeting for the other imaging technique. In both study designs the (significant) PCa detection rates are compared. An advantage of using these study designs is that there is no spectrum bias, i.e. the relevant biopsy population is being studied. Also, there is no observer bias, the investigator reading the images does not already know that there must be a tumor. Both spectrum bias and observer bias occur when translating results obtained from the correlation of imaging and radical prostatectomy specimens towards the primary diagnostic setting. Furthermore, the endpoint in this study design, (significant) PCa detection, is the most relevant endpoint in the clinic. We therefore believe that our trial will provide important and necessary data on one of the most relevant topics in PCa care. This data is gathered in a recommended, standardized fashion to minimize bias and allow data pooling.

Abbreviations

(mp)MRI: (multiparametric) Magnetic Resonance Imaging; AUC: Area Under the Curve; CDR: Cancer Detection Rate; CEUS: Contrast - Enhanced Ultrasound; CUDI: Contrast Ultrasound Dispersion Imaging; DRE: Digital Rectal Examination; EAU: European Association of Urology; IDM: Interdepartmental Monitoring; IRB: Institutional Review Board; PCa: Prostate Cancer; PSA: Prostate Specific Antigen; TIC: Time-Intensity-Curve; TRUS: Transrectal Ultrasound; UCA: Ultrasound Contrast Agent

Acknowledgements

Eigen (Grass Valley, USA) for providing the Artemis fusion system and technical support.

Funding

This trial is funded by the Dutch Cancer Society (grant number: UVA 2013-5941).

This funding source had no role in the design of this study and will not have any role during its execution, analyses, interpretation of the data, or decision to submit results.

Authors' contributions

AWP, HW and TI conceived the trial concept and designed the protocol for IRB approval. AWP and MJV, CKM, MRE and JdlR organised the trial logistics. HW is the principal investigator. MM and RJvS facilitate quantitative CEUS analysis and MRE oversees MRI acquisition and interpretation for this study. AWP, MJV and CKM drafted the manuscript. All authors reviewed and approved the final manuscript.

Competing interests

All authors of this manuscript declare no relationships with any companies, products or services related to the matter of this study.

Ethics approval and consent to participate

This trial will be conducted in accordance to the Good Clinical Practice standards, with the ethical principles that have their origins in the Declaration of Helsinki (Fortealeza, Brazil, October 2013). The trial protocol has been reviewed and approved by the IRB of the Academic Medical Center in Amsterdam, The Netherlands, under the ID 2015_263. The protocol is registered with The Dutch Central Committee on Research Involving Human Subjects (CCMO) under study ID: NL50791.018.14 and on the clinicaltrials.gov database (NCT02831920). Any amendments to the trial protocol will be submitted for review by the IRB. Trial registrations will be updated and participants will be informed about major amendments. Potential participants will be informed about the risks and benefits of participation both verbally by one of the investigators and in writing in the form of an extensive patient information brochure. Potential participants will be granted a minimum of 1 week to consider participation. Participants will only be included after written informed consent has been obtained. Patients can leave the study at any time for any reason if they wish to do so without any consequences. The investigator can decide to withdraw a subject from the study for urgent (medical) reasons. Patient data will be anonymized and stored in a secure database.

Author details

[1]Department of Urology, AMC University Hospital, Amsterdam, The Netherlands. [2]Department of Electrical Engineering, Eindhoven University of Technology, Eindhoven, The Netherlands. [3]Department of Radiology, AMC University Hospital, Amsterdam, The Netherlands.

References

1. Siegel R, Miller KD, Jemal A. Cancer Statistics, 2016. CA Cancer J Clin. 2016;66:7–30.
2. Ferlay J, Steliarova-Foucher E, Lortet-Tieulent J, Rosso S, Coebergh JW, Comber H, et al. Cancer incidence and mortality patterns in Europe: estimates for 40 countries in 2012. Eur J Cancer. 2013;49:1374–403.
3. Mottet N, Bellmunt J, Briers E, Bolla M, Cornford P, De Santis M et al. EAU Guidelines on Prostate Cancer - Update March 2016. European Association of Urology [Internet]. 2016 [cited 2017 March 21] Available from: http://uroweb.org/wp-content/uploads/EAU-Guidelines-Prostate-Cancer-2016-1.pdf . Accessed 21 Mar 2017.
4. Bjurlin MA, Carter HB, Schellhammer P, Cookson MS, Gomella LG, Troyer D, et al. Optimization of Initial Prostate Biopsy in Clinical Practice : Sampling, Labeling and Specimen Processing. JURO [Internet]. American Urological Association Education and Research, Inc.; 2013;189:2039–46. Available from: http://dx.doi.org/10.1016/j.juro.2013.02.072
5. Bjurlin MA, Meng X, Le Nobin J, Wysock JS, Lepor H, Rosenkrantz AB, et al. Optimization of prostate biopsy: The role of magnetic resonance imaging targeted biopsy in detection, localization and risk assessment. J Urol. 2014;192: 648–58. Available from: http://dx.doi.org/10.1016/j.juro.2014.03.117.
6. Vargas HA, Hötker AM, Goldman DA, Moskowitz CS, Gondo T, Matsumoto K, et al. Updated prostate imaging reporting and data system (PIRADS v2) recommendations for the detection of clinically significant prostate cancer using multiparametric MRI: critical evaluation using whole-mount pathology as standard of reference. Eur Radiol. 2016;26(6):1606-12.
7. Fütterer JJ, Briganti A, De Visschere P, Emberton M, Giannarini G, Kirkham A, et al. Can Clinically Significant Prostate Cancer Be Detected with Multiparametric Magnetic Resonance Imaging? A Systematic Review of the Literature. Eur Urol. 2015;68(6):1045-53.
8. Schoots IG, Roobol MJ, Nieboer D, Bangma CH, Steyerberg EW, Hunink MGM. Magnetic Resonance Imaging-targeted Biopsy May Enhance the Diagnostic Accuracy of Significant Prostate Cancer Detection Compared to Standard Transrectal Ultrasound-guided Biopsy: A Systematic Review and Meta-analysis. Eur. Urol. [Internet]. European Association of Urology; 2015;68:438–50. Available from: http://dx.doi.org/10.1016/j.eururo.2014.11.037
9. van Hove A, Savoie P-H, Maurin C, Brunelle S, Gravis G, Salem N, et al. Comparison of image-guided targeted biopsies versus systematic randomized biopsies in the detection of prostate cancer: a systematic literature review of well-designed studies. World J. Urol. [Internet]. 2014 [cited 2014 Sep 15];32: 847–58. Available from: http://www.ncbi.nlm.nih.gov/pubmed/24919965
10. Bjurlin MA, Mendhiratta N, Wysock JS, Taneja SS. Multiparametric MRI and targeted prostate biopsy: Improvements in cancer detection, localization, and risk assessment. Cent Eur J Urol. 2016;69:9–18.
11. Gayet M, Van Der Aa A, Beerlage HP, Schrier BP, Mulders PFA, Wijkstra H. The value of magnetic resonance imaging and ultrasonography (MRI/US)-fusion biopsy platforms in prostate cancer detection: A systematic review. BJU Int. 2016;117:392–400.
12. Postema A, Mischi M, de la Rosette J, Wijkstra H. Multiparametric ultrasound in the detection of prostate cancer: a systematic review. World J Urol. 2015; 33(11):1651-9.
13. Smeenge M, De La Rosette JJMCH, Wijkstra H. Current status of transrectal ultrasound techniques in prostate cancer. Curr. Opin. Urol. [Internet]. 2012 [cited 2013 Mar 31];22:297–302. Available from: http://www.ncbi.nlm.nih.gov/pubmed/22595778
14. Smeenge M, Barentsz J, Cosgrove D, De La Rosette J, De Reijke T, Eggener S, et al. Role of transrectal ultrasonography (TRUS) in focal therapy of prostate cancer: Report from a Consensus Panel. BJU Int. 2012;110:942–8.
15. Russo G, Mischi M, Scheepens W, De la Rosette JJ, Wijkstra H. Angiogenesis in prostate cancer: onset, progression and imaging. BJU Int. [Internet]. 2012 [cited 2013 Apr 2];110:E794–808. Available from: http://www.ncbi.nlm.nih.gov/pubmed/22958524
16. Postema A, Idzenga T, Mischi M, Frinking P, de la Rosette J, Wijkstra H. Ultrasound modalities and quantification: developments of multiparametric ultrasonography, a new modality to detect, localize and target prostatic tumors. Curr Opin Urol. 2015;25:191–7.
17. Kuenen MPJ, Saidov TA, Wijkstra H, Mischi M. Contrast-ultrasound dispersion imaging for prostate cancer localization by improved spatiotemporal similarity analysis. Ultrasound Med. Biol. [Internet]. 2013 [cited 2014 Apr 29];39:1631–41. Available from: http://www.ncbi.nlm.nih.gov/pubmed/23791350
18. Kuenen MPJ, Saidov T a, Wijkstra H, de la Rosette JJMCH, Mischi M. Spatiotemporal correlation of ultrasound contrast agent dilution curves for angiogenesis localization by dispersion imaging. IEEE Trans. Ultrason. Ferroelectr. Freq. Control [Internet]. 2013;60:2665–9. Available from: http://www.ncbi.nlm.nih.gov/pubmed/24297031
19. Valerio M, Donaldson I, Emberton M, Ehdaie B, Hadaschik BA, Marks LS, et al. Detection of clinically significant prostate cancer using magnetic resonance imaging-ultrasound fusion targeted biopsy: A systematic review. Eur Urol. 2015 Jul;68(1):8-19.
20. Postema AW, Frinking PJA, Smeenge M, De Reijke TM, De la Rosette JJMCH, Tranquart F, et al. Dynamic contrast-enhanced ultrasound parametric imaging for the detection of prostate cancer. BJU Int. 2016 Apr;117(4):598-603.
21. Kuru TH, Roethke MC, Rieker P, Roth W, Fenchel M, Hohenfellner M, et al. Histology core-specific evaluation of the European Society of Urogenital

Radiology (ESUR) standardised scoring system of multiparametric magnetic resonance imaging (mpMRI) of the prostate. BJU Int. 2013;112:1080–7.
22. Nam JM. Establishing equivalence of two treatments and sample size requirements in matched-pairs design. Biometrics. 1997;53:1422–30.
23. Liu JP, Hsueh HM, Hsieh E, Chen JJ. Tests for equivalence or non-inferiority for paired binary data. Stat Med. 2002;21:231–45.
24. Presti JC, O'Dowd GJ, Miller MC, Mattu R, Veltri RW. Extended peripheral zone biopsy schemes increase cancer detection rates and minimize variance in prostate specific antigen and age related cancer rates: results of a community multi-practice study. J Urol. 2003;169:125–9.
25. Frauscher F, Klauser A, Volgger H, Halpern EJ, Pallwein L, Steiner H, et al. Comparison of contrast enhanced color Doppler targeted biopsy with conventional systematic biopsy: impact on prostate cancer detection. J. Urol. [Internet]. United States; 2002;167:1648–52. Available from: http://www.ncbi.nlm.nih.gov/pubmed/11912381
26. Pelzer A, Bektic J, Berger AP, Pallwein L, Halpern EJ, Horninger W, et al. Prostate cancer detection in men with prostate specific antigen 4 to 10 ng/ml using a combined approach of contrast enhanced color Doppler targeted and systematic biopsy. J. Urol. [Internet]. 2005 [cited 2013 Dec 16]; 173:1926–9. Available from: http://www.ncbi.nlm.nih.gov/pubmed/15879783
27. Halpern EJ, Ramey JR, Strup SE, Frauscher F, McCue P, Gomella LG. Detection of prostate carcinoma with contrast-enhanced sonography using intermittent harmonic imaging. Cancer [Internet]. 2005 [cited 2013 May 21];104:2373–83. Available from: http://www.ncbi.nlm.nih.gov/pubmed/16240450
28. Bokor D, Chambers JB, Rees PJ, Mant TG, Luzzani F, Spinazzi A. Clinical safety of SonoVue, a new contrast agent for ultrasound imaging, in healthy volunteers and in patients with chronic obstructive pulmonary disease. Invest Radiol. 2001;36:104–9.
29. Cohen JL, Cheirif J, Segar DS, Gillam LD, Gottdiener JS, Hausnerova E, et al. Improved left ventricular endocardial border delineation and opacification with OPTISON (FS069), a new echocardiographic contrast agent: Results of a phase III multicenter trial. J Am Coll Cardiol. 1998;32:746–52.
30. Correas JM, Bridal L, Lesavre A, Méjean A, Claudon M, Hélénon O. Ultrasound contrast agents: Properties, principles of action, tolerance, and artifacts. Eur. Radiol. 2001;11:1316–28.
31. Jakobsen JA, Oyen R, Thomsen HS, Morcos SK. Safety of ultrasound contrast agents. Eur Radiol. 2005;15:941–5.
32. Becher H, Lofiego C, Mitchell A, Timperley J. Current indications for contrast echocardiography imaging. Eur J Echocardiogr. 2005;6:1–5.
33. Moore CM, Kasivisvanathan V, Eggener S, Emberton M, Futterer JJ, Gill IS, et al. Standards of reporting for MRI-targeted biopsy studies (START) of the prostate: Recommendations from an international working group. Eur Urol. 2013;64:544–52.

22

Association of early PSA decline and time to PSA progression in abiraterone acetate-treated metastatic castration-resistant prostate cancer

Masahiko Nakayama[1*], Hisanori Kobayashi[1], Tomihiro Takahara[1], Ryo Oyama[2], Keiichiro Imanaka[2] and Kazutake Yoshizawa[1]

Abstract

Background: Previous studies have demonstrated an association between prostate-specific antigen (PSA) kinetics and predictive value for treatment outcomes. Abiraterone acetate (AA) is a newly approved cytochrome-P450C17 inhibitor for treatment of metastatic castration-resistant prostate cancer (mCRPC), and few studies have evaluated PSA kinetics using AA so far. Results of a study evaluating PSA kinetics in the beginning of AA and enzalutamide responded chemotherapy-treated patients suggested different trends between the drugs. PSA kinetics of AA-treated patients has been reported using large datasets; however, no studies which have fully evaluated PSA kinetics in the beginning treatment. The present study aimed to assess the PSA kinetics and relationship between the PSA kinetics and PSA progression in chemotherapy-naïve and chemotherapy-treated mCRPC patients receiving AA.

Methods: We used two Japanese phase II trial datasets: JPN-201, chemotherapy-naïve mCRPC ($n = 48$) and JPN-202, chemotherapy-treated mCRPC ($n = 46$). PSA kinetic parameters were calculated using actual PSA values measured every 4 weeks, and a subgroup analysis was performed to evaluate the influence of early PSA response on time to PSA progression (TTPP). In addition, we used a Cox proportional hazard model to investigate the influence of variables on TTPP.

Results: PSA declined from week 4 but took more time to achieve nadir. PSA kinetic parameters were different between the datasets, mean time to PSA nadir was 5.3 ± 5.6 and 2.0 ± 3.4 months, and TTPP was 9.5 ± 7.4 and 3.8 ± 4.8 months in JPN-201 and JPN-202, respectively. In the subgroup analysis of week 4 PSA decline status, Kaplan–Meier curves for TTPP were similar between early responders and non-progression patients in JPN-201 (median, 9.2 vs. 6.5 months, respectively) but separated in JPN-202 (median, 3.7 vs. 1.9 months, respectively). According to univariate Cox regression analysis, achievement of PSA response (≥50 %) at week 12 was associated with TTPP in the both trials, but the hazard ratio of PSA decline (≥30 %) at week 4 was not significant in JPN-201.

Conclusions: Our results suggest that PSA kinetics were not comparable and early PSA response showed different association to TTPP according to prior history of chemotherapy.

Keywords: Abiraterone acetate, Castration-resistant prostate cancer, Kinetics, Prostate-specific antigen, Cox proportional hazard model

* Correspondence: mnakayam@its.jnj.com
[1]Medical Affairs Division, Janssen Pharmaceutical K.K., 5-2, Nishi-kanda, 3-Chome, Chiyoda-ku, Tokyo 101-0065, Japan
Full list of author information is available at the end of the article

Background

Globally, the estimated incidence of prostate cancer was approximately 1.4 million in 2013. There was a 3-fold increase in this incidence from 1990 to 2013, together with aging and population growth [1]. Since Huggins et al. discovered that prostate cancer growth is stimulated by androgens, castration has been the mainstay of advanced-stage prostate cancer treatment [2]; however, most patients develop resistance to castration.

Abiraterone acetate (AA) is a prodrug of abiraterone, which is a first-in-class inhibitor of cytochrome-P450C17 that plays a role in the mechanism of castration resistance by de novo androgen synthesis [3]. It is approved with prednisone for treatment of metastatic castration-resistant prostate cancer (mCRPC) worldwide. AA plus prednisone significantly prolonged overall survival (OS) compared with placebo plus prednisone for treatment of chemotherapy-naïve and chemotherapy-treated mCRPC in pivotal global trials [4, 5]. In Japan, two single-arm, open-label, phase II trials were separately conducted for the purpose of obtaining local registration [6, 7].

Prostate-specific antigen (PSA) is a reliable, sensitive, and easy to measure biomarker for prostate cancer and is therefore widely used for evaluation of treatment in practice [8, 9]. PSA kinetics has been studied in androgen deprivation therapy using anti-androgens or taxanes to analyze its predictive value for time-dependent outcomes such as OS and disease progression. Several studies have reported strength of PSA decline and its predictive value for OS, although certain results were controversial [9–11]. Recently, Caffo et al. reported the PSA kinetics of AA and enzalutamide responders and demonstrated different trends with regard to PSA kinetics between the drugs in chemotherapy-treated mCRPC patients [12]. However, patient number was limited, and PSA kinetics of chemotherapy-naïve mCRPC patients was not reported. Xu et al. also reported PSA kinetics of AA-treated mCRPC patients separately by chemotherapy-naïve and -treated populations. However, PSA kinetics within 12 weeks was not evaluated because the original trials measured PSA values every 12 or 16 weeks [13]. Thus, PSA kinetics in AA-treated mCRPC patients has not been fully clarified so far.

Moreover, the Prostate Cancer Clinical Trial Working Group (PCWG2) advises to ignore early PSA changes to avoid detecting continuing rise of PSA level and increasing in size before it regress [8]. However, some researchers reported early PSA decline, and its predictive value was possibly different by patient backgrounds and treatment [12, 14, 15]. In addition, the clinical practice in Japan, most of mCRPC patients are primary followed by monthly PSA testing, so, there is a potential of over use of early response as predictive factor for efficacy regardless the PCWG2 criteria.

The aims of the present study were to assess the PSA kinetic profile, and the relationship between PSA kinetics calculated based on actual PSA values measured 4 weeks and 12 weeks and PSA progression in chemotherapy-naïve and chemotherapy-treated mCRPC patients receiving AA.

Methods

Data source

This post-hoc study was conducted using datasets from two Japanese phase II trials of AA for mCRPC: JPN-201 (ClinicalTrials.gov Identifier, JNJ-212082-JPN-201) that included chemotherapy-naïve patients ($n = 48$) and JPN-202 (ClinicalTrials.gov Identifier, JNJ-212082-JPN-202) that included patients who received docetaxel-based chemotherapy ($n = 46$). Results from the original trials are available elsewhere [6, 7]. Major inclusion criteria were as follows: men with mCRPC aged ≥ 20 years with a PSA level of ≥ 5 ng/mL and an Eastern Cooperative Oncology Group Performance Status (ECOG-PS) score of 0 or 1 for JPN-201 and 0 to 2 for JPN-202, histologically or cytologically confirmed adenocarcinoma of the prostate without neuroendocrine differentiation or small cell histology, and testosterone levels of ≤ 50 ng/dL by medical or surgical castration. Eligible patients were orally administered AA 1000 mg with 10-mg prednisolone per day. For patients with medical castration, castration was maintained by using a luteinizing hormone-releasing hormone (LHRH) agonist throughout the study. PSA was assessed at baseline and every 28 days after the AA dose.

The primary endpoint of the original trials was the proportion of patients achieving a PSA decline of ≥ 50 % from baseline within 12 weeks of therapy in accordance with the Prostate-Specific Antigen Working Group criteria (PSAWG) [16].

An independent ethics committee or institutional review board approved the protocols of original trials and informed consent forms, and the trials were conducted in accordance with the ethical principles in the Declaration of Helsinki and consistent with the Good Clinical Practices and applicable regulatory requirements. All patients or their legally acceptable representatives provided written informed consent, which included consent for post-hoc analysis before entering the original trials.

PSA values used in the study and definitions of PSA kinetic parameters

We used PSA values obtained after each 28-day cycle from baseline (day 0) to end of treatment (EOT) or study cutoff date (the longest duration was 785 days) to calculate the PSA kinetic parameters.

The following PSA kinetic parameters were calculated, as defined in the present study:

(1) Maximum percentage PSA decline (%; defined as nadir PSA value/baseline PSA value × 100)
(2) Time to PSA nadir (months; defined as duration from baseline to PSA nadir)
(3) Nadir PSA value (ng/mL; defined as the minimum PSA value during the treatment period)
(4) EOT PSA value (ng/mL; defined as the last PSA value at EOT)
(5) PSA response (≥50 %) according to PCWG2 criteria
(6) PSA response (≥30, 50, and 90 %) at week 12 according to PCWG2 criteria
(7) Time to PSA progression (TTPP; months, defined as duration from baseline to the day of PSA progression according to PCWG2 criteria)

The purpose of the original studies was to demonstrate similarity with global trials, response criteria needed to be identical with global trials used. In the present study, we referred PCWG2 criteria instead of PSAWG criteria, because it no longer used in the current clinical practice.

Statistical analysis

Findings from JPN-201 and JPN-202 were separately analyzed. Patient demographics, baseline characteristics, and PSA kinetic parameters were descriptively summarized using mean, standard deviation (SD), and percentage values. The percentage PSA change was longitudinally described based on mean (SD) and 95 % confidence intervals (CI) at each time point to characterize the post-treatment PSA kinetics.

We analyzed the impact of early PSA decline on TTPP. Because treatment was repeated every 28 days, and PSA was measured on the first day of each cycle in JPN-201 and JPN-202, the PSA value at week 4 was the earliest PSA value available to assess PSA transition. We subdivided the percent PSA change at week 4 into the following three subgroups: (1) PSA decline ≤ −30 % (30 %-decline), (2) PSA > −30 and < 25 % (non-decline), and (3) PSA elevation ≥ 25 % (25 %-elevation). Furthermore, TTPP was analyzed based on PSA response (≥50 %) at week 12 according to the PCWG2 criteria. In addition, impact of the PSA kinetic parameters on TTPP was investigated using a Cox proportional hazard model to obtain the hazard ratio (HR) and its 95 % CI. TTPP curves were developed using Kaplan–Meier method.

All statistical analyses were performed using R version 3.1.0 (a language and environment for statistical computing; R Foundation for Statistical Computing, Vienna, Austria).

Results

Baseline demographics and characteristics

In the present study, data from a total of 94 patients were analyzed: 48 patients from JPN-201 and 46 from JPN-202. Baseline demographics and characteristics are summarized in Table 1. In JPN-201, the median age was 70 years, 83.3 of the patients had ECOG-PS scores of 0, and 89.6 % had a Gleason score of ≥ 8. In JPN-202, the median age was 71 years, 52.2, 34.8, and 13.0 % of the patients had ECOG-PS scores of 0, 1, and 2, respectively, and 78.3 % had a Gleason score of ≥ 8.

In JPN-202, all patients had received docetaxel-based chemotherapy at study entry.

Abiraterone compliance, dose reducations and interaptions

In JPN-201, 91.7 % (44/48) had > 90 % compliance with AA. Dose reductions were required for 3 (6.3 %) patients. Dose interruptions were required for 21 (45.7 %) patients, once for 13 and 9 patients required 2 or more dose interruptions.

In JPN-202, 93.5 % (43/46) had > 90 % compliance with AA. Dose reductions were required for 6 (13.0 %) patients. Dose interruptions were required for 22 (47.8 %) patients, 8 patients required 2 or more dose interruptions.

No patients discontinued study treatment because of poor compliance in the both trials.

PSA kinetic parameter values

PSA values were well followed up, PSA progression was confirmed 75 (36/48) and 10 % (5/48) was censored within the first year in JPN-201. In JPN-202, PSA progression was confirmed 93 (43/46) and 4 % (2/46) was censored within the first year.

In JPN-201, PSA rapidly decreased from week 4 onwards, and the mean PSA decline from baseline value was 51.6 % (SD: 41.2) (Fig. 1a). Figure 1b depicts the percentage change of PSA transition in each patient. The PSA kinetic parameters are shown in Table 2. At week 4, 36 patients achieved a 30 %-decline, 9 patients showed a non-decline, and 3 patients showed a 25 %-elevation. PSA responses (≥50 %) were confirmed in 28 of 36 patients who achieved 30-decline, 2 patients who showed a non-decline, and none of the 25 %-elevation patients. Figure 2a shows the TTPP according to the week 4 percent PSA change subgroups. The median TTPP was 9.2 months for 30 %-decline, 6.5 months for non-decline, and 1.0 month for 25 %-elevation. In addition, of the 9 non-decline patients, 1 continued to have a PSA response and 6 showed PSA progression at EOT. Other 2 patients were censored by discontinuing of the treatment. Figure 2b shows TTPP according to the PSA response (≥50 %) at week 12. The median TTPP was 11.1 months for responders, 1.9 month for patients with PSA progression, and 6.5 months for others (non-response and non-progression).

Table 1 Baseline patient demographics and characteristics

	Chemotherapy-naive JPN-201 ($n = 48$)	Chemotherapy-treated JPN-202 ($n = 46$)
Median age (range), years	70 (46–89)	71 (51–83)
Gleason score		
< 7	0 %	0 %
7	8.3 %	17.4 %
≥ 8	89.6 %	78.3 %
Unknown	2.1 %	4.3 %
ECOG-PS score		
0	83.3 %	52.2 %
1	16.7 %	34.8 %
2	–	13.0 %
Extent of disease		
Bone	91.7 %	95.7 %
Hepatic	2.1 %	4.3 %
Lymphatic	39.6 %	37.0 %
Pulmonary	0 %	10.9 %
Other	0 %	6.5 %
Median months from initiating LHRH agonist to first dose (range)	21.91 (6.2–191.6)	41.23 (4.4–182.8)
Median baseline PSA (range), ng/mL	31.40 (6.0–469.0)	147.00 (7.2–1450.0)
Median baseline hemoglobin (range), g/dL	12.85 (10.2–15.2)	11.80 (9.0–14.9)
Median LDH (range), IU/L	212.0 (164–1045)	211.0 (122–723)
Median alkaline phosphatase (range), IU/L	292.0 (139–2643)	327.0 (69–2991)
No. of previous chemotherapy regimens		
1	–	39.1 %
2	–	60.9 %

ECOG-PS Eastern Corporative Oncology Group Performance Status, *LDH* lactate dehydrogenase, *LHRH* luteinizing hormone-releasing hormone, *PSA* prostate-specific antigen

In JPN-202, the mean PSA decline at week 4 was 14.9 % (SD: 59.1) (Fig. 1c). Figure 1d depicts the percentage change of PSA transition for each patient. The PSA kinetic parameters are shown in Table 2. At week 4, 21 patients achieved a 30 %-decline, 14 patients showed a non-decline and 11 showed a 25 %-elevation. PSA responses (≥50 %) were confirmed in 13 of 21 30 %-decline patients, while none of the patients had PSA responses in the other subgroups. Figure 3a shows the TTPP according to the subgroups; the median TTPP was 3.7 months for 30 %-decline, 1.9 months for non-decline, and 1.0 month for 25 %-elevation. All non-30 %-decline patients had PSA progression at EOT. Figure 3b shows the TTPP according to PSA response (≥50 %) at week 12. The median TTPP was 4.6 months for responders, 1.9 months for patients with PSA progression, and 4.6 months for others (non-response and non-progression).

Results of univariate Cox analyses

Table 3 shows the results of univariate Cox regression analyses for TTPP. In JPN-201, all variables showed significance except PSA decline (≥30 %) at week 4. In JPN-202, all variables showed significance except nadir PSA value and PSA response (≥90 %) at week 12.

Discussion

In this post-hoc analysis, we first assessed the PSA kinetic profile in AA plus prednisolone-treated mCRPC patients. There was a clear difference in the PSA kinetic profile between chemotherapy-naïve and chemotherapy-treated patients. The majority of chemotherapy-naïve patients showed a rapid PSA decline at week 4, and additional 4 months were needed to reach PSA nadir. On the other hand, the majority of chemotherapy-treated patients showed non-decline or 25 % elevation at week 4, and the mean time to reach PSA nadir was 2.0 months. Moreover, the percent change in the PSA values in chemotherapy-treated patients tended to be larger, and most of the patients experienced PSA progression within a year after treatment initiation (Fig. 1). The mean TTPP was approximately 4 months, which was

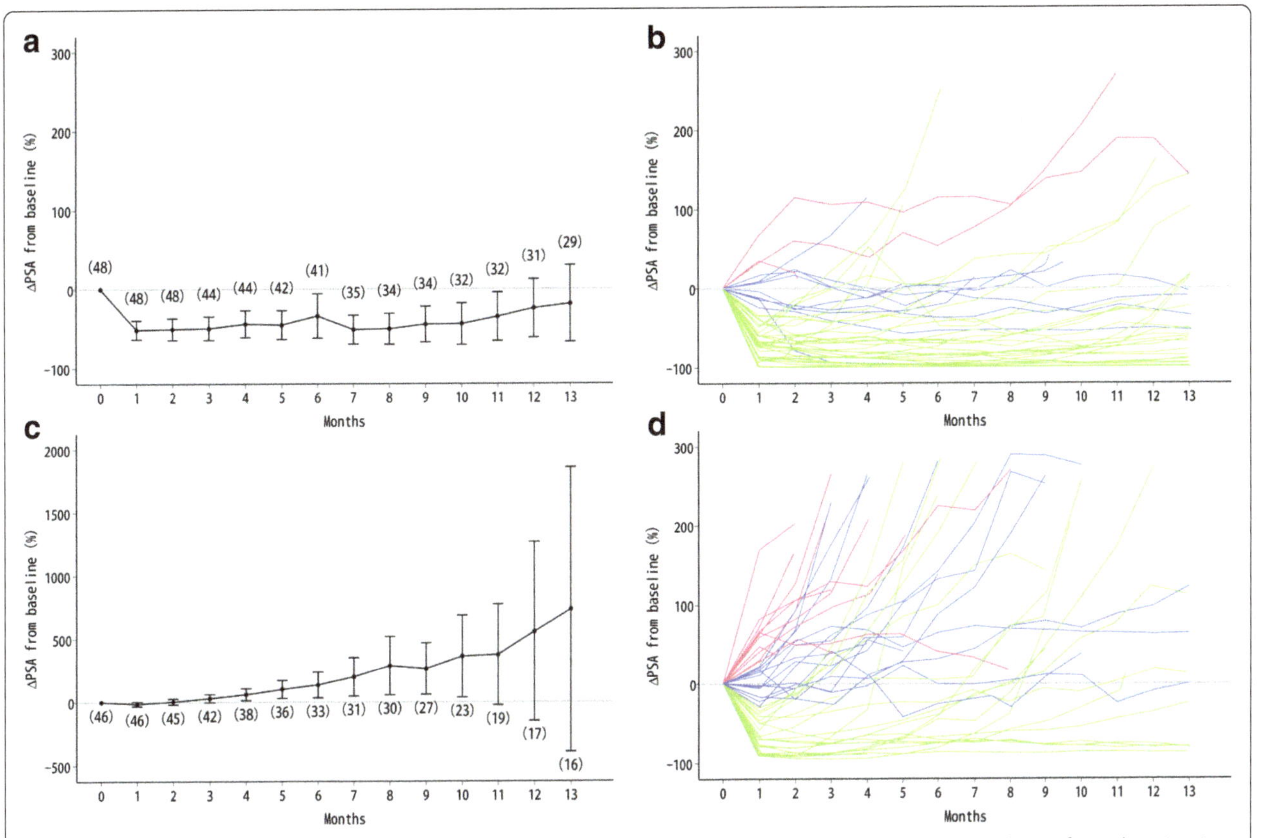

Fig. 1 Percent PSA transition from baseline to month 13. **a** Mean percent PSA change in JPN-201, (n). **b** Percent PSA change for each patient in JPN-201; green, PSA ≤ −30 % (30 %-decline); blue, −30 % < PSA < 25 % (non-decline); red, PSA ≥ 25 % (25 %-elevation) according to PSA change at week 4. **c** Mean percent PSA change in JPN-202, (n). **d** Percent PSA change for each patient in JPN-202; green, PSA ≤ −30 % (30 %-decline); blue, −30 % < PSA < 25 % (non-decline); red, 25 % ≥ PSA (25 %-elevation) according to PSA change at week 4. Data are expressed as mean ± 95 % CI. Note: PSA changes of ≥ 300 % and those after month 13 are not shown

approximately half of the value reported in JPN-201 (9.5 months). Differences in characteristics of patient populations with mCRPC may impact the PSA kinetic profile, and such PSA kinetic differences could mainly be associated with previous history of chemotherapy. The mechanisms related to the differences in PSA kinetic profiles between chemotherapy-naïve and chemotherapy-treated patients are unclear; however, it is recommended that PSA kinetics would be separately evaluated according to prior history of chemotherapy. Caffo et al. reported that the time to PSA nadir in responders among chemotherapy-treated mCRPC patients was 15.5 weeks with AA but 7.0 weeks with enzalutamide [12]. Moreover, the anti-tumor effects of both drugs are

Table 2 PSA kinetic parameters, mean ± SD (95 % CI)

	JPN-201 (*n* = 48) Chemotherapy-naive	JPN-202 (*n* = 46) Chemotherapy-treated
Maximum % PSA decline	64.4 ± 38.3 (53.3–75.5)	19.7 ± 59.4 (2.0–37.3)
Time to PSA nadir (months)	5.3 ± 5.6 (3.7–6.9)	2.0 ± 3.4 (1.0–3.0)
Nadir PSA value (ng/mL)	19.5 ± 28.3 (11.3–27.7)	184.9 ± 282.3 (101.0–268.7)
PSA response (≥30 %) at week 12, n (%; 95 % CI)	35 (72.9; 58.2–84.7)	15 (32.6; 19.5–48.0)
PSA response (≥50 %) at week 12, n (%; 95 % CI)	29 (60.4; 45.3–74.2)	13 (28.3; 16.0–43.5)
PSA response (≥90 %) at week 12, n (%; 95 % CI)	9 (18.8; 8.9–32.6)	2 (4.3; 0.5–14.8)
PSA response (≥50 %) in treatment period, n (%; 95 % CI)	30 (62.5; 47.48–76.0)	13 (28.3; 16.0–43.5)
Time to PSA progression (months)	9.5 ± 7.4 (7.4–11.6)	3.8 ± 4.8 (2.4–5.2)

PSA prostate-specific antigen, *CI* confidence interval, *SD* standard deviation

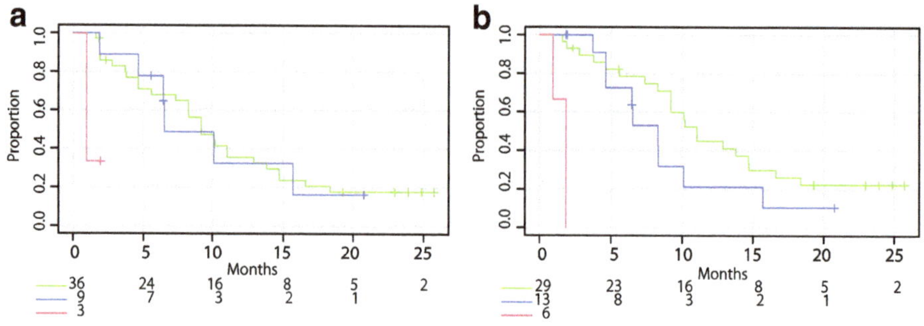

Fig. 2 Kaplan–Meier curves for time to PSA progression in JPN-201. **a** green, PSA ≤ −30 % (30 %-decline); blue, −30 % < PSA < 25 % (non-decline); red, PSA ≥ 25 % (25 %-elevation) according to PSA change at week 4. **b** green, PSA response (≥50 %); blue, PSA non-response/progression; red, PSA progression according to PSA response at week 12

derived from different mechanisms of action; abiraterone inhibits androgen synthesis at non-gonadal sites (adrenal gland and intratumorally) to reduce androgens to below castrate concentrations, while enzalutamide, an anti-androgen, directly binds androgen receptors to inhibit androgen receptor nuclear translocation [17]. These differences in the mechanisms of action might affect PSA kinetics.

In the present study, some patients showed a continuous stable level of PSA (Fig. 1b). In JPN-201, of the 9 (19 %) patients categorized as non-decline, most did not show large PSA elevation within 12 months. The TTPP curves were similar between non-decline and 30 %-decline patients (Fig. 2a). Thus, for chemotherapy-naïve patients without PSA progression at week 4, there would be a clinically similar chance of benefit from AA treatment. This is also supported by the result of Cox regression analysis, HR was significant for PSA response (≥50 %) at week 12 but not for PSA decline (≥30 %) at week 4 (Table 3).

On the other hand, in JPN-202, the non-decline TTPP curve was shorter than that of 30 %-decline and differed from that of 25 %-elevation (Fig. 3a). A half of the non-decline patients had rapid PSA progression; however, another half of the patients showed continuous stable levels of PSA (Fig. 1d), suggesting that patients with non-decline still had some potential of obtaining a clinical benefit from the treatment. The TTPP curves based on PSA response at week 12 were close between responders and patients with non-progression (Fig. 3b). Overall, further observation is recommended for patients in both population regardless obtaining PSA elevation at week 4.

In addition, temporal PSA elevation was recently reported with docetaxel treatment [18], which led to the phenomenon being referred to as "PSA flare," indicating a PSA elevation with initiation of an LHRH agonist. PSA flares were also reported with AA treatment [19, 20]. According to the definition by Olbert et al., wherein a PSA flare is defined as initially rising PSA under therapy, dropping thereafter to values below baseline, 3 of 9 non-decline patients (Fig. 1b; blue lines) in JPN-201and 1 of 21 in JPN-202 (Fig. 1d; blue lines) were considered to have a PSA flare. PSA transition in such patients showed slow PSA elevations for 2 months, which declined below baseline levels within 1 to 2 months after the peak level. In taxane-based chemotherapy, the pattern of flare-up was slightly different. In the chemotherapy-

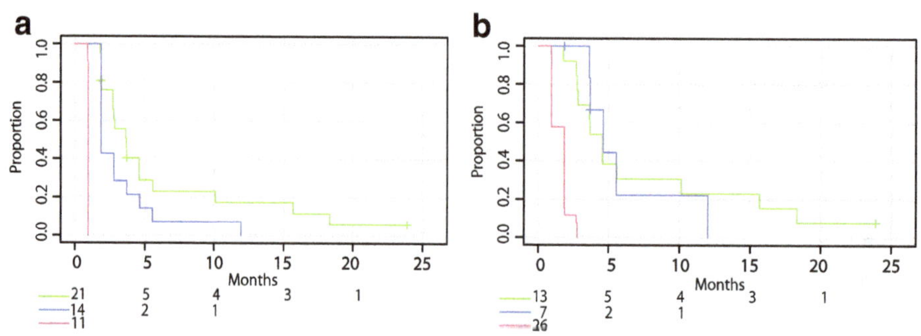

Fig. 3 Kaplan–Meier curves for time to PSA progression in JPN-202. **a** green, PSA ≤ −30 % (30 %-PSA-decline); blue, −30 % < PSA < 25 % (non-decline); red, PSA ≥ 25 % (25 %-elevation) according to PSA change at week 4. **b** green, PSA response (≥50 %); blue, PSA non-response/progression; red, PSA progression according to PSA response at week 12

Table 3 Results of univariate Cox analysis for time to PSA progression

	JPN-201		JPN-202	
	Chemotherapy-naive		Chemotherapy-treated	
	HR	95 % CI	HR	95 % CI
Maximum % PSA decline	0.975	0.964–0.986	0.981	0.975–0.987
Time to PSA nadir (months)	0.818	0.741–0.903	0.153	0.081–0.291
Nadir PSA value (ng/mL)	1.012	1.002–1.022	1.001	0.999–1.002
% PSA decline at week 4	0.989	0.981–0.998	0.980	0.973–0.986
% PSA decline at week 12	0.981	0.974–0.989	0.998	0.984–0.992
PSA decline (≥30 %) at week 4				
Non-decline (reference)	–	–	–	–
Decline	0.753	0.341–1.664	0.342	0.180–0.648
PSA response (≥30 %) at week 12				
Non-responder (reference)	–	–	–	–
Responder	0.331	0.158–0.692	0.335	0.167–0.674
PSA response (≥50 %) at week 12				
Non-responder (reference)	–	–	–	–
Responder	0.394	0.119–0.781	0.298	0.141–0.627
PSA response (≥90 %) at week 12				
Non-responder (reference)	–	–	–	–
Responder	0.357	0.137–0.930	0.807	0.193–3.369

CI confidence interval, *HR* hazard ratio, *PSA* prostate-specific antigen

related PSA flare, a peak PSA level was reached within 1 month after the first dose, and peak PSA levels were detected 1 to 2 months earlier than in the present study [18, 21, 22].

In general, elevated or stable PSA levels are a key decision factor for treatment change in routine clinical practice. Based on the aforementioned results, careful consideration is recommended for evaluation of the efficacy and decision for treatment change in AA treatment.

Some limitations of the present study are as follows: TTPP is a well-known surrogate endpoint for OS and is easy to follow-up in clinical practice [8]. In the present study, investigation of OS was inappropriate because patient number and number of events were limited. Therefore, we alternatively evaluated TTPP. Nonetheless, the primary endpoint in both JPN-201 and JPN-202 was PSA response rate at week 12; however, patient number was insufficient to apply statistical testing to analyze TTPP between the subgroups. Especially, patient number of non-30 %-decline was limited (11 in chemotherapy-naïve and 25 in chemotherapy-treated population). Moreover, in clinical practice, a wide variety of prior therapies, patient conditions, and concomitant use of drugs may have a potential impact on PSA kinetic profiles; it will therefore be important to reconfirm these results in clinical practice.

Conclusions

Our results suggest that PSA kinetics and impact of early PSA decline on TTPP were not comparable and early PSA response showed slightly different association to TTPP according to prior history of chemotherapy. However, this is simply a descriptive study for which practice changing assessment of response or predictor of failure just cannot be made, further studies are warranted to confirm these results.

Abbreviations

AA, abiraterone acetate; CI, confidence interval; ECOG-PS, Eastern Cooperative Oncology Group Performance Status; EOT, end of treatment; HR, hazard ratio; LHRH, luteinizing hormone-releasing hormone; mCRPC, metastatic castration-resistant prostate cancer; OS, overall survival; PCWG2, Prostate Cancer Clinical Trials Working Group; PSA, prostate-specific antigen; PSAWG, Prostate-Specific Antigen Working Group; SD, standard deviation; TTPP, time to prostate-specific antigen progression

Acknowledgements

We would like to thank all the patients and their families and investigators who participated in JPN-201 and JPN-202. The names of the independent ethics committee or institutional review board approved the original trials were; Hokkaido University Hospital IRB, Gunma University Hospital IRB, Kumagaya General Hospital IRB, Asahi General Hospital IRB, Toho University Sakura Medical Center IRB, The Institutional Review Board of National Cancer Center, Kyorin University Hospital IRB, Kitasato University Hospital IRB, Yokosuka Kyosai Hospital IRB, Yokohama City University Hospital IRB, Niigata University Medical & Dental Hospital IRB, Ishikawa Prefectural Central Hospital IRB, Osaka City University Hospital IRB, Kurashiki Central Hospital IRB, Kagawa University Hospital IRB, National Shikoku Cancer Center IRB, Kyushu University Hospital IRB, Osaka

Medical Center for Cancer and Cardiovascular Diseases IRB, Kinki University Hospital IRB, Hara Sansin Hospital IRB and Gifu University Hospital IRB for JPN-201. For JPN-202, Hokkaido University Hospital IRB, Gunma University Hospital IRB, Kumagaya General Hospital IRB, Asahi General Hospital IRB, Toho University Sakura Medical Center IRB, Tokyo Women's University Hospital IRB, Kyorin University Hospital IRB, Kitasato University Hospital IRB, Yokosuka Kyosai Hospital IRB, Yokohama City University Hospital IRB, Niigata University Medical & Dental Hospital IRB, Ishikawa Prefectural Central Hospital IRB, Osaka City University Hospital IRB, Kurashiki Central Hospital IRB, Kagawa University Hospital IRB, National Shikoku Cancer Center IRB, Kyushu University Hospital IRB and Kinki University Hospital IRB.

Funding
The original trials (JNJ-212082-JPN-201 and JNJ-212082-JPN-202) were conducted and funded by Janssen Pharmaceutical K.K.

Availability of data and materials
Janssen pharmaceutical, a pharmaceutical company of Johnson and Johnson, has a rights to the raw data of JNJ-212082-JPN-201 and JNJ-212082-JPN-202. As part of our commitment to the implementation of the joint EFPIA/PhRMA principles for responsible sharing of clinical trial data, researchers who desire access to data from our clinical trials can make a request on "http://www.clinicaltrialstudytransparency.com".

Authors' contributions
KY, TT, HK and MN were involved in the conception and design of the study. RO was responsible for the overall study project. MN and HK were responsible for statistical analysis. MN and KY drafted the manuscript and KI was responsible for medical and urological interpretation of the analyzed data of the study. All authors read and approved the final version of the manuscript.

Competing interests
Masahiko Nakayama, Hisanori Kobayashi, Tomihiro Takahara, Kazutake Yoshizawa, Ryo Oyama, and Keiichiro Imanaka are employees of Janssen Pharmaceutical K.K.

Ethics approval and consent to participate
An independent ethics committee or institutional review board approved the protocols, and the trials were conducted in accordance with the ethical principles in the Declaration of Helsinki and consistent with the Good Clinical Practices and applicable regulatory requirements. All patients provided written informed consent before entering the original trials.

Author details
[1]Medical Affairs Division, Janssen Pharmaceutical K.K., 5-2, Nishi-kanda, 3-Chome, Chiyoda-ku, Tokyo 101-0065, Japan. [2]Research and Development Division, Janssen Pharmaceutical K.K., 5-2, Nishi-kanda, 3-Chome, Chiyoda-ku, Tokyo 101-0065, Japan.

References

1. Fitzmaurice C, Dicker D, Pain A, Hamavid H, Moradi-Lakeh M, MacIntyre MF, Allen C, Hansen G, Woodbrook R, Wolfe C, et al. The global burden of cancer 2013. JAMA Oncol. 2015;1(4):505–27.
2. Huggins C, Masina MH, Eichelberger L, Wharton JD. Quantitative studies of prostatic secretion : I. Characteristics of the normal secretion; the influence of thyroid, suprarenal, and tstis extirpation and androgen substitution on the prostatic output. J Exp Med. 1939;70(6):543–56.
3. Barrie SE, Potter GA, Goddard PM, Haynes BP, Dowsett M, Jarman M. Pharmacology of novel steroidal inhibitors of cytochrome P450(17) alpha (17 alpha-hydroxylase/C17-20 lyase). J Steroid Biochem Mol Biol. 1994; 50(5–6):267–73.
4. de Bono JS, Logothetis CJ, Molina A, Fizazi K, North S, Chu L, Chi KN, Jones RJ, Goodman OB, Jr., Saad F, et al. Abiraterone and increased survival in metastatic prostate cancer. N Engl J Med. 2011;364(21):1995–2005.
5. Ryan CJ, Smith MR, de Bono JS, Molina A, Logothetis CJ, de Souza P, Fizazi K, Mainwaring P, Piulats JM, Ng S, et al. Abiraterone in metastatic prostate cancer without previous chemotherapy. N Engl J Med. 2013;368(2):138–48.
6. Satoh T, Uemura H, Tanabe K, Nishiyama T, Terai A, Yokomizo A, Nakatani T, Imanaka K, Ozono S, Akaza H. A phase 2 study of abiraterone acetate in Japanese men with metastatic castration-resistant prostate cancer who had received docetaxel-based chemotherapy. Jpn J Clin Oncol. 2014;44(12):1206–15.
7. Matsubara N, Uemura H, Satoh T, Suzuki H, Nishiyama T, Uemura H, Hashine K, Imanaka K, Ozono S, Akaza H. A phase 2 trial of abiraterone acetate in Japanese men with metastatic castration-resistant prostate cancer and without prior chemotherapy (JPN-201 study). Jpn J Clin Oncol. 2014;44(12):1216–26.
8. Scher HI, Halabi S, Tannock I, Morris M, Sternberg CN, Carducci MA, Eisenberger MA, Higano C, Bubley GJ, Dreicer R, et al. Design and end points of clinical trials for patients with progressive prostate cancer and castrate levels of testosterone: recommendations of the Prostate Cancer Clinical Trials Working Group. J Clin Oncol. 2008;26(7):1148–59.
9. Armstrong AJ, Eisenberger MA, Halabi S, Oudard S, Nanus DM, Petrylak DP, Sartor AO, Scher HI. Biomarkers in the management and treatment of men with metastatic castration-resistant prostate cancer. Eur Urol. 2012;61(3):549–59.
10. Collette L, Burzykowski T, Carroll KJ, Newling D, Morris T, Schroder FH. Is prostate-specific antigen a valid surrogate end point for survival in hormonally treated patients with metastatic prostate cancer? Joint research of the European Organisation for Research and Treatment of Cancer, the Limburgs Universitair Centrum, and AstraZeneca Pharmaceuticals. J Clin Oncol. 2005;23(25):6139–48.
11. Halabi S, Armstrong AJ, Sartor O, de Bono J, Kaplan E, Lin CY, Solomon NC, Small EJ. Prostate-specific antigen changes as surrogate for overall survival in men with metastatic castration-resistant prostate cancer treated with second-line chemotherapy. J Clin Oncol. 2013;31(31):3944–50.
12. Caffo O, Veccia A, Maines F, Bonetta A, Spizzo G, Galligioni E. Potential value of rapid prostate-specific antigen decline in identifying primary resistance to abiraterone acetate and enzalutamide. Future Oncol. 2014;10(6):985–93.
13. Xu XS, Ryan CJ, Stuyckens K, Smith MR, Saad F, Griffin TW, Park YC, Yu MK, Vermeulen A, Poggesi I, et al. Correlation between prostate-specific antigen kinetics and overall survival in abiraterone acetate-treated castration-resistant prostate cancer patients. Clin Cancer Res. 2015; 21(14):3170–7.
14. Guccione JR, Ledet EM, Stolten MD, Steinberger AE, Chow LD, Cotogno P, Lewis BE, Sartor AO. Early assessment of PSA response in CRPC patients treated with enzalutamide (Enza) or abiraterone (Abi). ASCO Meeting Abstracts. 2016;34(2_suppl):249.
15. Conteduca V, Crabb SJ, Scarpi E, Hanna C, Maines F, Joyce H, Fabbri P, Derosa L, Massari F, Lolli C, et al. Association between early PSA increase and clinical outcome in patients treated with enzalutamide for metastatic castration resistant prostate cancer. ASCO Meeting Abstracts. 2016;34(2_suppl):231.
16. Bubley GJ, Carducci M, Dahut W, Dawson N, Daliani D, Eisenberger M, Figg WD, Freidlin B, Halabi S, Hudes G, et al. Eligibility and response guidelines for phase II clinical trials in androgen-independent prostate cancer: recommendations from the Prostate-Specific Antigen Working Group. J Clin Oncol. 1999;17(11):3461–7.
17. Hoffman-Censits J, Kelly WK. Enzalutamide: a novel antiandrogen for patients with castrate-resistant prostate cancer. Clin Cancer Res. 2013; 19(6):1335–9.
18. Olbert PJ, Hegele A, Kraeuter P, Heidenreich A, Hofmann R, Schrader AJ. Clinical significance of a prostate-specific antigen flare phenomenon in patients with hormone-refractory prostate cancer receiving docetaxel. Anticancer Drugs. 2006;17(8):993–6.
19. Burgio SL, Conteduca V, Rudnas B, Carrozza F, Campadelli E, Bianchi E, Fabbri P, Montanari M, Carretta E, Menna C, et al. PSA flare with abiraterone in patients with metastatic castration-resistant prostate cancer. Clin Genitourin Cancer. 2015;13(1):39–43.
20. Narmala SK, Boulmay BC. PSA flare after initiation of abiraterone acetate. J Community Support Oncol. 2014;12(5):191–2.
21. Nelius T, Klatte T, de Riese W, Filleur S. Impact of PSA flare-up in patients with hormone-refractory prostate cancer undergoing chemotherapy. Int Urol Nephrol. 2008;40(1):97–104.
22. Angelergues A, Maillet D, Flechon A, Ozguroglu M, Mercier F, Guillot A, Le Moulec S, Gravis G, Beuzeboc P, Massard C, et al. Prostate-specific antigen flare induced by cabazitaxel-based chemotherapy in patients with metastatic castration-resistant prostate cancer. Eur J Cancer. 2014;50(9):1602–9.

23

Level of invasion into fibromuscular band is an independent factor for positive surgical margin and biochemical recurrence in men with organ confined prostate cancer

Aram Kim[4], Myong Kim[1], Se Un Jeong[2], Cheryn Song[1], Yong Mee Cho[2], Jae Yoon Ro[3] and Hanjong Ahn[1*]

Abstract

Background: This study aimed investigate the effect of the level of invasion into fibromuscular band (FMB) of prostate on the positive surgical margin (PSM) and biochemical recurrence (BCR) after radical prostatectomy (RP) in patients with organ-confined (pT2) prostate cancer.

Methods: The clinical and pathological data of 461 consecutive patients with pT2 prostate cancer were evaluated regarding the level of invasion into FMB. The relationship between levels of invasion into FMB and PSM / BCR was assessed.

Results: The rate of PSM at an FMB level of at 2 was 18.8%, which was significantly greater than the rates at levels 0 (5.4%) and 1 (7.8%). The level of FMB ($p = 0.007$) and percentage of tumor volume ($p = 0.012$) were identified as independent factors predictive of a positive surgical margin in a multivariate analysis. The 5-year BCR-free survival rates for a level 0–1 FMB with negative surgical margin, level 0–1 FMB with positive surgical margin, level 2 FMB with negative surgical margin, and level 2 FMB with positive surgical margin were 96.6%, 86.4%, 85.6%, and 72.9%, respectively ($p < 0.001$). A level 2 FMB ($p = 0.050$), positive surgical margin ($p = 0.001$), and surgical Gleason score ($p = 0.001$) were identified as independent predictors of a BCR of pT2 prostate cancer.

Conclusions: Among patients with negative surgical margins, the surgical Gleason score and level of FMB independently affected the incidence of a BCR of pT2 prostate cancer. The level of FMB was an independent predictor of both a positive surgical margin and a BCR of pT2 disease. Accordingly, the level of FMB might help to further stratify the prognosis of patients with pT2 disease.

Keywords: Organ confined prostate cancer, Biochemical recurrence, Positive surgical margin, Fibromuscular band, Predictive factor

Background

All oncologic surgeries aim to completely remove cancers. Therefore, the presence of a positive surgical margin (PSM) after radical prostatectomy (RP) for prostate cancer is considered an adverse event in curing this cancer, with outcome associated with prostate specific antigen (PSA) biochemical recurrence (BCR) and poor outcome [1, 2]. The reported rates of PSMs among pathologically localized prostatectomy specimens vary from 6.5% to 38% in contemporary series of RP [1, 3]. The rate of PSM for pT2 prostate cancers is thought to reflect the surgeon's experience [4, 5]. However, tumor-behavioral factors might also influence the rate of PSM for organ-confined prostate cancer. A large-volume tumor adjacent to the prostatic capsule may be prone to a PSM if the surgeon rigorously attempts to preserve the nerves and maximize the remaining functioning urethra. The level of prostatic capsular invasion, which focuses on the extra-prostatic extension (EPE), was reported to affect the incidence of BCR [6]. However, recent articles

* Correspondence: hjahn@amc.seoul.kr
[1]Department of Urology, Asan Medical Center, University of Ulsan College of Medicine, 88 Olympic-Ro 43 Gil Songpa-Gu, Seoul 05505, Republic of Korea
Full list of author information is available at the end of the article

have avoided the term "prostatic capsule" [6–8], as the prostate does not have a true capsule at the apex, anterior side, and base. Therefore, we instead revisited the level of invasion into fibromuscular band (FMB) as an independent factor for a PSM or BCR in patients with organ-confined prostate cancer. We hypothesized that the level of invasion into FMB would be an independent tumor-behavioral factor that could affect the rates of PSM and BCR in patients with pT2 prostate cancer.

Methods

Patient selection

We reviewed 473 patients with pT2 prostate cancer who had undergone RP (robotic: 369, open: 104) at our hospital from January 2010 to March 2014. We excluded four patients who received neoadjuvant treatment and eight patients for whom complete clinical data were unavailable or who were lost to follow-up. Eventually, 461 patients were enrolled, with a median follow-up of 51.2 (range: 1.9–74.9) months. The serum PSA levels were measured at 3-month intervals during the first year after RP, 6-month intervals during years 2–5, and annually thereafter. A BCR was defined as a PSA level > 0.2 ng/mL.

Pathologic evaluation and determination of the level of invasion into fibromuscular band

All surgical specimens were assessed microscopically after histological sectioning. Each specimen was weighed, and the external surface was covered in India ink prior to fixation in 10% formalin. Each specimen was examined in 3–5 mm sections from the base to the apex, perpendicular to the major. Subsequently, the sections were divided into halves or quadrants to fit the cassettes routinely used for paraffin embedding, and slide-mounted thin sections were stained with hematoxylin-eosin. Primary and secondary Gleason scores were assigned to the total cancer within the specimen, according to the revised (2005) criteria for Gleason scoring [9]. Each specimen was staged according to the 2010 American Joint Committee on Cancer staging system [10]. The presence of cancer cells in the inked surface of RP specimen was considered a positive surgical margin [11]. The percentage of tumor volume (PTV) was estimated by the sum of visually determined tumor foci relative to the prostate gland on every section, and categorized into three groups: < 5%, 5–15.0%, and > 15.0%. The levels of EPE were classified as 0, 1, and 2 according to the classification by Wheeler et al. (Fig. 1) [12]. In level 0, the cancer cells are located in the prostatic stroma with a normal gland. Level 1 involves cancer cells within the prostatic stroma but beyond the boundary of normal gland. Level 2 involves cancer cells confined to the prostate, within a layer more fibrous than muscular. We used the highest level of FMB if there were several tumors in prostate and the levels of FMB were evaluated and confirmed by 2 pathologists.

Statistical analysis

The patients' clinical and pathological characteristics were compared according to the levels of EPE, using the χ^2 test (categorical variables) and Student's *t*-test (continuous variables). Uni- and multivariate binary logistic regression analyses were performed to determine the pre- and post-operative variables predictive of a PSM. The 5-year BCR-free survival rate after RP was estimated using the Kaplan–Meier method. Cox proportional hazard analyses were performed to identify the prognostic factors affecting the incidence of BCR. All statistical analyses were performed using commercially available software (SPSS® version 21.0, IBM, Chicago, IL, USA), and a p value < 0.05 was considered statistically significant.

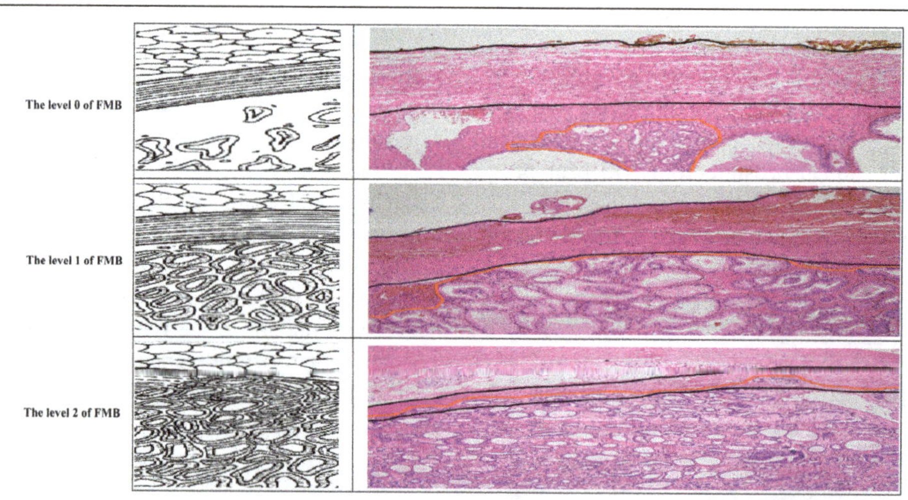

Fig. 1 Illustration and microscopic images of the level of invasion into fibromuscular band (black line: fibromuscular band; red line: prostate cancer)

Results

Comparison of clinical features according to the level of invasion into fibromuscular band

The patients' clinical and pathological characteristics are summarized in Table 1. A higher clinical T stage, percentage of positive cores, and biopsy Gleason score were more frequently observed among patients with level 2 FMB, compared to those with levels 0 and 1. The PTV increased significantly according to the level of FMB, and higher surgical Gleason scores were more frequent with a level 2 FMB than with a level 0 or 1 FMB (all $p < 0.001$). Other parameters such as the PSA and prostate size did not differ significantly among the three groups (p range, 0.426–0.672; Table 1).

Associations between the level of invasion into fibromuscular band and PSM after RP

The rates of PSM at a level 2 FMB (18.7%) were significantly greater than those at levels 0 (5.4%) and 1 (7.8%) ($p = 0.001$), whereas this parameter did not differ significantly between levels 0 and 1 ($p = 0.495$; Table 1). In a univariate analysis with postoperative variables, the PTV (p = 0.001) and level of FMB ($p = 0.001$) were significant factors affecting the PSM. The PTV ($p = 0.012$) and level of EPE ($p = 0.007$) were also identified as independent factors in a multivariate analysis (Table 2).

Associations between the level of invasion into fibromuscular band and BCR-free survival after RP

During the follow-up period, 29 patients (6.2%) experienced a BCR at a mean interval of 28.8 months after RP. Overall, the 5-year BCR-free survival rate was 92.4%. The 5-year BCR-free survival rates of patients with level 0–1 FMB and level 2 FMB were 95.4% and 84.2%, respectively ($p = 0.002$; Fig. 2a), and those of patients with a negative surgical margin and PSM were 94.4% and 78.5%, respectively ($p < 0.001$; Fig. 2b). The 5-year BCR-free survival rates of patients with Gleason scores of 6, 3 + 4, 4 + 3 and 8–10 were 97.6%, 94.5%, 86.7%, and 76.6%, respectively (p < 0.001).

When patients were stratified by margin status and level of FMB (level 0–1 vs. level 2), the 5-year BCR-free survival rates of those with a level 0–1 FMB and negative surgical margin, level 0–1 FMB and PSM, level 2 FMB and negative surgical margin, and level 2 FMB and PSM were 96.6%, 86.4%, 85.6%, and 72.9%, respectively ($p < 0.001$; Fig. 2c). Patients with a level 0–1 FMB and PSM did not significantly differ from those with a level 2 FMB and negative surgical margin in terms of survival ($p = 0.578$). Among the subgroups with surgical Gleason scores greater than 4 + 3, the corresponding survival rates were 88.4%, 87.2%, 76.2%, and 53.3%, respectively ($p = 0.012$; Fig. 2d).

A multivariate analysis of postoperative variables predictive of a BCR identified the surgical Gleason

Table 1 Clinical and pathological characteristics of the patients with pT2 prostate cancer

Level of FMB	Total	Level 0	Level 1	Level 2	*p* value
No. of patients	461	74	243	144	
Mean PSA (ng/mL)	6.6	6.5	6.5	7.0	0.672
Prostate size (cc)	36.0	37.8	35.2	36.5	0.426
Mean % of positive biopsy cores	20.2	13.0	19.0	26.2	< 0.001
Clinical stage					0.031
cT1	257	53	130	73	
≥ cT2	204	21	113	71	
Biopsy Gleason score, No.					< 0.001
6	197	50	104	43	
3 + 4	160	19	84	57	
4 + 3	71	2	38	31	
8–10	33	3	17	13	
Surgical Gleason score, No.					< 0.001
6	124	41	65	18	
3 + 4	205	26	110	69	
4 + 3	99	4	51	44	
8–10	33	3	17	13	
Mean PTV	8.7	3.5	8.4	11.5	< 0.001
Rate of PSM, N (%)	50 (10.8%)	4 (5.4%)	19 (7.8%)	27 (18.7%)	0.001

FMB fibromuscular band, *PSA* prostate specific antigen, *PTV* percentage of tumor volume, *PSM* positive surgical margin

Table 2 Risk factors for PSM after radical prostatectomy in pT2 prostate cancer

	Univariate analysis		Multivariate analysis	
	OR (95% CI)	*p* value	OR (95% CI)	*p* value
PSA	1.036 (0.994–1.080)	0.092		
Level of FMB		0.001		0.007
Level 0–1	Reference		Reference	
Level 2	2.817 (1.561–5.083)		2.303 (1.252–4.235)	
PTV		0.001		0.012
Lesser than 5%	Reference		Reference	
5–15.0%	1.793 (0.814–3.948)	0.147	1.600 (0.720–3.557)	0.249
Greater than 15.0%	4.147 (1.863–9.231)	< 0.001	3.293 (1.447–7.498)	0.005
Surgical Gleason score		0.130		
6	Reference			
3 + 4	2.178 (0.909–5.219)	0.081		
4 + 3	3.092 (1.218–7.849)	0.018		
8–10	2.266 (0.621–8.267)	0.215		

PSA prostate specific antigen, *FMB* fibromuscular band, *PTV* percentage of tumor volume, *PSM* positive surgical margin

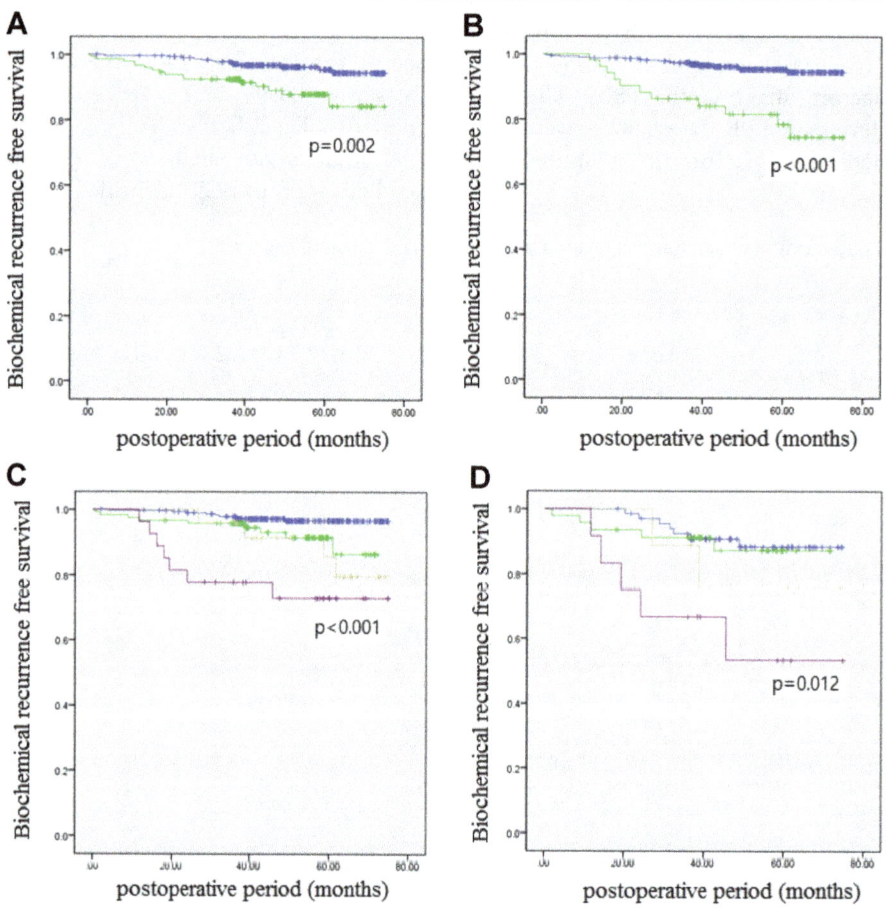

Fig. 2 Biochemical recurrence-free survival over time in patients with pT2 prostate cancer and (**a**) a level 0–1 FMB (Blue) vs. level 2 FMB (Green); **b** negative surgical margin (Blue) vs. positive surgical margin (Green); **c** level 0–1 FMB and NSM (Blue) vs. level 0–1 FMB and PSM (Green) vs. level 2 FMB and NSM (Yellow) vs. level 2 FMB and PSM (Purple); **d** Among patients with a surgical Gleason score > 4 + 3, a level 0–1 FMB and NSM (Blue) vs. level 0–1 FMB and PSM (Green) vs. level 2 FMB and NSM (Yellow) vs. level 2 FMB and PSM (Purple)

score ($p = 0.001$), PSM (p = 0.001), and level 2 FMB ($p = 0.050$) as independent predictors (Table 3). Among the subgroups with negative surgical margins, the level of FMB remained an independent prognostic factor for a BCR ($p = 0.045$), along with the surgical Gleason score (p = 0.001) and PSA level ($p < 0.001$).

Discussion

Although the effect of a PSM on long-term cancer-related mortality remains controversial [2, 13], this factor has been proposed as an important predictor of disease progression [14, 15] and one of the strongest determinants of the possibility of benefitting from adjuvant radiotherapy [1]. Among pT2 prostate cancers, a PSM has been considered an iatrogenic factor because these tumors are confined to the prostate; therefore, the surgeons' experience might be important for reducing the incidence of PSM in a prostate-confined cancer [4, 5]. Previous studies have reported dramatically different rates of PSM according to the surgeons' clinical experience [16], and found that the learning curves for surgical margins after open or laparoscopic RP plateaued at approximately 200–250 cases [17, 18]. We also reported a similar experience regarding the learning curves for surgical margins in a robotic RP series, wherein we demonstrated that the robotic RP reached a comparable PSM rate for pT3 disease with a surgical experience exceeding 500 cases [19]. However, even after transcending this learning curve for surgical margins, surgeons are among organ-confined prostate disease. Tumor-behavioral factors, such as the extent of EPE, have been identified as risk factors for a PSM, along with the preoperative PSA level and Gleason score [4, 20]. However, it remains unclear whether the tumor-behavioral factor itself is important in terms of the PSM. We previously identified the PTV as an independent risk factor for a PSM ($p = 0.035$), and both the PTV ($p < 0.001$) and surgical Gleason score (≥8; $p = 0.021$) as independent predictors of a BCR of organ-confined prostate cancer [21].

In this study, we hypothesized that the level of invasion into FMB might be another important tumor-behavioral factor associated with the risks of PSM and BCR after a RP of organ-confined disease. Our current results demonstrated that the level of invasion into FMB was an independent risk factor for a PSM (level 2 PCI; $p = 0.007$), along with the tumor volume ($p = 0.013$; Table 2). Accordingly, the level of invasion into FMB, tumor volume, and surgical Gleason score are tumor-behavioral factors that might promote a PSM after RP for organ-confined prostate cancer. On the whole, these results agree with those in our previous reports [21]. However, the significance of PTV for BCR was not consistent with our previous study, which included an older cohort (2000–2007) and used specialized method of PTV estimation [21]. The mean PTV was higher in our previous study than in the present study (12.1% vs. 8.7%).

We believe that the level of invasion into FMB has important clinical implications for organ-confined prostate cancer. Although a previous study reported that higher levels of prostatic capsular invasion were associated with a more adverse prognosis among patients with prostate

Table 3 Risk factors for BCR after radical prostatectomy (RP) in pT2 prostate cancer

	Univariate analysis		Multivariate analysis	
	HR (95% CI)	*p* value	HR (95% CI)	*p* value
Level of FMB		0.003		0.050
Level 0–1	Reference		Reference	
Level 2	3.067 (1.471–6.393)		2.124 (1.001–4.508)	
Surgical Gleason score		< 0.001		0.001
6	Reference		Reference	
3 + 4	2.417 (0.1513–11.383)	0.264	1.878 (0.395–8.923)	0.428
4 + 3	7.909 (1.770–35.348)	0.007	5.585 (1.229–25.384)	0.026
8–10	14.099 (2.929–67.876)	0.001	10.311 (2.119–50.175)	0.004
PTV		0.084		
Lesser than 5%	Reference			
5–15.0%	2.421 (0.872–6.723)	0.090		
Greater than 15.0%	3.364 (1.150–9.841)	0.027		
Surgical Margin Status		< 0.001		0.001
Negative	Reference		Reference	
Positive	4.813 (2.268–10.213)		3.607 (1.683–7.726)	

BCR biochemical recurrence, *FMB* fibromuscular band, *PTV* percentage of tumor volume

cancer, the authors did not demonstrate whether the level of prostatic capsular invasion was an independent prognostic factor for a BCR of pT2 prostate cancer [6]. In our study, we used the term "fibromuscular band (FMB)" which was commonly accepted instead of "prostatic capsule" [6] and identified the level of invasion into FMB as an independent predictor of a BCR (Table 3). The 5-year BCR-free survival rate among patients with a level 2 FMB and negative surgical margin was similar to that of patients with a level 0–1 FMB group and PSM (86.4% vs. 85.6%; $p = 0.578$; Fig. 2c). Especially, patients with pT2 disease, a level 2 FMB, PSM, and a surgical Gleason score ≥ 4 + 3 had a worse 5-year BCR-free survival rate, compared to patients with a level 0–1 EPE, PSM, and surgical Gleason score ≥ 4 + 3, although this difference failed to reach statistical significance (53.3% vs. 76.2%; $p = 0.225$). The recent American Urology Association (AUA)/American Society for Therapeutic Radiology and Oncology (ASTRO) guideline mandated the use of adjuvant radiation therapy for patients with pT3 prostate cancer, based on the results from several randomized controlled trials [22]. Moreover, several studies of non-organ confined prostate cancer demonstrated that adjuvant radiotherapy significantly reduced the risk of BCR and improved metastasis-free and overall survival [23–25]. Although RP provides decent overall long-term oncologic control and favorable survival rates in patients with organ-confined prostate cancer, we note that the clinical courses might vary depending on the presence of other risk factors. Given the BCR-free survival rates reported for the control arms of previous studies [23–25], we believe that a certain subgroup of patients with pT2 disease will require adjuvant radiotherapy to reduce the risk of BCR after RP. The group with the worst prognosis in the present study, those with pT2 disease, a level 2 FMB, PSM, and surgical Gleason score ≥ 4 + 3, had a 5-year BCR-free survival rate of 53.3%, similar to that of patients with T3b disease in a previous study [26]. We believe that these patients should therefore be considered candidates for adjuvant radiotherapy after RP.

The present study had a retrospective design and relatively small sample size, and there were other limitations, such as a critical reproducibility of the level of invasion into FMB. Pathologists must re-evaluate the level of invasion into FMB, as well as the levels of all tumors. The highest level of FMB should be used for cases involving multiple tumors in the prostate. Furthermore, the effect of the level of invasion into FMB according to the tumor location remains controversial, and additional studies are needed. Despite these limitations, our study attempted to revisit the concept of the level of invasion into FMB as a tumor-behavioral factor in a contemporary RP cohort. External validation studies with larger cohorts or prospectively designed studies are needed to confirm the clinical implications of our findings.

Conclusions

The level of invasion into FMB is an independent tumor-behavioral factor for PSM and BCR in organ-confined prostate cancer. Patients with a level 2 FMB had a higher risk of BCR after RP. Therefore, the level of invasion into FMB might be used to stratify patients with pT2 disease and a poor prognosis.

Abbreviations

BCR: Biochemical recurrence; EPE: Extra-prostatic extension; FMB: Fibromuscular band; PSA: Prostate specific antigen; PSM: Positive surgical margin; PTV: Percentage of tumor volume; RP: Radical prostatectomy

Acknowledgments

Not applicable

Funding

No fund

Authors' contributions

AK collected data, design of the study, analysis interpretation of data and drafted the manuscript. MK and CS contributed to surgeries, the conception and design of the study, SJ contributed to acquisition and analysis of pathologic data and interpretation. YC and JR contributed to slide review and data analysis. All authors read and approved the final manuscript. HA contributed to Study design, data interpretation, drafting the manuscript, final approval of the version to be published.

Competing interests

The authors declare that they have no competing interests.

Author details

[1]Department of Urology, Asan Medical Center, University of Ulsan College of Medicine, 88 Olympic-Ro 43 Gil Songpa-Gu, Seoul 05505, Republic of Korea. [2]Department of Pathology, Asan Medical Center, University of Ulsan College of Medicine, Seoul 05505, Republic of Korea. [3]Department of Pathology and Genomic Medicine, Houston Methodist Hospital, Weill Medical College of Cornell University, Houston, TX 10065, USA. [4]Department of Urology, Konkuk University Medical Center, Konkuk University School of Medicine, Seoul 05030, Republic of Korea.

References

1. Yossepowitch O, et al. Positive surgical margins after radical prostatectomy: a systematic review and contemporary update. Eur Urol. 2014;65(2):303–13.
2. Chalfin HJ, et al. Impact of surgical margin status on prostate-cancer-specific mortality. BJU Int. 2012;110(11):1684–9.

3. Yossepowitch O, et al. Positive surgical margins in radical prostatectomy: outlining the problem and its long-term consequences. Eur Urol. 2009;55(1): 87–99.
4. Eastham JA, et al. Variations among individual surgeons in the rate of positive surgical margins in radical prostatectomy specimens. J Urol. 2003; 170(6 Pt 1):2292–5.
5. Chun FK, et al. Surgical volume is related to the rate of positive surgical margins at radical prostatectomy in European patients. BJU Int. 2006;98(6): 1204–9.
6. Wheeler TM, et al. Clinical and pathological significance of the level and extent of capsular invasion in clinical stage T1-2 prostate cancer. Hum Pathol. 1998;29(8):856–62.
7. Ayala AG, et al. The prostatic capsule: does it exist? Its importance in the staging and treatment of prostatic carcinoma. Am J Surg Pathol. 1989;13(1):21–7.
8. Paluru S, Epstein JI. Does the distance between tumor and margin in radical prostatectomy specimens correlate with prognosis: relation to tumor location. Hum Pathol. 2016;56:11–5.
9. Epstein JI, et al. The 2005 International Society of Urological Pathology (ISUP) consensus conference on Gleason grading of prostatic carcinoma. Am J Surg Pathol. 2005;29(9):1228–42.
10. Edge, S.B., et al., *Prostate*, in *AJCC cancer staging manual*, American joint committee on Cancer, Editor. 2010, Springer: New York. p. 457–468.
11. Epstein JI, et al. Prognostic factors and reporting of prostate carcinoma in radical prostatectomy and pelvic lymphadenectomy specimens. Scand J Urol Nephrol Suppl. 2005;216:34–63.
12. Wheeler TM. Anatomic considerations in carcinoma of the prostate. Urol Clin North Am. 1989;16(4):623–34.
13. Stephenson AJ, et al. Do margins matter? The influence of positive surgical margins on prostate cancer-specific mortality. Eur Urol. 2014;65(4):675–80.
14. Stephenson AJ, et al. Location, extent and number of positive surgical margins do not improve accuracy of predicting prostate cancer recurrence after radical prostatectomy. J Urol. 2009;182(4):1357–63.
15. Eastham JA, et al. Prognostic significance of location of positive margins in radical prostatectomy specimens. Urology. 2007;70(5):965–9.
16. Roder MA, et al. Risk factors associated with positive surgical margins following radical prostatectomy for clinically localized prostate cancer: can nerve-sparing surgery increase the risk? Scand J Urol. 2014;48(1):15–20.
17. Secin FP, et al. The learning curve for laparoscopic radical prostatectomy: an international multicenter study. J Urol. 2010;184(6):2291–6.
18. Vickers A, et al. The learning curve for surgical margins after open radical prostatectomy: implications for margin status as an oncological end point. J Urol. 2010;183(4):1360–5.
19. Park J, et al. Comparison of oncological outcomes between retropubic radical prostatectomy and robot-assisted radical prostatectomy: an analysis stratified by surgical experience. World J Urol. 2014;32(1):193–9.
20. Wieder JA, Soloway MS. Incidence, etiology, location, prevention and treatment of positive surgical margins after radical prostatectomy for prostate cancer. J Urol. 1998;160(2):299–315.
21. Song C, et al. Tumor volume, surgical margin, and the risk of biochemical recurrence in men with organ-confined prostate cancer. Urol Oncol. 2013; 31(2):168–74.
22. Wiegel T, et al. Adjuvant radiotherapy versus wait-and-see after radical prostatectomy: 10-year follow-up of the ARO 96-02/AUO AP 09/95 trial. Eur Urol. 2014;66(2):243–50.
23. Bolla M, et al. Postoperative radiotherapy after radical prostatectomy for high-risk prostate cancer: long-term results of a randomised controlled trial (EORTC trial 22911). Lancet. 2012;380(9858):2018–27.
24. Thompson IM, et al. Adjuvant radiotherapy for pathological T3N0M0 prostate cancer significantly reduces risk of metastases and improves survival: long-term followup of a randomized clinical trial. J Urol. 2009; 181(3):956–62.
25. Wiegel T, et al. Phase III postoperative adjuvant radiotherapy after radical prostatectomy compared with radical prostatectomy alone in pT3 prostate cancer with postoperative undetectable prostate-specific antigen: ARO 96-02/AUO AP 09/95. J Clin Oncol. 2009;27(18):2924–30.
26. Steuber T, et al. Comparative assessment of the 1992 and 2002 pathologic T3 substages for the prediction of biochemical recurrence after radical prostatectomy. Cancer. 2006;106(4):775–82.

Anti-tumor effects of a recombinant anti-prostate specific membrane antigen immunotoxin against prostate cancer cells

Ping Meng[1†], Qing-chuan Dong[2†], Guang-guo Tan[3], Wei-hong Wen[4], He Wang[5], Geng Zhang[1], Yan-zhu Wang[1], Yu-ming Jing[1], Chen Wang[6], Wei-jun Qin[1*] and Jian-lin Yuan[1*]

Abstract

Background: To evaluate anti-prostate cancer effects of a chimeric tumor-targeted killer protein.

Methods: We established a novel fusion gene, immunocasp-3, composed of NH2-terminal leader sequence fused with an anti-prostate-specific membrane antigen (PSMA) antibody (J591), the furin cleavage sequences of diphtheria toxin (Fdt), and the reverse coding sequences of the large and small subunits of caspase-3 (revcaspase-3). The expressing level of the immunocasp-3 gene was evaluated by using the reverse transcription-PCR (RT-PCR) and western blot analysis. Cell viability assay and cytotoxicity assay were used to evaluate its anti-tumor effects in vitro. Apoptosis was confirmed by electron microscopy and Annexin V-FITC staining. The antitumor effects of immunocasp-3 were assessed in nude mice xenograft models containing PSMA-overexpressing LNCaP cells.

Results: This study shows that the immunocasp-3 proteins selectively recognized and induced apoptotic death in PSMA-overexpressing LNCaP cells *in vitro*, where apoptotic cells were present in 15.3% of the cells transfected with the immunocasp-3 expression vector at 48 h after the transfection, in contrast to 5.5% in the control cells. Moreover, LNCaP cells were significantly killed under the condition of the co-culture of the immunocasp-3-secreting Jurkat cells and more than 50% of the LNCaP cells died when the two cell lines were co-cultured within 5 days. In addition, The expression of immunocasp-3 also significantly suppressed tumor growth and greatly prolonged the animal survival rate *in vivo*.

Conclusion: A novel fusion gene, immunocasp-3, may represent a viable approach to treating PSMA-positive prostate cancer.

Keywords: Gene therapy, Prostate cancer, Prostate-specific membrane antigen, Recombinant protein, Apoptosis

Background

Prostate cancer is one of the most prevalent malignancy among males in Western countries [1]. Androgen ablation therapy are typically used to treat metastatic prostate cancer and advanced prostate cancer [2]. However, most of prostate cancer eventually develop to castration resistant prostate cancers(CRPC),then progressing rapidly [3]. Therefore, it is urgent to develop new molecule-targeted therapies.

* Correspondence: weijunqfmmu@163.com; jianliny@fmmu.edu.cn
†Equal contributors
[1]Department of Urology, Xijing Hospital, Fourth Military Medical University, Xi'an, Shaanxi, China
Full list of author information is available at the end of the article

Prostate-specific membrane antigen (PSMA) is a type II membrane glycoprotein of 100 kD, containing a transmembrane domain,a short intracellular segment and an extensive extracellular domain [4]. The expression of PSMA was independent of androgen, which was increased along with disease progression and reached to highest level in CRPC [5–7]. Moreover, the expression of PSMA is abundant in new vessels associated with the tumor but not in normal vessels [8–11]. Considering these points, the combination of gene therapy with anti-PSMA antibody represents an ideal treatment measure.

Caspase-3, one of critical cysteine protease family members, takes an important part in the signal transduction pathways that mediate apoptosis in mammalian cells [12]. Cleavage of immunotoxins was mediated by Furin, which was a rate-limiting step for several secreted proteins to produce cytotoxic activity [13]. Wang tao *et al.* described the construction and characterization of e23sFv-Fdt-revcaspase 3 containing the furin cleavage sequences (Diphtheria toxin, $A_{187}GNRVRRSVG_{196}$, Fdt) and concluded that the activity of immunocasp-3 proteins is comparable to that of PEA II-caspase 3, as they contain much less exogenous fragments [14].

To develop a more effective and specific agent for antitumor therapy, we established a novel fusion gene, immunocasp-3 in this work, which was composed of NH2-terminal leader sequence fused with an anti-PSMA antibody (J591), the furin cleavage sequences of diphtheria toxin (Fdt), and the reverse coding sequences of the large and small subunits of caspase-3 (revcaspase-3) (Fig. 1a). The antitumor activities of immunocasp-3 and immunocasp-3 -secreting lymphocytes were evaluated *in vitro* and *in vivo*.

Methods

Cells lines

Two human prostate adenocarcinoma cell lines (LNCaP cells and PC-3 cells) and human Jurkat cells (American Type Culture Collection, Rockville, MD) were cultured in RPMI 1640 medium supplemented with 10% heat-inactivated fetal bovine serum. The response to PSMA for LNCaP and PC-3 cells was positive and negative, respectively, which has been confirmed in the previous study [15].

Antibodies and plasmids

The hybridoma of J591 was purchased from the American Type Culture Collection (Rockville, MD). The plasmid pCMV-Fdt-revcaspase 3 was provided by Dr. Angang Yang (Fourth Military Medical University, Xi An, China).

Mice

Four-to-six-week-old male nude mice, obtained from the Laboratory Animal Research Center of Fourth Military Medical University. All animal experiments were fully approved by the Administrative Committee of Experimental Animal Care and Use of Fourth Military Medical University, and conformed to the National Institute of Health guidelines on the ethical use of animals.

Plasmids construction

A set of primers to amply the whole variant region sequences of heavy chain(VH) and light chain (VL) of murine antibodies were used to acquire VH and VL gene from hybridoma J591. HindIII, NotI site sequences, and a signal peptide sequence (MKHLWFFLLLVAAPRWVLS) were incorporated into J591 fragments by PCR. Fdt-revcaspase 3 was amplified by PCR using a pCMV-Fdt-revcaspase 3 plasmid as the template. The establishment of the recombinant genes was involved in the sequential fusion of the genes, which could encode J591, Fdt, and revcaspase 3. The recombinant genes were cloned downstream in the expression vector pCMV (Fig. 1a). The vector sequences were validated by DNA sequencing.

Cell transfection

Twenty-four hours prior to transfection, LNCaP cells and PC-3 cells were seeded in 24-well plates at a density of 1×10^5 cells per well. The transfection was performed by using Lipofectamine 2000 (Invitrogen, Carlsbad, CA) according to the standard procedure of the kit. the cells were selected in the medium consisting of 800 μg/ml G418 (Invitrogen, Carlsbad, CA) for two to three weeks. The cells were cultured in the medium consisting of 800 μg/ml G418 (Invitrogen, Carlsbad, CA) for two more weeks to select stable transfection.

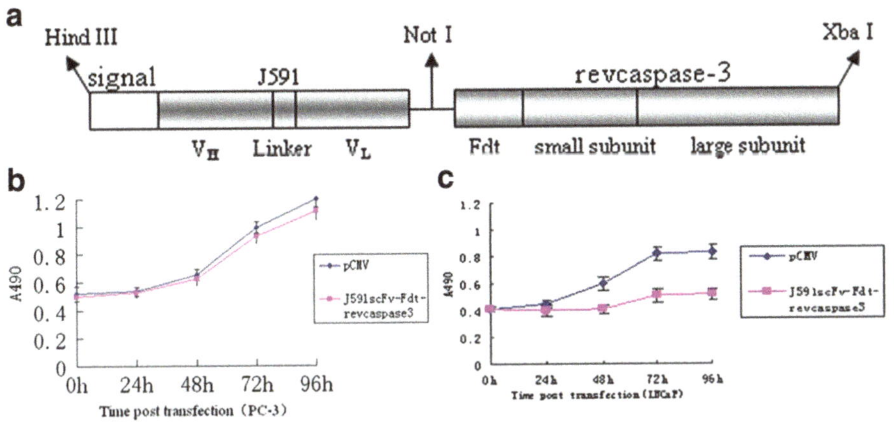

Fig. 1 Expression of immunocasp-3 in PC-3 and LNCaP cells. **a**: Schematic diagram of immunocasp-3 comprising signal sequence, an anti-PSMA antibody (J591), the furin cleavage sequences of diphtheria toxin (Fdt), and reversed caspase-3 (revcaspase-3). MTT assay of PC-3 (**b**) and LNCaP cells (**c**) transfected with immunocasp-3

Cell viability assay

The viability of the cells was assessed using the 3-(4,5-dimethylthiazol-2-yl)-2,5-diphenyltetrazolium bromide (MTT) reduction assay. In the MTT assay, the yellow tetrazolium salt (MTT) is reduced in metabolically active cells to form insoluble purple formazan crystals, which are solubilized by the addition of a detergent. The color can then be quantitated by spectrophotometry. The cells transfected with the immunocasp-3 gene were cultured in 96-well plates for 24 to 96 h. Cells were then incubated with 20 μL of MTT (1.5 mg/mL; Sigma-Aldrich) per well for 4 h at 37 °C. Cells were centrifuged at 800 rpm for 10 min, and then 150 μL of DMSO was added and mixed by gentle pipetting to solubilize the cells. The optical density of the solution was read at 490 nm using a Universal Microplate Reader (Bio-Tek Instruments, Inc.).

Western blot analysis

We separated The lysates of transfected cells and the serum-free supernatant fluids of cells transfected with immunocasp-3 permanently by SDS-PAGE. Then proteins of cells were blotted onto polyvinylidene difluoride membranes (Amersham Pharmacia Biotech), and then we incubated these membranes with primary antibodies which recognize caspase-3 (1:500; BD PharMingen) at 4 °C in PBST overnight. Next, we washed out the primary antibodies and changed to horseradish peroxidase-conjugated secondary antibody (1:2,000; ZhongShan), incubating for 2 h at room temperature. Immunoreactive bands were detected by chemiluminescence kit (Pierce).

Electron microscopy

Pellets of cells were fixed with with 2.5% glutaraldehyde in 0.1 mol/L sodium phosphate buffer (pH 7.4) for 2 h at 4 °C. Then after being washed 3 times, and they were fixed at second time in 1% osmic acid in phosphate buffer before scrapping, dehydration, and embedding. Ultrathin sections mounted on 200 mesh grid were examined in a GEM-2000EX electron microscope.

Cytotoxicity assay in vitro

Transwell filters (Costar), (diameter: 12 mm, pore size: 0.40 μm), which separate the cells but not large molecules, were used for the cocultivation assay. Tumor cells overexpressing PSMA (LNCaP) and control cells expressing undetectable PSMA (PC-3) were placed at the bottom chamber, and the transfected Jurkat cells were placed at the top chamber. Viable cells at the bottom chambers were numbered by trypan blue exclusion at the indicated time points after cocultivation. The percentages of cell killing were calculated as follows: 1 - (the number of cells cocultured with stably transfected Jurkat/the number of cells cocultured with Jurkat controls) × 100%.

Antitumor activity of immunocasp-3 in vivo

Four-to-six-week-old male nude mice were inoculated with 2×10^6 human prostate cancer LNCaP cells by administering a subcutaneous injection of the cells in the right hind flank. Tumors were allowed to grow until they reached a diameter of 5–7 mm (day 0). The mice were then randomly divided into different treatment groups of 5 mice each. One group of mice received 6 doses (twice a week) of 10 μg of pCMV-J591-Fdt-revcaspase 3 mixed with lipofectamine as intramuscular injections administered in the right posterior limb. Another group of 5 mice received 3 weekly intravenous injections of 2×10^6 Jurkat-J591-Fdt-revcaspase 3 cells. The control group was injected with either liposome-mixed empty pCMV vector or unmodified Jurkat cells. Tumor growth was monitored with measurement of 2 perpendicular tumor diameters every 3 days using a caliper, and the volume of the tumor in mice was calculated by formula: tumor volume = $(\text{width})^2 \times \text{length}/2$. The survival time of the mice was assessed. The mice were then sacrificed by cervical dislocation and dissected, tissues were washed and fixed in 10% neutral-buffered formalin, and then embedded in paraffin. These paraffin-embedded tissue sections were dewaxed, hydrated, incubated in 0.3% methanol-H_2O_2 for 20 min to remove endogenous peroxidase and then stained with rabbit anti-human active caspase-3, as described above.

Statistical analysis

Statistical analysis was performed using the SPSS12.0 software package for Windows (SPSS). Survival rates were analyzed by the Kaplan-Meier method, and intergroup comparisons were made using the log-rank test. Statistical significance was defined as $P \leq 0.05$.

Results

Immunocasp-3 fusion proteins expressed in PC-3 and Jurkat cells

PC-3 cells were transiently transfected with the immunocasp-3 expression vector or the pCMV void vector. Translocation was evaluated indirectly by measuring the degree of caspase-3-induced cytotoxicity. The proliferation properties of immunocasp-3-expressing PC-3 cells were similar to those of cells transfected with the pCMV void vector, which suggests that the expression of the immunocasp-3 fusion protein was not toxic (Fig. 1b).

$CD4^+$ Jurkat cells were then transfected with the immunocasp-3 expression vector and stable-expression cells were selected by the G418 selection method; the expression of the vector was expected to induce these cells to secrete the targeted protein, which in turn would kill PSMA-overexpressing tumor cells. The expression of the immunocasp-3 gene was detected by reverse transcription-PCR (RT-PCR) with primers specific to

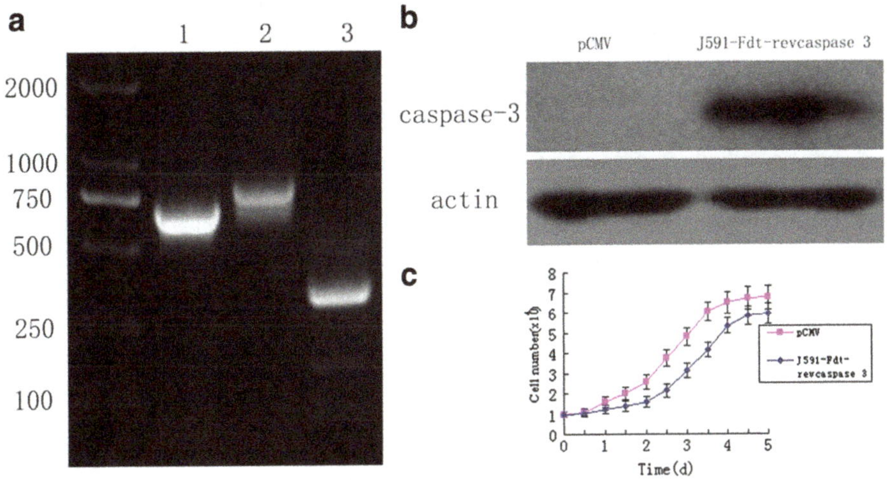

Fig. 2 Detection of immunocasp-3 protein secreted by genetically modified Jurkat cells. **a**: Genomic DNA was isolated from the immunocasp-3-modified Jurkat cell clones and analyzed by PCR: J591 (lane 1); revcaspase-3 (lane 2); β-actin (lane 3), respectively. **b**: Western blot analysis of the concentrated cell culture medium obtained from Jurkat cells stably transfected with the immunocasp-3 gene. Blots were probed with the anti-caspase-3 antibody. **c**: Growth and proliferation characteristics of Jurkat cells transfected with immunocasp-3 or unmodified Jurkat cells

anti-PSMA antibody fragment (J591) and Fdt-revcaspase 3 (Fig. 2a). The expression and secretion of fusion proteins were confirmed by western blot for cell culture supernatants (Fig. 2b). Consequently, the immunocasp-3-modified Jurkat cells remained alive and showed similar growth and proliferation properties to those of unmodified cells (Fig. 2c), suggesting that the expression of the chimeric protein is associated with low toxicity.

Immunocasp-3 fusion proteins specifically kill PSMA-overexpressing tumor cells in vitro

Fusion proteins were transiently expressed in PSMA-positive LNCaP and PSMA-negative PC-3 cells. Cell death was observed apparently in LNCaP (Fig. 1c) cells but not in PC-3 cells at 48 h after transfection. Cytotoxicity was not due to the immunocasp-3 secretion, but rather the result of PSMA expression on the surface of LNCaP cells. Typical apoptotic changes were observed

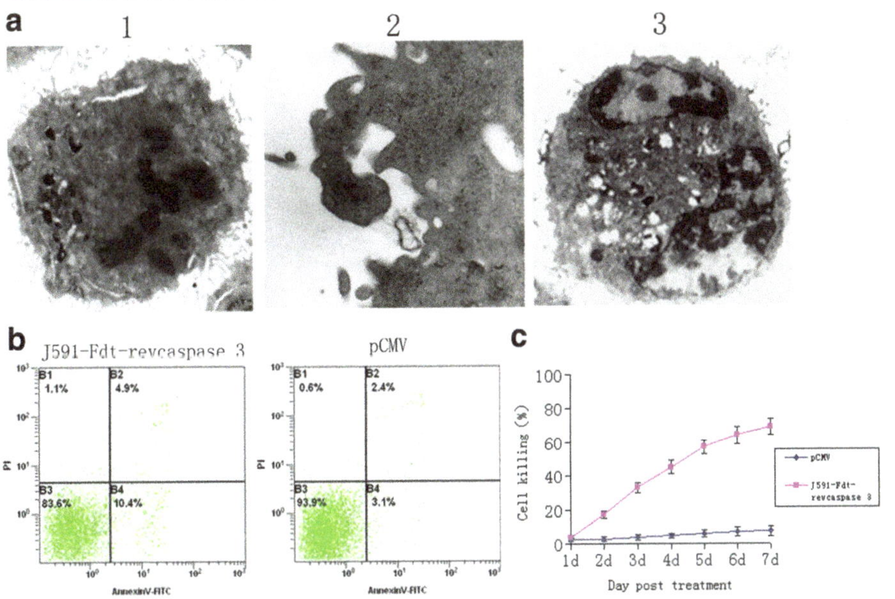

Fig. 3 Immunocasp-3 fusion proteins inhibit the growth of LNCaP cells. **a**: Electronic microscopy of LNCaP 48 h after transfection of immunocasp-3. **b**: 48 h after transfection, LNCaP cells were subjected to Annexin V-FITC staining concomitant with 4,6-diamidino-2-phenylindole nucleus staining and analyzed by flow cytometry. **c**: LNCaP cells were cocultured with immunocasp-3-expressing Jurkat cells for the indicated time points, and the percentages of killing were calculated

in cells expressing immunocasp-3 by the electronic microscope, including chromatin condensation and margination at the nuclear periphery, cellular shrinkage and blebbing, and formation of apoptotic bodies (Fig. 3a). Moreover, using FITC-annexin V staining of the cells, it was revealed that apoptotic cells were present in 15.3% of the cells transfected with the immunocasp-3 expression vector at 48 h after the transfection (Fig. 3b), in contrast to 5.5% in the control cells, a percentage which was higher than that in the control cells. The genetically modified Jurkat cells were then cocultivated in vitro with PSMA-positive LNCaP and PSMA-negative PC-3 cells. The ratio of Jurkat: target cells was adjusted to 3:1, basing on pilot experiments of optimal ratio for cell killing. As shown in Fig. 3c, a significant number of LNCaP cells, but not PC-3 cells, were killed by immunocasp-3-secreting Jurkat cells. More than 50% of the cells had died within 5 days of coculture, and additional killing of PSMA-overexpressing tumor cells was seen after longer times.

Taken together, we conclude that immunocasp-3 proteins are capable of recognizing and killing PSMA-positive LNCaP cells, but not PSMA-negative PC-3 cells in vitro.

Immunocasp-3 fusion proteins effectively suppress the growth of PSMA-overexpressing tumor cells in vivo and prolongs survival in nude mice

The in vivo antitumor activity of immunocasp-3 in nude mice xenograft models containing PSMA-overexpressing LNCaP cells were assessed by measuring the tumor size and animal survival rate. LNCaP cells were subcutaneously inoculated into nude mice to form solid tumors. Murine xenograft models were randomly divided into two treatment groups. One group of mice were received 6 doses of 10 μg of pCMV-J591-Fdt-revcaspase 3, or empty pCMV every 3 days over the course of the study. Another group of prostate cancer-bearing mice received 3 weekly intravenous. injections of 2×10^6 Jurkat cells expressing J591-Fdt-revcaspase-3 or unmodified Jurkat cells. Both the vector-lipofectamine-treated group and Jurkat-cell-treated groups showed greater decrease in tumor volume and longer survival time than controls (Fig. 4a and b). Meanwhile, Jurkat-cell-treated group was more efficient

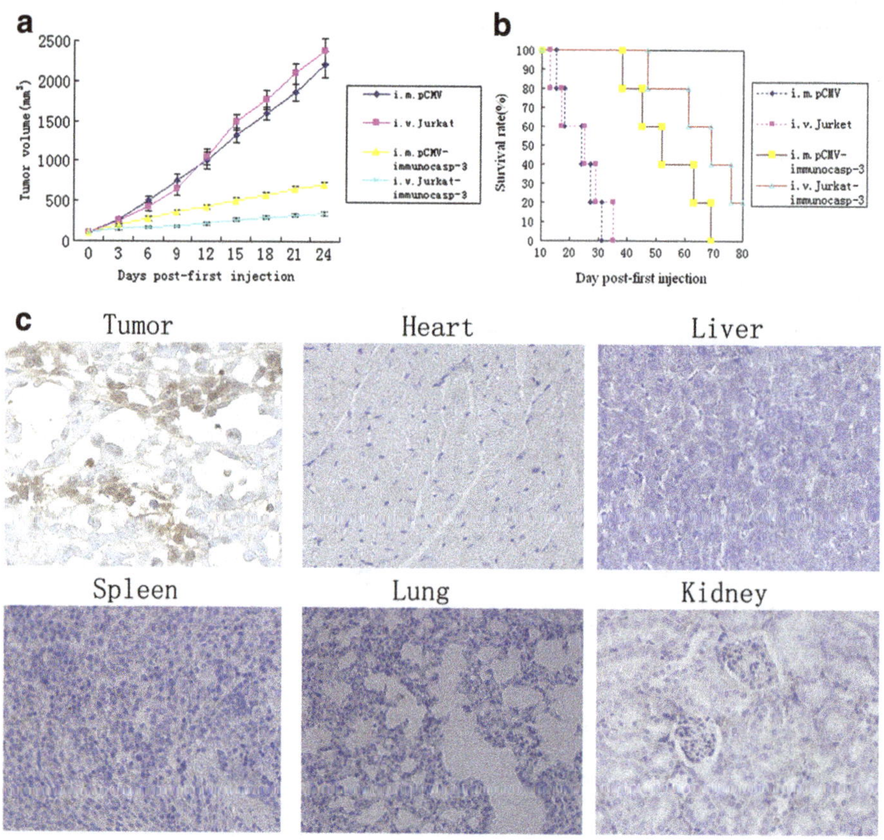

Fig. 4 The antitumor activity of immunocasp-3 on PSMA-overexpressing tumors in vivo. **a**: Tumor volume and tumor growth curves in mice injected with lipofectamine-encapsulated immunocasp-3 gene or pCMV plasmid or with immunocasp-3 gene-modified Jurkat cells or control Jurkat cells. **b**: Survival of mice after treatment, as described in **a.** **c**: Nude mice with LNCaP tumor received 3 weekly intravenous. injections of 2×10^6 immunocasp-3 gene-modified Jurkat cells. Tissues were then subjected to immunohistochemical analysis with an anti-caspase-3 antibody

than the vector-lipofectamine group in reducing tumor size ($P < 0.05$), suggesting that this strategy of gene administration results in more effective and stable antitumor activities in LNCaP xenografts. Immunohistochemical analysis also confirmed the presence of caspase-3 activity in tumors treated with Jurkat cells expressing J591-Fdt-revcaspase 3, but not in the normal tissues (Fig. 4c).

Discussion

Many strategies have been designed to kill cancer cells [16–18]. Because of its restricted and abundant surface expression on prostate cancer cells, PSMA constitutes an attractive target for immunotherapies against prostate cancer. Many papers have already reported that the combination of gene therapy and anti-PSMA antibody receives an ideal therapeutic result [19–24]. Indeed, the antibody used in this study, J591, has been previously used for the treatment of prostate cancer cells [23, 25–29].

Wild-type caspase-3 consists of an NH2-terminal prodomain, a large subunit, and a small subunit. However, active caspase-3, which is constructed with the reverse order of the subunits [30], can induce apoptosis of tumor cells without apoptotic signals; these properties make active caspase-3 an attractive candidate molecule for gene therapy. In this study, the caspase 3 gene was generated by reversing the order of the coding sequences for the large and small subunits [31]. To achieve successful proapoptotic gene therapy for prostate cancer cells, it is necessary to devise a gene construct that expresses the proapoptotic gene selectively in the prostate cells. Therefore, we generated a novel immunocasp-3 gene by fusing a leader sequence, an anti-PSMA antibody (J591) and the furin cleavage sequences of diphtheria toxin (Fdt) to the active revcaspase-3 [14]. The results of our in vitro and in vivo studies revealed that the resultant protein, immunocasp-3, killed PSMA-overexpressing tumor cells, but not PSMA-negative cells. PC-3 cells are PSMA-negative tumor cells. Immunocasp-3 fusion proteins secreted in the culture media cannot enter PC-3 cells via receptor-mediated endocytosis, and thus cause no damage. Our results showed that PC-3 cells expressing recombinant Immunocasp-3 fusion proteins proliferate normally. Once internalized by PSMA-overexpressing tumor cells such as LNCaP cells, immunocasp-3 proteins are exposed to a low-pH environment in the endosome, where the peptide bond in the Fdt domain is cleaved by furin. Then immunocasp-3 proteins release COOH-terminal fragments, which consequently translocate to the cytosol and induce PSMA-overexpressing tumor cells to apoptosis. Both injection of lipofectamine-encapsulated immunocasp-3 and infusion of immunocasp-3 gene-modified Jurkat cells could suppress tumors due to continuous secretion of the killer protein and its diffusion through lymph fluid and blood. However, compared with direct injections of lipofectamine-encapsulated immunocasp-3, the applyment of immunocasp-3 gene-modified Jurkat cells may be a more effective and convenient therapeutic method, which simplified the procedure like protein purification. Moreover, caspase-3 proteins were endogenous human proteins that not only kill prostate cancer cells in a physiological manner, but also resulted in relatively weak immunogenicity and minor general toxicity over repeated administrations. However, because of immunogenicity of murine antibodies, fully human antibodies could become necessary.

Conclusions

The newly immunocasp-3 is both highly specific and effective against PSMA-overexpressing prostate cancer cells. Treatment using this gene merits further investigation and consideration as a molecularly targeted therapeutic measure for prostate cancers.

Abbreviations

MTT: 3-(4,5-dimethylthiazol-2-yl)-2,5-diphenyltetrazolium bromide; PSMA: Anti-prostate-specific membrane antigen; SPSS: Statistical software package for social sciences; VH: Heavy chain; VL: Light chain

Acknowledgements

The authors would like to acknowledge Dr. Angang Yang of the Department of Biochemistry and Molecular Biology, Fourth Military Medical University.

Funding

This study was supported by grants from the National Nature Science Foundation of China (No. 30872582, 81172146, 81372771 and 81301187).

Authors' contributions

YJL, WWH and QWJ created the study design. MP, DQC and TGG performed the cell experiment and drafted the manuscript. WH and ZG constructed the plasmids. WYZ, WC and JYM performed the animal experiment. All the authors read and approved the final manuscript.

Competing interests

The authors declare that they have no competing interests.

Author details

[1]Department of Urology, Xijing Hospital, Fourth Military Medical University, Xi'an, Shaanxi, China. [2]Department of Urology Surgery, Peoples' Hospital of Shaanxi Province, Xi'an, Shaanxi, China. [3]Department of Pharmaceutical Analysis, School of Pharmacy, Fourth Military Medical University, Xi'an, Shaanxi, China. [4]Department of Immunology, Fourth Military Medical University, Xi'an, Shaanxi, China. [5]Department of Urology, Tangdu Hospital, The Fourth Military Medical University, Xi'an, Shaanxi, China. [6]State Key Laboratory of NBC Protection for Civilian, Beijing, China.

References

1. Siegel R, Naishadham D, Jemal A. Cancer statistics, 2013. CA Cancer J Clin. 2013;63(1):11–30.
2. Klein EA, Kupelian PA. Localized prostate cancer: radiation or surgery? Urol Clin North Am. 2003;30(2):315–30. ix.
3. Denmeade SR, Isaacs JT. A history of prostate cancer treatment. Nat Rev Cancer. 2002;2(5):389–96.
4. Israeli RS, Powell CT, Corr JG, Fair WR, Heston WD. Expression of the prostate-specific membrane antigen. Cancer Res. 1994;54(7):1807–11.
5. Chandran SS, Banerjee SR, Mease RC, Pomper MG, Denmeade SR. Characterization of a targeted nanoparticle functionalized with a urea-based inhibitor of prostate-specific membrane antigen (PSMA). Cancer Biol Ther. 2008;7(6):974–82.
6. Chang SS, Reuter VE, Heston WD, Gaudin PB. Comparison of anti-prostate-specific membrane antigen antibodies and other immunomarkers in metastatic prostate carcinoma. Urology. 2001;57(6):1179–83.
7. Marchal C, Redondo M, Padilla M, Caballero J, Rodrigo I, Garcia J, Quian J, Boswick DG. Expression of prostate specific membrane antigen (PSMA) in prostatic adenocarcinoma and prostatic intraepithelial neoplasia. Histol Histopathol. 2004;19(3):715–8.
8. Liu H, Moy P, Kim S, Xia Y, Rajasekaran A, Navarro V, Knudsen B, Bander NH. Monoclonal antibodies to the extracellular domain of prostate-specific membrane antigen also react with tumor vascular endothelium. Cancer Res. 1997;57(17):3629–34.
9. Chang SS, Reuter VE, Heston WD, Bander NH, Grauer LS, Gaudin PB. Five different anti-prostate-specific membrane antigen (PSMA) antibodies confirm PSMA expression in tumor-associated neovasculature. Cancer Res. 1999;59(13):3192–8.
10. Chang SS, O'Keefe DS, Bacich DJ, Reuter VE, Heston WD, Gaudin PB. Prostate-specific membrane antigen is produced in tumor-associated neovasculature. Clin Cancer Res. 1999;5(10):2674–81.
11. Kinoshita Y, Kuratsukuri K, Landas S, Imaida K, Rovito Jr PM, Wang CY, Haas GP. Expression of prostate-specific membrane antigen in normal and malignant human tissues. World J Surg. 2006;30(4):628–36.
12. Thornberry NA, Lazebnik Y. Caspases: enemies within. Science. 1998; 281(5381):1312–6.
13. Chiron MF, Fryling CM, FitzGerald D. Furin-mediated cleavage of Pseudomonas exotoxin-derived chimeric toxins. J Biol Chem. 1997;272(50): 31707–11.
14. Wang T, Zhao J, Ren JL, Zhang L, Wen WH, Zhang R, Qin WW, Jia LT, Yao LB, Zhang YQ, et al. Recombinant immunoproapoptotic proteins with furin site can translocate and kill HER2-positive cancer cells. Cancer Res. 2007; 67(24):11830–9.
15. Ikegami S, Yamakami K, Ono T, Sato M, Suzuki S, Yoshimura I, Asano T, Hayakawa M, Tadakuma T. Targeting gene therapy for prostate cancer cells by liposomes complexed with anti-prostate-specific membrane antigen monoclonal antibody. Hum Gene Ther. 2006;17(10):997–1005.
16. Portsmouth D, Hlavaty J, Renner M. Suicide genes for cancer therapy. Mol Aspects Med. 2007;28(1):4–41.
17. Springer CJ, Niculescu-Duvaz I. Prodrug-activating systems in suicide gene therapy. J Clin Invest. 2000;105(9):1161–7.
18. Yazawa K, Fisher WE, Brunicardi FC. Current progress in suicide gene therapy for cancer. World J Surg. 2002;26(7):783–9.
19. Zhao FJ, Zhang S, Yu ZM, Xia SJ, Li H. Specific targeting of prostate cancer cells in vitro by the suicide gene/prodrug system, uracil phosphoribosyltransferase/5-fluorouracil, under the control of prostate-specific membrane antigen promoter/enhancer. Prostate Cancer Prostatic Dis. 2009;12(2):166–71.
20. Kularatne SA, Zhou Z, Yang J, Post CB, Low PS. Design, synthesis, and preclinical evaluation of prostate-specific membrane antigen targeted (99 m)Tc-radioimaging agents. Mol Pharm. 2009;6(3):790–800.
21. Wolf P, Alt K, Buhler P, Katzenwadel A, Wetterauer U, Tacke M, Elsasser-Beile U. Anti-PSMA immunotoxin as novel treatment for prostate cancer? High and specific antitumor activity on human prostate xenograft tumors in SCID mice. Prostate. 2008;68(2):129–38.
22. Wolf P, Gierschner D, Buhler P, Wetterauer U, Elsasser-Beile U. A recombinant PSMA-specific single-chain immunotoxin has potent and selective toxicity against prostate cancer cells. Cancer Immunol Immunother. 2006;55(11):1367–73.
23. Fracasso G, Bellisola G, Cingarlini S, Castelletti D, Prayer-Galetti T, Pagano F, Tridente G, Colombatti M. Anti-tumor effects of toxins targeted to the prostate specific membrane antigen. Prostate. 2002;53(1):9–23.
24. Huang X, Bennett M, Thorpe PE. Anti-tumor effects and lack of side effects in mice of an immunotoxin directed against human and mouse prostate-specific membrane antigen. Prostate. 2004;61(1):1–11.
25. Tagawa ST, Beltran H, Vallabhajosula S, Goldsmith SJ, Osborne J, Matulich D, Petrillo K, Parmar S, Nanus DM, Bander NH. Anti-prostate-specific membrane antigen-based radioimmunotherapy for prostate cancer. Cancer. 2010;116(4 Suppl):1075–83.
26. Wolf P, Freudenberg N, Buhler P, Alt K, Schultze-Seemann W, Wetterauer U, Elsasser-Beile U. Three conformational antibodies specific for different PSMA epitopes are promising diagnostic and therapeutic tools for prostate cancer. Prostate. 2010;70(5):562–9.
27. Liu C, Hasegawa K, Russell SJ, Sadelain M, Peng KW. Prostate-specific membrane antigen retargeted measles virotherapy for the treatment of prostate cancer. Prostate. 2009;69(10):1128–41.
28. Moffatt S, Papasakelariou C, Wiehle S, Cristiano R. Successful in vivo tumor targeting of prostate-specific membrane antigen with a highly efficient J591/PEI/DNA molecular conjugate. Gene Ther. 2006;13(9):761–72.
29. Bander NH, Trabulsi EJ, Kostakoglu L, Yao D, Vallabhajosula S, Smith-Jones P, Joyce MA, Milowsky M, Nanus DM, Goldsmith SJ. Targeting metastatic prostate cancer with radiolabeled monoclonal antibody J591 to the extracellular domain of prostate specific membrane antigen. J Urol. 2003; 170(5):1717–21.
30. Srinivasula SM, Ahmad M, MacFarlane M, Luo Z, Huang Z, Fernandes-Alnemri T, Alnemri ES. Generation of constitutively active recombinant caspases-3 and −6 by rearrangement of their subunits. J Biol Chem. 1998; 273(17):10107–11.
31. Jia LT, Zhang LH, Yu CJ, Zhao J, Xu YM, Gui JH, Jin M, Ji ZL, Wen WH, Wang CJ, et al. Specific tumoricidal activity of a secreted proapoptotic protein consisting of HER2 antibody and constitutively active caspase-3. Cancer Res. 2003;63(12):3257–62.

25

Abiraterone acetate for chemotherapy-naive metastatic castration-resistant prostate cancer

Liancheng Fan[†], Baijun Dong[†], Chenfei Chi[†], Yanqing Wang[†], Yiming Gong[†], Jianjun Sha, Jiahua Pan, Xun Shangguan, Yiran Huang, Lixin Zhou[*] and Wei Xue[*]

Abstract

Background: To evaluate the efficacy and safety of abiraterone acetate (AA) plus prednisone compared with prednisone alone in Asian patients with chemotherapy-naive metastatic castration-resistant prostate cancer (mCRPC), and to identify predictive factors.

Methods: We reviewed the medical records of 60 patients with chemotherapy-naive mCRPC at Renji Hospital who were treated with AA plus prednisone ($n = 43$) or prednisone alone ($n = 17$). All patients were assessed for prostate-specific antigen (PSA) response, PSA progression-free survival (PSA PFS), radiographic progression-free survival (rPFS), and overall survival (OS). The ability of several parameters to predict PSA PFS, rPFS, and OS was studied.

Results: The median follow-up time was 14.0 months (range 7.0–18.5 months), at which time 19 death events had been reported: 11 in the AA + prednisone group and 8 in the prednisone group. The AA + prednisone group had significantly longer median PSA PFS (10.3 vs 3.0 months, $P < 0.001$), rPFS (13.9 vs 3.9 months, $P < 0.001$), and OS (23.3 vs 17.5 months, $P = 0.016$) than the prednisone-alone group. The most frequently reported grade 3 or 4 adverse event in both the AA + prednisone and prednisone-alone groups was elevated alanine aminotransferase level in 5 of 43 patients (11.6%) and 2 of 17 patients (11.8%), respectively. No adverse events led to discontinuation of therapy. In multivariate analysis, time from androgen deprivation therapy (ADT) to castration resistance of ≤18 months was a determinant of shorter OS ($P = 0.007$).

Conclusions: These results support the favourable safety and efficacy profile of AA for the treatment of Asian patients with chemotherapy-naive mCRPC. Longer duration of ADT response was significantly associated with longer survival.

Keywords: Abiraterone, Metastatic castration-resistant prostate cancer, Chemotherapy-naive, Response to previous therapy

* Correspondence: zhou_li_xin@hotmail.com; xuewei@renji.com
[†]Liancheng Fan, Baijun Dong, Chenfei Chi, Yanqing Wang and Yiming Gong contributed equally to this work.
Department of Urology, School of Medicine, Renji Hospital, Shanghai Jiao Tong University, Shanghai 200127, China

Background

Prostate cancer (PC), particularly metastatic castration-resistant prostate cancer (mCRPC), accounts for a large proportion of the global cancer burden [1]. Although most men with PC initially respond to androgen-deprivation therapy (ADT), the response is not sustained and almost all patients eventually progress to a lethal castration-resistant phenotype within 18–24 months [2].

Chemotherapy has been the standard treatment for mCRPC since 2004 [3–5]. More recently, the treatment paradigm had been dramatically altered by the advent of several AR pathway-targeted agents, new-generation chemotherapies, and immunotherapies [6]. Abiraterone acetate (AA) is a potent and selective inhibitor of CYP17, a key enzyme in androgen biosynthesis [7]. AA blocks the transformation of cholesterol to androgens in the testicles, adrenal glands, and tumor, which reduces serum testosterone to undetectable levels [7–9]. The COU-AA-301 and COU-AA-302 trials demonstrated a significantly increased median overall survival (OS) of patients with ECOG-PS (Eastern Cooperative Oncology Group performance status) scores of 0 or 1 when treated both after and before chemotherapy with AA compared with placebo [10–13].

Currently, AA is not commonly used in clinical practice in Asian countries, and little is known about the clinical outcomes of Asian populations with chemotherapy-naive mCRPC treated with AA in real-world clinical practice. Moreover, AA is usually used to treat patients whose ECOG-PS is 2 in clinical practice, unlike the setting of previous clinical trials that included only patients with ECOG-PS of ≤1 [10–13] [14]. In addition, the response rates to AA are currently unpredictable. Thus, the ability to accurately predict response to AA would facilitate clinical decision-making, especially if alternative treatments such as chemotherapy are being considered.

In the present study, we evaluated the efficacy and safety of AA in the treatment of chemotherapy-naive mCRPC patients (ECOG-PS ≤2) at our centre in China and analysed factors predicting the outcome.

Methods

Patient population

Sixty chemotherapy-naive mCRPC patients have written consent and were enrolled in our study between September 2012 and March 2016. We have calculated the sample size of this study based on the previous similar studies [15, 16]. Approval for this study was obtained from the Committee for Ethics of Renji Hospital. Of the 60 patients, 43 have received AA and prednisone and 17 have received prednisone alone. These patients were consecutively enrolled in this study.

Briefly, eligibility criteria were age ≥ 18 years with histologically or cytologically confirmed adenocarcinoma of the prostate; prostate-specific antigen (PSA) progression in accordance with Prostate Cancer Clinical Trials Working Group 2 (PCWG2) criteria or radiographic progression in soft tissue or bone with or without PSA progression; ongoing ADT with a serum testosterone level of < 50 ng/dL (1.7 nmol/L); previous ADT followed by PSA progression after discontinuing the anti-androgen therapy. Patients who had received therapy with ketoconazole for more than 7 days were excluded.

Patients in the AA + prednisone group received AA 1 g orally twice daily (administered as four 250 mg tablets) plus prednisone 5 mg orally twice daily. Patients in the prednisone-alone group received prednisone 5 mg orally twice daily.

Procedures

Radiographic examination with computed tomography and bone scanning were performed every 8 weeks for the first 24 weeks and every 12 weeks thereafter. Clinical safety assessments included laboratory monitoring of blood chemistry, haematological values, kidney function, serum lipids, and PSA at baseline and at monthly visits thereafter.

Efficacy outcomes

The definitions of PSA and radiographic progressive disease were in accordance with the PCWG-2 criteria [17]. The co-primary end points were PSA response rate (proportion of patients achieving ≥50% PSA decline according to Prostate Specific Antigen Working Group criteria), PSA progression-free survival (PSA PFS), radiographic progression-free survival (rPFS), and OS. OS was defined as the time from the first dose to the last follow-up (March 2016) or death. PSA PFS and rPFS were defined as the time from first dose to PSA progression or radiographic progression, respectively, as previously described [17], or the time to last follow-up or death.

Safety analysis

Clinical assessments were conducted at monthly visits and included medical history, vital sign measurements, physical examination, review of concomitant therapy and procedures, and review of adverse events (AEs).

Statistical analysis

The cut-off date for analysis was 17 March 2016. At that time, there had been 11 deaths in the AA + prednisone group (25.58%) and 8 deaths in the prednisone group (47.06%). The median follow-up time was estimated by the Kaplan–Meier method, with death as a censoring

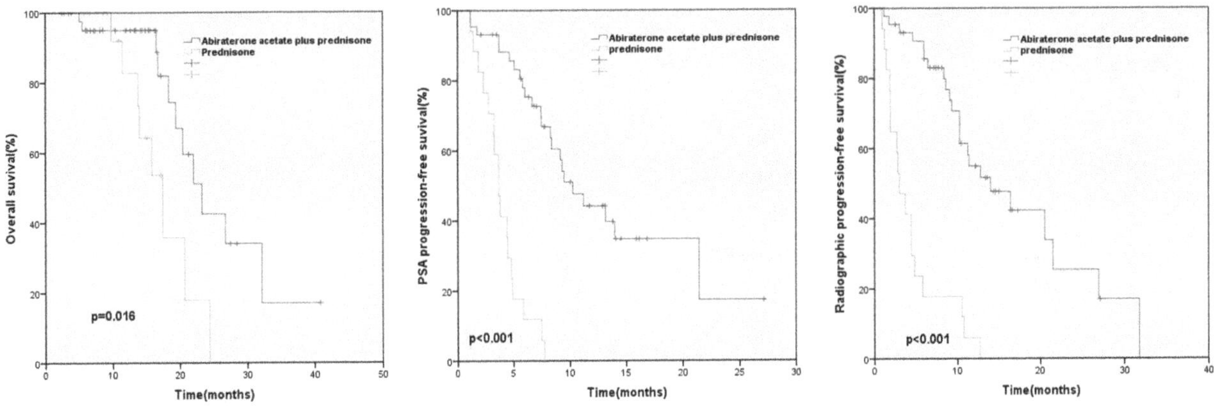

Fig. 1 mCRPC patients in the AA + prednisone group had significantly longer survivals than those in prednisone group

event. Continuous variables, except time from ADT to castration resistance, are reported as the medians with interquartile ranges (IQR) and were analysed by the Wilcoxon signed rank test. The time from ADT to castration resistance was dichotomised by calculating the area under the receiver operating characteristic (ROC) curve to identify the optimal cut-off time. Categorical variables were analysed by chi-square tests. Survival distributions, including PSA PFS, rPFS, and OS, were estimated by the Kaplan–Meier method, and treatment differences were compared using the log-rank test. X^2-test was used to compare group differences in PSA response rates. An exploratory multivariate analysis for OS, PSA PFS, and rPFS was performed using the Cox proportional hazards model, adjusting for known baseline prognostic factors. All tests were two-sided. Differences were considered to be statistically significant at $P < 0.05$. SPSS version 19.0 software was used for all analyses.

Results

Efficacy outcomes

Sixty patients diagnosed with chemotherapy-naive mCRPC at Renji Hospital between September 2012 and March 2016 were enrolled (Raw data was shown in Additional file 1). At the time of follow-up, treatment was ongoing for 20 patients(46.5%) in the AA + prednisone group and no patients (0%) in the prednisone-alone group. The main reason for discontinuation was disease progression for both groups, and no patients stopped treatment because of side effects.

At the median follow-up time of 14.0 months (IQR: 7.0–18.5), 19 deaths had been observed: 11 of 43 patients (25.6%) in the AA + prednisone group and 8 of 17 patients (47.1%) in the prednisone-alone group. PSA progression and radiographic progression were observed in the same number of patients in the AA + prednisone group (both 22 of 43 patients [51.2%]) and in the prednisone-alone group(both 17 of 17 patients [100%]).

The median PSA PFS was significantly longer for the AA + prednisone group than the prednisone-alone group (10.3 months [7.7–12.9]vs 3.0 months [1.7–4.4],$P < 0.001$), as was the median rPFS (13.9 months [8.4–19.5]vs 3.9 months [3.0–4.4],$P < 0.001$), and the median OS (23.3 months [18.8–27.7]vs 17.5 months [13.2–21.8],$P = 0.016$) (Fig. 1). The PSA response rate (≥50% decline) of the AA + prednisone group (27 of 43 patients [62.8%]) was more than five times that of the prednisone-alone group (2 of 17patients [11.8%]). Table 1 summarises the survival outcomes of patients in the AA + prednisone and prednisone-alone groups.

Patient characteristics

In the AA-prednisone group ($n = 43$), the median age was 67 years (63–76). Of the 43 patients, 35 (81.4%) had ECOG-PS scores of 0 or 1,and 8 (18.6%) had an ECOG-PS of 2. Gleason scores were available for all 43 patients; 15 (34.88%) had Gleason scores of < 7 and 28 (65.2%) had 8–10, respectively. The baseline PSA at treatment initiation was 41.5 (range 15.9–239) ng/mL.

Table 1 Comparison of survival outcomes between the AA + prednisone and prednisone-alone groups

	Median OS, months(IQR)	Median PSA PFS,months(IQR)	Median rPFS, months(IQR)	PSA response rate
AA				
+ prednisone group	23.3 (18.8~ 27.7)	10.3 (7.7~ 12.9)	13.9 (8.4~ 19.5)	62.79% (27 of 43)
Prednisone-alone group	17.5 (13.2~ 21.8)	3.0 (1.7~ 4.4)	3.9 (3.0~ 4.4)	11.76% (2 of 17)
P value	0.016	< 0.001	< 0.001	< 0.001

Abbreviations: *AA* abiraterone acetate, *OS* overall survival, *PSA PFS* PSA progression free survival, *rPFS* radiographic progression free survival, *IQR* interquartile range

Table 2 Clinical characteristics of mCRPC patients ($n = 60$)

Parameters	AA group No. of patients(%)	Prednisone-alone group No. of patients(%)	*P* value
Age (median, IQR) years	67(63–76)	67(62.5~ 74.5)	0.8
ECOG PS			1.0
0	22(51.2%)	9(53.0%)	
1	13(30.2%)	5(29.4%)	
2	8(18.6%)	3(17.6%)	
PSA (median, IQR) μg/L	41.6 (15.9~ 239)	46.1(38.0~ 92.4)	0.7
Gleason Score			0.6
≤7	15(4.9%)	7(41.2%)	
>7	28(65.1%)	10(58.8%)	
Metastatic site			
Bone metastasis	42(97.7%)	17(100%)	1
Lymph node metastasis	18(41.9%)	5(29.4%)	0.4
Lung metastasis	1(2.3%)	0(0%)	1
The number of bone metastasis			0.7
0	1(2.3%)	0(0%)	
1~ 3	13(30.2%)	4(23.5%)	
4~ 10	11(25.6%)	3(17.7%)	
> 10	18(41.9%)	10(58.8%)	
PSA PFS(percentage)	23(53.5%)	17(100%)	
rPFS(percentage)	23(53.5%)	8(47.1%)	
OS(percentage)	11(25.6%)	8(47.1%)	
Follow-up time (median, IQR) months	14.2 (7.2–18.4)	13.8 (9.0–17.4)	

Abbreviations: *HR* hazard ratio, *CI* confidence interval, *PSA* prostate-specific antigen, *ALP* alkaline phosphatase, *Hb* hemoglobin, *Alb* albumin, *ECOG PS* Eastern Collaborative Oncology Group performance status, *ADT* androgen deprivation therapy, *IQR* interquartile range

All 43 patients had confirmed metastases; 42 (97.7%) had bone metastases, 17 (39.6%) had lymph node involvement, and 1 (2.3%) had lung metastases. Eleven patients (25.6%)were symptomatic prior to initiation of AA + prednisone therapy.

In the prednisone-alone group ($n = 17$), the median age was 67 years (62.5–74.5), 14 (82.4%) patients had ECOG-PS scores of 0 or 1, and 3 patients (17.6%) had ECOG-PS scores of 2. Seven patients (41.2%) had a Gleason score < 7 and 10 (58.8%) had scores between 8 and 10. The baseline PSA at treatment initiation was 46.6 (range 38–92.4)ng/dL. All 17 patients had confirmed bone metastases and 5 (29.4%)had lymph node involvement. As shown in Table 2, there were no significant differences in the clinical characteristics between patients in the AA + prednisone and prednisone-only groups in this study.

Prognostic factors for chemotherapy-naive mCRPC patients treated with AA

From the ROC curve analysis of the association between OS and the time from ADT to castration resistance, the optimal cut-off value was 18 months (Fig. 2). In univariate analysis, four variables were significant determinants of PSA PFS and OS and three were significant determinants of rPFS (Table 3). Several covariates were important predictors of outcomes in the multivariate survival models (Table 4). Short time from ADT to castration resistance (≤18 months) was a significant

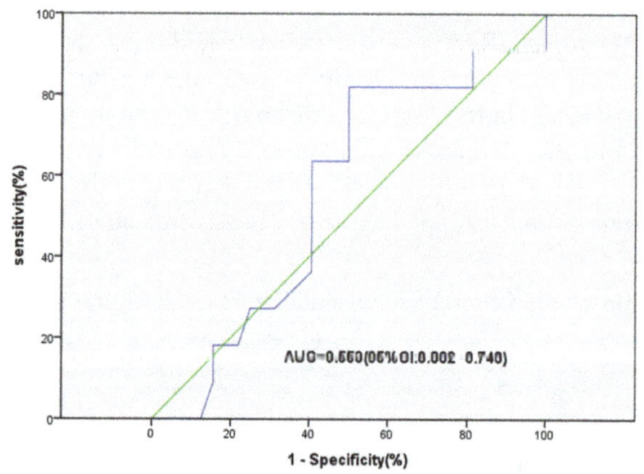

Fig. 2 Receiver operating characteristic curve analysis of the optimal cut-off for the time from ADT to castration resistance

Table 3 Univariate analyses of clinical parameters in mCRPC patients

Parameters	PSA PFS		OS		rPFS	
	HR (95% CI)	*P*-value	HR (95% CI)	P-value	HR (95% CI)	P-value
Age (years)	1.0 (0.9–1.0)	0.1	1.00 (0.9–1.1)	1.0	1.0 (0.9–1.0)	0.06
PSA (μg/L) (> 10 vs ≤10)	3.8 (0.9–16.2)	0.035	26.5 (0.01–49,948.6)	0.08	3.0 (0.7–12.7)	0.09
Gleason Score (> 7 vs ≤7)	0.8 (0.4–1.9)	0.65	1.07 (0.3–3.83)	0.92	0.9 (0.38–2.21)	0.84
ALP (≤120 vs > 120 U/L)	0.3 (0.1–0.7)	0.01	0.2 (0–0.9)	0.05	0.3 (0.09–0.66)	0.01
Hb(g/L)	1.0 (0.97–1.01)	0.34	1.0 (0.90–0.99)	0.029	1.0 (0.95–1.01)	0.14
Alb(g/L)	0.9 (0.8–1.0)	0.15	0.8 (0.6–1.0)	0.04	0.9 (0.8–1.0)	0.05
Time from ADT to castration resistance (≤18 vs > 18 months)	2.9 (1.2–7.1)	0.02	11.2 (2.2–57.7)	0.002	4.0 (1.5–10.7)	0.004
ECOG PS	2.9 (1.4–5.7)	0.004	1.6 (0.6–4.2)	0.34	3.6 (1.7–7.9)	0.001

Abbreviations: *HR* hazard ratio, *CI* confidence interval, *PSA* prostate-specific antigen, *ALP* alkaline phosphatase, *Hb* hemoglobin, *Alb* albumin, *ECOG PS* Eastern Collaborative Oncology Group performance status, *ADT* androgen deprivation therapy, *OS* overall survival, *PSA PFS* PSA progression free survival, *rPFS* radiographic progression free survival

determinant of OS (hazard ratio [HR] = 12.8, 95% confidence interval [CI]: 2.0–83.1, P = 0.007); ECOG-PS score (HR = 2.6, 95% CI 1.2–5.5, P = 0.012), baseline PSA level (HR = 4.9, 95% CI: 1.0–23.0, P = 0.043), and short time from ADT to castration resistance (≤18 months) (HR = 3.4, 95% CI: 1.2–9.4, P = 0.02) were significant determinants of PSA PFS; and ECOG-PS (HR = 3.3, 95%CI: 1.5–7.2, P = 0.003) was also a significant determinant of rPFS.

Safety assessments

The most frequently reported grade 3 or 4 AE(reported in ≥3% of patients) in the AA + prednisone group were elevated alanine aminotransferase (ALT) levels (5 patients [11.6%]), hypokalaemia (4 patients [9.3%]), and hyperglycaemia (2 patients[4.7%]). In the prednisone group, the most frequently reported grade 3 or 4 AEs (reported in ≥3% of patients) were elevated ALT (2 patients [11.8%]), hypokalaemia, (2 patients [11.8%]), and hyperglycaemia(1 patient [5.9%]). None of the AEs resulted in discontinuation of therapy (Table 5).

Discussion

The results of this study support the favourable safety and efficacy profile of AA for the treatment of Asian patients with chemotherapy-naive mCRPC. In addition, we observed that longer (≥18 months) duration of the ADT response was a significant determinant of survival of chemotherapy-naive mCRPC patients treated with AA. These results could serve to guide clinicians in determining whether patients with shorter (< 18 months) times from ADT to castration resistance might benefit more from chemotherapy than from AA.

An international collaborative study (COU-AA-302) confirmed that AA was effective for the treatment of chemotherapy-naive mCRPC patients, and significantly improved rPFS and OS with an acceptable AE profile [10]. In the current study, we demonstrated that AA is equally effective in the treatment of chemotherapy-naive mCRPC of Chinese ethnicity. To our knowledge, this is the first report of the long-term (follow-up > 12 months) efficacy and safety of AA in the treatment of Asian patients with chemotherapy-naive mCRPC.

The median OS and rPFS of our AA cohort (23.27 and 13.93 months, respectively) were shorter than those in the COU-AA-302 trial (34.7 and 16.5 months, respectively) [12] (Table 6). In this regard, a recent study reported a median OS of 18.1 months for chemotherapy-naive Asian mCRPC patients treated with

Table 4 Multivariate analyses of clinical parameters in mCRPC patients

Parameters	PSA PFS		OS		rPFS	
	HR (95% CI)	P-value	HR (95% CI)	P-value	HR (95% CI)	P-value
PSA (μg/L) (> 10 vs ≤10)	4.9 (1.1–23.0)	0.04				
ALP (≤120 vs > 120 U/L)	0.6 (0.2–1.9)	0.37	0.1 (0–1.2)	0.07	0.4 (0.1–1.1)	0.08
Hb(g/L)			1.0 (0.9–1.0)	0.17		
Alb(g/L)			1.1 (0.8–1.5)	0.68		
Time from ADT to castration resistance (≤18 vs > 18 months)	3.4 (1.2–9.4)	0.02	12.8 (2.0–83.1)	0.007	2.6 (0.9~ 7.6)	0.08
ECOG PS	2.6 (1.2–5.5)	0.012			3.3 (1.5–7.2)	0.003

Abbreviations: *HR* hazard ratio, *CI* confidence interval, *PSA* prostate-specific antigen, *ALP* alkaline phosphatase, *Hb* hemoglobin, *Alb* albumin, *ECOG PS* Eastern Collaborative Oncology Group performance status, *ADT* androgen deprivation therapy, *OS* overall survival, *PSA PFS* PSA progression free survival, *rPFS* radiographic progression free survival

Table 5 Grade 3 or 4 adverse events with an incidence of > 3%

Grade 3/4 AEs(reported in ≥3% of patients)	AA group	Prednisone-alone group
ALT increased	11.6% (5 of 43)	11.8% [2 of 17]
Hypokalaemia	9.3% (4 of 43)	11.8% [2 of 17]
Hyperglycaemia	4.7% (2 of 43)	5.9% [1 of 17]

Abbreviations: *ALT* Alanine aminotransferase, *AA* abiraterone acetate

AA, which is much shorter than the 34.7 months reported in the COU-AA-302 study [15]. Furthermore, a recent publication described the results of a bridging study of Asian patients in a randomised, double-blind, placebo-controlled phase 3 clinical trial of AA for mCRPC after docetaxel failure [18]. That study demonstrated a median PSA PFS of 5.5 months after treatment with AA + prednisone, which was also inferior to the PSA PFS outcome in the COU-AA-301 trial (median 8.5 months) [11]. We postulate that inclusion of chemotherapy-naive patients with poor prognostic features in our study could have accounted for the unsatisfactory survival results compared with the COU-AA-302 trial. Of note, in our study, chemotherapy-naive patients with an ECOG-PS score of 2, who were specifically excluded in the COU-AA-302 trial, had significantly inferior survival compared with patients with COG PS 0 and 1. The relative infrequency of post-AA treatment of our patient cohort compared with the COU-AA-302 trial cohort (11.6% versus 67% of patients, respectively) might also have contributed to the shorter survival time reported here (Table 7). Finally, the fact that our patient cohort included symptomatic patients, whereas the COU-AA-302 trial included only asymptomatic or mildly symptomatic patients, could also be a reason for the inferior survival in our study.

In the COU-AA-302 study, dose reduction and discontinuation because of treatment-related AEs were 7 and 7% of patients, respectively [13]. Patients In our study experienced very few AEs overall, and none resulted in discontinuation of drug therapy. Although the AEs may have been surveyed less vigorously in our study compared with clinical trials, AA appeared to be well tolerated by the Asian patients comprising our study.

In the present study, multivariate analysis indicated that shorter time (< 18 months) between ADT and castration resistance predicted worse survival outcome in the patients treated with AA + prednisone. Indeed, Cox regression analysis demonstrated that this was an independent prognostic factor for both OS and PSA PFS. Data from an earlier study showed that the duration of prior ADT is an independent prognostic factor for OS of chemotherapy-naive mCRPC patients(P = 0.002) [19]. However, the time from ADT to castration resistance is probably a better reflection of sensitivity to ADT. We should note that duration of prior hormonal therapy (HT) was defined as the total time to castration resistance plus the time with castration resistance on HT.

Studies of other HTs suggested that a short response to first-line ADT predicts a poor response to subsequent HT [20–22]. In a retrospective study of 436 patients with CRPC treated with secondary HT, the median duration of secondary HT treatment was longer for patients who received primary ADT for > 24 months than for those who received primary ADT for < 24 months ($P < 0.0001$) [20]. In addition, a report of 61 patients with chemotherapy-pretreated CRPC who were treated by AA revealed that duration of the ADT response was an independent predictor of OS($P = 0.006$) [16]. This is consistent with a European consensus statement that short duration of ADT response could identify patients with increased risk of primary resistance to AR pathway-targeted therapies [23]. Polymorphisms in genes in the androgen metabolic pathway were reported to be significantly associated with time to progression on ADT, suggesting that shorter time to castration resistance may be associated with poorer response to ADT rather than to chemotherapy. This might also explain how the duration of response to previous ADT may influence the prognosis of CRPC patients treated with AA [24, 25].

Azad et al. [26] studied the prognostic significance of ECOG-PS and found that it was a significant predictor of PFS ($P = 0.043$), OS ($P < 0.001$), and PSA decline (P = 0.002). Our results showing that ECOG-PS was a significant determinant of rPFS and PSA PFS are consistent with that study.

It is interesting to note that treatment with AA early in the disease course may contribute to better survival. Considering the results of our multivariate analysis showing that ECOG-PS score was a significant

Table 6 Comparison of survival outcomesin the COU-AA-302 study and our study

	Median OS, months	Median PSA PFS, months	Median rPFS, months
Present study (AA plus prednisone group)	23.3	10.3	13.9
COU-AA-302 study	34.7	–	16.5

Abbreviations: *OS* overall survival, *PSA PFS PSA* progression free survival, *rPFS* radiographic progression free survival, *AA* abiraterone acetate

Table 7 Subsequent therapy for prostate cancer

	Percentage of patients (AA group in the present trial) (*N* = 43)	Percentage of patients (COU-AA-302 trial) (*N* = 546)
Patients with subsequent therapy	14.0%(6 of 43)	67% (365 of 546)
AA	2.3% (1 of 43)	13%(69 of 546)
Docetaxel	2.3% (1 of 43)	57%(311 of 546)
Estramustine phosphate	4.7% (2 of 43)	0
Radium-223	7% (3 of 43)	4%(20 of 546)

Abbreviations: *AA* abiraterone acetate

determinant of both rPFS (HR = 2.606, $P = 0.012$) and PSA PFS (HR = 3.379, $P = 0.02$) and that baseline PSA level was a significant determinant of rPFS (HR = 4.914, $P = 0.043$), we postulate that better physical status may contribute to better survival outcomes of mCRPC patients treated with AA. We also found that just as comparative experimental results between COU-AA-301 trial and COU-AA-302 trial [10–13], the survival outcome of patients in our study was superior to that of Asian mCRPC patients treated with AA after docetaxel failure [18] in spite of being lack of OS because of short follow-up period (12.9 months) and limited number of observed death events (PSA PFS 10.27 months vs 5.5 months). These findings strengthen the rationale for the use of AA early in the clinical course of Asian mCRPC patients.

The study had some limitations. First, this study was a retrospective study which had a small sample size and was completed at a single centre. However, we consider this limitation would not influence the ability to capture the real survival outcome of AA in this study. Second, the number of patients in the AA + prednisone and prednisone-alone groups were unequal, which may have biased the results. Finally, the follow-up time was short and we do not know if the inferior survival outcomes reported here will continue at later follow-up times. In addition, another follow-up study will be planned in the future to evaluate the effect of sequential therapies.

The prognostic factors identified here should be validated, and we encourage others to continue the analysis of patients with mCRPC in different treatment settings, such as second-line chemotherapy, enzalutamide, or radium-223, for example. Such studies will aid in the development of optimised therapy sequences. Additionally, identifying patient subgroups who obtain the most benefit from AA could be important in maximising its cost-effectiveness [27–30].

Conclusion

The AA plus prednisone treatment significantly prolonged PSA PFS, rPFS and OS in Asian patients with chemotherapy-naive mCRPC. The tolerance of patients was satisfactory and it is an effective and safe option for treating chemotherapy-naive mCRPC patients. Longer duration of ADT response was significantly associated with longer survival of chemotherapy-naive mCRPC patients treated with AA. This might help guide the selection of the best therapy for mCRPC.

Abbreviations

(PC): Prostate cancer; (PCWG2): Prostate Cancer Clinical Trials Working Group 2; AA: Abiraterone acetate; ADT: Androgen deprivation therapy; AEs: Adverse events; ALT: Alanine aminotransferase; ECOG-PS: Eastern Cooperative Oncology Group performance status; HR: Hazard ratio; IQR: Interquartile ranges; mCRPC: Metastatic castration-resistant prostate cancer; OS: Overall survival; PSA PFS: PSA progression-free survival; PSA: Prostate-specific antigen; ROC: Receiver operating characteristic; rPFS: Radiographic progression-free survival

Acknowledgements

None.

Funding

This study was supported by National Natural Science Foundation of China (91129725,81572536), Science and Technology Commission of Shanghai Municipality (14140901700), the Joint research foundation of Shanghai Shenkang hospital development center on innovative medical technology (SHDC12015125), Shanghai Municipal Education Commission(15ZZ058), Shanghai Municipal Education Commission-Gaofeng Clinical Medicine Grant Support (20152215), Key Disciplines Group Construction Project of Pudong Health Bureau of Shanghai (PWZxq2014–05), and the Shanghai Jiao Tong University School of Medicine Translational Research Innovation Fund (15ZH4002).

Authors' contribution

LF, BD, CC and YW carried out this study, participated in the statistical analysis and drafted the manuscript. WX and LZ participated in the design of the study and performed the statistical analysis. JS, JP, XS and YH contributed to acquisition of data and interpretation of data. All authors read and approved the final manuscript.

Competing interest

The authors declare that they have no competing interests.

References

1. Ferlay J, Shin HR, Bray F, Forman D, Mathers C, Parkin DM. Estimates of worldwide burden of cancer in 2008: GLOBOCAN 2008. Int J Cancer. 2010; 127:2893–917.
2. Sharifi N, Dahut WL, Steinberg SM, et al. A retrospective study of the time to clinical endpoints for advanced prostate cancer. BJU Int. 2005;96:985–9.
3. Tannock IF, de Wit R, Berry WR, et al. Docetaxel plus prednisone or mitoxantrone plus prednisone for advanced prostate cancer. N Engl J Med. 2004;351:1502–12.
4. Petrylak DP, Tangen CM, Hussain MH, et al. Docetaxel and estramustine compared with mitoxantrone and prednisone for advanced refractory prostate cancer. N Engl J Med. 2004;351:1513–20.
5. de Bono JS, Oudard S, Ozguroglu M, et al. Prednisone plus cabazitaxel or mitoxantrone for metastatic castration-resistant prostate cancer progressing after docetaxel treatment: a randomised open-label trial. Lancet. 2010;376: 1147–54.
6. Basch E, Loblaw DA, Oliver TK, et al. Systemic therapy in men with metastatic castration-resistant prostate cancer:American Society of Clinical Oncology and Cancer Care Ontario clinical practice guideline. J Clin Oncol. 2014;32:3436–48.
7. Attard G, Reid AH, A'Hern R, et al. Selective inhibition of CYP17 with abiraterone acetate is highly active in the treatment of castration-resistant prostate cancer. J Clin Oncol. 2009;27:3742–8.
8. Ang JE, Olmos D, de Bono JS. CYP17 blockade by abiraterone: further evidence for frequent continued hormone-dependence in castration-resistant prostate cancer. Br J Cancer. 2009;100:671–5.
9. Attard G, Reid AH, Yap TA, et al. Phase I clinical trial of a selective inhibitor of CYP17, abiraterone acetate, confirms that castration-resistant prostate cancer commonly remains hormone driven. J Clin Oncol. 2008;26:4563–71.
10. de Bono JS, Logothetis CJ, Molina A, et al. Abiraterone and increased survival in metastatic prostate cancer. N Engl J Med. 2011;364:1995–2005.
11. Fizazi K, Scher HI, Molina A, et al. Abiraterone acetate for treatment of metastatic castration-resistant prostate cancer: final overall survival analysis of the COU-AA-301 randomised, double-blind, placebo-controlled phase 3 study. Lancet Oncol. 2012;13:983–92.
12. Ryan CJ, Smith MR, de Bono JS, et al. Abiraterone in metastatic prostate cancer without previous chemotherapy. N Engl J Med. 2013;368:138–48.
13. Ryan CJ, Smith MR, Fizazi K, et al. Abiraterone acetate plus prednisone versus placebo plus prednisone in chemotherapy-naive men with metastatic castration-resistant prostate cancer (COU-AA-302): final overall survival analysis of a randomised, double-blind, placebo-controlled phase 3 study. Lancet Oncol. 2015;16:152–60.
14. Clayton R, Wu J, Heng DY, et al. A multicentre analysis of abiraterone acetate in Canadian patients with metastatic castration-resistant prostate cancer. Can Urol Assoc J = Journal de l'Association des urologues du Canada. 2014;8:E583–90.
15. Poon DM, Chan K, Lee SH, et al. Abiraterone acetate in metastatic castration-resistant prostate cancer - the unanticipated real-world clinical experience. BMC Urol. 2016;16:12.
16. Davies RS, Smith C, Button MR, et al. What predicts minimal response to Abiraterone in metastatic castrate-resistant prostate Cancer? Anticancer Res. 2015;35:5615–21.
17. Scher HI, Halabi S, Tannock I, et al. Design and end points of clinical trials for patients with progressive prostate cancer and castrate levels of testosterone: recommendations of the prostate Cancer clinical trials working group. J Clin Oncol. 2008;26:1148–59.
18. Sun Y, Zou Q, Sun Z, et al. Abiraterone acetate for metastatic castration-resistant prostate cancer after docetaxel failure: a randomized, double-blind, placebo-controlled phase 3 bridging study. Int J Urol. 2016;23:404–11.
19. Bellmunt J, Kheoh T, Yu MK, et al. Prior endocrine therapy impact on Abiraterone acetate clinical efficacy in metastatic castration-resistant prostate Cancer: post-hoc analysis of randomised phase 3 studies. Eur Urol. 2015.
20. Nakabayashi M, Werner L, Oh WK, Regan MM, Kantoff PW, Taplin ME. Secondary hormonal therapy in men with castration-resistant prostate cancer. Clin Genitourin Cancer. 2011;9:95–103.
21. Nakabayashi M, Xie W, Regan MM, Jackman DM, Kantoff PW, Oh WK. Response to low-dose ketoconazole and subsequent dose escalation to high-dose ketoconazole in patients with androgen-independent prostate cancer. Cancer. 2006;107:975–81.
22. Loriot Y, Eymard JC, Patrikidou A, et al. Prior long response to androgen deprivation predicts response to next-generation androgen receptor axis targeted drugs in castration resistant prostate cancer. Eur J Cancer. 2015;51: 1946–52.
23. Fitzpatrick JM, Bellmunt J, Fizazi K, et al. Optimal management of metastatic castration-resistant prostate cancer: highlights from a European expert consensus panel. Eur J Cancer. 2014;50:1617–27.
24. Ross RW, Oh WK, Xie W, et al. Inherited variation in the androgen pathway is associated with the efficacy of androgen-deprivation therapy in men with prostate cancer. J Clin Oncol. 2008;26:842–7.
25. Yang M, Xie W, Mostaghel E, et al. SLCO2B1 and SLCO1B3 may determine time to progression for patients receiving androgen deprivation therapy for prostate cancer. J Clin Oncol. 2011;29:2565–73.
26. Azad AA, Eigl BJ, Leibowitz-Amit R, et al. Outcomes with abiraterone acetate in metastatic castration-resistant prostate cancer patients who have poor performance status. Eur Urol. 2015;67:441–7.
27. Liancheng Fan, Rui Wang, Chenfei Chi, Wen Cai, Yong Zhang, Hongyang Qian, Xiaoguang Shao, Yanqing Wang, Fan Xu, Jiahua Pan, Yinjie Zhu, Xun Shangguan, Lixin Zhou, Baijun Dong, Wei Xue. Systemic immune-inflammation index predicts the combined clinical outcome after sequential therapy with abiraterone and docetaxel for metastatic castration-resistant prostate cancer patients. The Prostate. 2018;78(4):250-56.
28. Baijun Dong, Liancheng Fan, Yanqing Wang, Chenfei Chi, Xiaowei Ma, Rui Wang, Wen Cai, Xiaoguang Shao, Jiahua Pan, Yinjie Zhu, Xun Shangguan, Zhixiang Xin, Jianian Hu, Shaowei Xie, Xiaonan Kang, Lixin Zhou, Wei Xue. Influence of abiraterone acetate on neuroendocrine differentiation in chemotherapy-naive metastatic castration-resistant prostate cancer. The Prostate. 2017;77(13):1373-380.
29. Liancheng Fan, Yanqing Wang, Chenfei Chi, Jiahua Pan, Shangguan Xun, Zhixiang Xin, Jianian Hu, Lixin Zhou, Baijun Dong, Wei Xue. Chromogranin A and neurone-specific enolase variations during the first 3 months of abiraterone therapy predict outcomes in patients with metastatic castration-resistant prostate cancer. BJU International. 2017;120(2):226-32.
30. Liancheng Fan, Xiao Wang, Chenfei Chi, Yanqing Wang, Wen Cai, Xiaoguang Shao, Fan Xu, Jiahua Pan, Yinjie Zhu, Xun Shangguan, Zhixiang Xin, Jianian Hu, Shaowei Xie, Rui Wang, Lixin Zhou, Baijun Dong, Wei Xue. Prognostic nutritional index predicts initial response to treatment and prognosis in metastatic castration-resistant prostate cancer patients treated with abiraterone. The Prostate. 2017;77(12):1233-241.

26

Obesity is associated with increased risk of invasive penile cancer

Kerri T. Barnes[1], Bradley D. McDowell[2], Anna Button[2], Brian J. Smith[3], Charles F. Lynch[2,4] and Amit Gupta[1,4*]

Abstract

Background: To validate the association between obesity and penile cancer at a population level, we conducted a matched case–control study linking the Iowa Department of Motor Vehicles Drivers' License Database (DLD) with cancer surveillance data collected by the State Health Registry of Iowa (SHRI).

Methods: All men diagnosed with invasive penile squamous cell carcinoma from 1985 to 2010 were identified by SHRI. Two hundred sixty-six cancer cases and 816 cancer-free male controls, selected from the Iowa DLD, were matched within 5-year age and calendar year strata. Body mass index (BMI) was calculated using self-reported height and weight from the DLD.

Results: Conditional logistic regression was used to evaluate the association between BMI and the risk of developing invasive penile cancer. Obesity was significantly associated with an increased risk of developing penile cancer. For every five-unit increase in BMI the risk of invasive penile cancer increased by 53 % (OR 1.53, 95 % CI 1.29-1.81, $p < 0.0001$).

Conclusion: We previously reported an association between obesity and higher risk of invasive penile cancer and advanced cancer stage at diagnosis in a hospital-based retrospective study. This population-based study confirms an association between obesity and invasive penile cancer.

Keywords: Penile cancer, Obesity, Epidemiologic study, Case control study

Background

Penile cancer accounts for 0.4–0.6 % of malignancies in the United States and Western Europe [1]. Lack of neonatal circumcision, poor genital hygiene, phimosis, human papilloma virus (HPV) infection and smoking are all risk factors for invasive penile cancer [2]. In a hospital-based retrospective study, we reported an association between obesity and higher risk of having invasive penile cancer after controlling for race and smoking status [3]. In order to validate the association between obesity and penile cancer at the population level, we conducted a matched case–control study linking the Iowa Department of Motor Vehicles Drivers' License Database (DLD) with the State Health Registry of Iowa (SHRI), which is a member of the Surveillance, Epidemiology, and End Results (SEER) Program [4].

* Correspondence: amit-gupta-1@uiowa.edu
[1]Department of Urology, University of Iowa, 200 Hawkins Dr., 3 RCP, Iowa City, IA 52242-1089, USA
[4]Department of Epidemiology, University of Iowa, Iowa City, IA, USA
Full list of author information is available at the end of the article

Methods

Institutional Review Board approval was obtained for this study. Cancer cases were ascertained by the SHRI as part of its surveillance mandate. All male Iowa residents diagnosed at 18+ years of age between 1985 and 2010 with microscopically-confirmed invasive penile squamous cell carcinoma were identified. These criteria yielded an initial cohort of 278 cases. The DLD was obtained from the Iowa Department of Motor Vehicles. This database contains full name, date of birth, license issue date, and self-reported height and weight. Each person in the database may have multiple records that correspond to successive license renewals.

Data from the SHRI (for diagnoses made between 1985 and 2010) and the DLD (for licenses issued in 1985, 1993, 2008 and 2012) were linked using full name, social security number and date of birth. Of the 278 initially identified penile cancer cases, 266 (96 %) were successfully matched to one or more records in the DLD. A control group of males were randomly selected from the Iowa DLD, and SHRI records were checked to confirm that these men had not been diagnosed with cancer. These controls were randomly selected from within 5-year calendar year strata from 1985 to 2012 (according to time of diagnosis for cases and time of DL issuance for controls) and 5-year age strata for ages 30 through 90+. Matching was done in a 3:1 ratio, yielding 798 controls.

Body mass index (BMI) was calculated using self-reported height and weight from the DLD and categorized as at or below normal weight (<25), overweight (25–29.9), or obese (≥30) according to World Health Organization (WHO) criteria [5]. Because DL issuance dates (and corresponding BMIs) do not often coincide closely with dates of diagnoses (Table 1), linear mixed effects regression was used to estimate BMI at the time of diagnosis for each case. All available BMIs calculated from the DLD information were included in the regression analysis and modeled as a function of (1) fixed effects for linear temporal trends prior to and after diagnosis and (2) random effects for case-specific mean differences. The regression-derived estimates of BMI at diagnosis were then used in the subsequent analysis of cancer risk. This was not necessary for controls since their BMIs were calculated directly from DLs selected to coincide with the diagnosis dates of their matched cases. Conditional logistic regression was used to evaluate the association between BMI and risk of developing invasive penile cancer, while adjusting for the 5-year age and calendar year matching strata which controlled for changes in association over time. Estimated effects of BMI are reported as odds ratios, along with 95 % confidence intervals. All statistical tests were two-sided and assessed for significance at the 0.05 level.

Results

The mean age of cases and controls were 68.3 and 69.3 years, respectively. In the mixed effects regression analysis for penile cancer patients, BMIs increased at an estimated rate of 1.0 unit every 10 years (95 % CI: 0.7 - 1.3; $p < 0.0001$). A non-significant decreased rate of 0.1 units (95 % CI: -0.4 - 0.5; $p = 0.52$) was estimated for the change in BMI after diagnosis.

Penile cancer cases were significantly more likely to be overweight or obese as compared to controls (Table 2). Based on conditional logistic regression, as compared to men with a normal weight (BMI <25), the risk of invasive penile cancer increased with increasing obesity, with an odds ratio of 2.64 (95 % CI 1.81-3.86; $p = 0.0103$) for overweight men and 3.24 (95 % CI 2.07-5.08; $p = 0.0002$) for obese men. When BMI was treated as a continuous variable, the risk of invasive penile cancer increased by an estimated 53 % (OR 1.53, 95 % CI 1.29-1.81, $p < 0.0001$ for every five-unit increase in BMI [Table 2]).

Table 1 Summary of the number and timing of drivers' licenses available for penile cancer cases relative to diagnosis

DL Issued	N	Number of licenses		Years to closest license	
		Mean (SD)	Range	Mean (SD)	Range
Before diagnosis	262	1.5 (0.7)	1–4	8.8 (6.7)	0–25
After diagnosis	90	1.3 (0.6)	1–4	6.6 (5.6)	1–22
Before or after	266	1.9 (0.9)	1–5	6.6 (5.9)	0–25

A sensitivity analysis was performed to assess the effect of using regression-derived estimates of BMI at diagnosis. This was accomplished by repeating the risk analysis using observed BMIs from the subset of cases who had DL issue dates prior to and within 5 years of diagnosis. Estimated odds ratios were higher in the sensitivity analysis, albeit with wider confidence intervals; thus suggesting that risk estimates are not artificially inflated by the use of case-estimated BMIs.

Discussion

In this population-based case–control study, we found increasing BMI was associated with higher risk of developing invasive penile cancer. These results are consistent with our previous hospital-based study, which showed the odds of having invasive penile cancer doubled with each five-unit increase in BMI [3]. To our knowledge, this is the first population-based case–control study investigating the role of BMI in penile cancer incidence. Strengths of this study include the ability to capture a large number of penile cancer cases given its rarity and utilizing two large population-based databases (SHRI and the Iowa DLD) which are not subject to referral bias.

The link between obesity and cancer is gaining acceptance and it was recently reported that 3.6 % of all new cancers in 2012 were attributable to high BMI [6]. We hypothesize the association as it relates to penile cancer is secondary to obesity-related mechanisms such as impaired genital hygiene and self-examination, buried penis with smegma accumulation and functional phimosis; all risk factors for development of penile cancer. Obesity may also lead to diabetes, which increases the risk of phimosis and the risk of penile cancer [7]. Other, more systemic obesity-associated carcinogenesis mechanisms, such as chronic inflammation, oxidative stress and insulin resistance may also play a role in the development of penile cancer [8].

This study is limited by the inability to control for other risk factors of penile cancer such as circumcision status, smoking history and race. As circumcision is not associated with obesity, and 93 % of Iowa residents are Caucasian [9], these factors are unlikely to confound these results. Also, smoking is inversely associated with obesity [10], and any confounding due to smoking will bias the study towards the null and unlikely to explain our findings. Furthermore, in our previous case series these factors were controlled for and an association was

Table 2 BMI summary statistics for cases vs controls. For cases, the predicted date-of-diagnosis BMI was used

	Cases	Controls	OR (95 % CI)	*p*-value
Body Mass Index Categories	N (%)	N (%)		
<25	44 (16.5)	279 (35.0)	1.0	Ref
25–29.9 (overweight)	153 (57.5)	377 (47.2)	2.64 (1.81–3.86)	0.0103
≥30 (obese)	69 (26.0)	142 (17.8)	3.24 (2.07–5.08)	0.0002
	Mean (SD)	Mean (SD)		
Body Mass Index (kg/m^2)	28.4 (3.6)	26.8 (4.5)	1.53 (1.29–1.81)*	<0.0001

*Estimated effect for a 5-unit increase in BMI as a continuous variable

still found [3]. A second limitation is the use of self-reported height and weight. This has been reported to underestimate obesity prevalence's in men [11]; however, this underreporting should be consistent between cases and controls and will bias the study towards the null, minimizing the difference seen. Therefore, our results could actually underestimate the effects of obesity on penile cancer risk. Furthermore, the use of the Iowa DLD as a population-based sampling frame has been shown to include 97 % of men on the state's tumor registry, therefore not excluding the less affluent who may be at highest risk of penile cancer [12]. Finally, temporal differences in BMI and the time of diagnosis necessitated the use of case-estimated BMIs; however, a sensitivity analysis indicated that this did not artificially inflate risk estimates.

Conclusions

Many adverse health consequences result from obesity, including increased risk for several cancers. This study shows that obesity is associated with an increased risk of developing invasive penile cancer. Penile cancer is a morbid condition and therapeutic options for advanced cancer are limited. Obesity may represent a modifiable risk factor for the development of penile cancer. Greater emphasis on education of obese men about this risk might encourage weight loss and persuade them to perform periodic genital self-examination and seek care early.

Abbreviations

BMI, body mass index; DLD, drivers' license database; HPV, human papilloma virus; SEER, surveillance, epidemiology, and end results; SHRI, State Health Registry of Iowa; WHO, World Health Organization

Acknowledgements

None.

Funding

This work was made possible by the University of Iowa Holden Comprehensive Cancer Center Population Research Core which is supported in part by P30 CA086862 and the Iowa Cancer Registry which is supported in part by HSN261201000032C.

Authors' contributions

KTB participated in project design and development, data collection/management, and manuscript writing/editing. BDM participated in project design and development, data collection/management, data analysis, and manuscript editing. AB participated in project design and development, data collection/management, data analysis, and manuscript editing. BJS participated in project design and development, data collection/management, data analysis, and manuscript editing. CFL participated in project design and development and manuscript editing. AG participated in project design and development, data collection/management, data analysis, and manuscript writing/editing. All authors have read, edited and approved the final version of the manuscript.

Competing interests

The authors declare that they have no competing interests.

Author details

[1]Department of Urology, University of Iowa, 200 Hawkins Dr., 3 RCP, Iowa City, IA 52242-1089, USA. [2]Holden Comprehensive Cancer Center, University of Iowa, Iowa City, IA, USA. [3]Department of Biostatistics, University of Iowa, Iowa City, IA, USA. [4]Department of Epidemiology, University of Iowa, Iowa City, IA, USA.

References

1. Siegal R, Ma J, Zou Z, Jemal A. Cancer statistics, 2014. CA Cancer J Clin. 2014;64:9–29.
2. Daling J, Madeleine M, Johnson L, et al. Penile cancer: importance of circumcision, HPV and smoking in in situ and invasive disease. Int J Cancer. 2005;116:606–16.
3. Barnes KT, Smith BJ, Lynch CF, Gupta A. Obesity and invasive penile cancer. Eur Urol. 2013;63:588–9.
4. State Health Registry of Iowa. Iowa Cancer Registry. http://www.public-health.uiowa.edu/shri/. Accessed 9 October 2014.
5. World Health Organization. Global Database on Body Mass Index. BMI Classification. http://apps.who.int/bmi/index.jsp?introPage=intro_3.html. Accessed 9 October 2014.
6. Arnold M, Pandeya N, Byrnes G, et al. Global burden of cancer attributable to high body-mass index in 2012: a population-based study. Lancet Oncol. 2015;16:36–46.
7. Bromage S, Crump A, Pearce I. Phimosis as a presenting feature of diabetes. BJU Int. 2008;101:338–40.
8. Basen-Engquist K, Chang M. Obesity and cancer risk: recent review and evidence. Curr Oncol Rep. 2011;13:71–6.
9. U.S. Census Bureau. State and County Quick Facts. http://quickfacts.census.gov/qfd/states/19000.html. Accessed 1 November 2014.

10. Flegal K, Troiano R, Pamuik E, Kuczmarski RJ, Campmbell SM. The influence of smoking cessation on the prevalence of overweight in the United States. NEJM. 1995;333:1165–70.
11. Morris D, Schubert S, Ngo D, Moore JM. DMV records are valuable for monitoring obesity in Oregon. Oregon Health Authority Environmental Public Health Tracking. http://public.health.oregon.gov/HealthyEnvironments/TrackingAssessment/EnvironmentalPublicHealthTracking/Documents/Reports/EPHT_DMV_obesity_tracking.pdf. Accessed 13 December 2014.
12. Lynch C, Logsden-Sackett N, Edwards S, Cantor KP. The driver's license list as a population-based sampling frame in Iowa. Am J Public Health. 1994;84:469–72.

Global expression of *AMACR* transcripts predicts risk for prostate cancer – a systematic comparison of AMACR protein and mRNA expression in cancerous and noncancerous prostate

Saeid Alinezhad[1*], Riina-Minna Väänänen[1], Natalia Tong Ochoa[1], Emily A. Vertosick[2], Anders Bjartell[3], Peter J Boström[4], Pekka Taimen[5] and Kim Pettersson[1]

Abstract

Background: The high false negative rates for initial prostate biopsies refer a large number of the men for repeat biopsies each year. Therefore, biomarkers associated with high risk of the presence of malignancy in histologically benign biopsies could provide a tool to discriminate the patients who need repeat biopsy or intensive follow-up from those who do not. Here we examined the diagnostic applicability of alpha-methylacyl CoA racemase (*AMACR)* and androgen receptor (*AR)* mRNA expression and AMACR protein levels in benign and cancerous prostatic tissue.

Methods: *AMACR* and *AR* mRNA levels were measured with quantitative, reverse-transcription PCR (qRT-PCR) assays in 79 radical prostatectomy (RP) cases (including 69 benign (RP-Be) and 69 cancerous (RP-PCa) samples) and 19 benign prostate samples obtained from cystoprostatectomies. To further determine the detailed areas of altered *AMACR* expression, *AMACR* mRNA level measurement and protein staining were performed for three cross-sectioned RP cases.

Results: The median *AMACR* and *AR* expression levels were 194.6 ($p < 0.0001$) and 6.6 ($p = 0.0004$) times higher in RP-PCa samples than in the benign cystoprostatectomy (CP) samples, respectively. There was no statistically significant difference between RP-PCa and RP-Be samples, except for *AMACR/KLK3* (Kallikrein-Related Peptidase 3) ratio, which was significantly higher in RP-PCa samples than in RP-Be samples ($p = 0.016$). In the systematic study of cross-sections, *AMACR* mRNA was detected in all of the studied areas including histologically benign tissue, but at significantly higher levels in carcinoma areas ($p < 0.001$). AMACR protein expression was detected in 80 % (28/35) of the areas that contained carcinoma and in 37 % (44/119) of the benign and PIN areas from the same patients.

Conclusions: *AMACR* transcripts were detected in all RP-PCa and RP-Be samples but not in non-cancerous CP samples, which suggest a global increase of *AMACR* expression in cancerous prostates. Therefore patients with false negative biopsies might benefit from an *AMACR* mRNA measurement when assessing their cancer risk.

Keywords: Prostate cancer, mRNA expression, Biomarker, AMACR, Radical prostatectomy and cystoprostatectomy

* Correspondence: saeali@utu.fi
[1]Division of Biotechnology, University of Turku, Tykistökatu 6A 6th floor, 20520 Turku, Finland
Full list of author information is available at the end of the article

Background

Prostate cancer (PCa) is the most common cancer in men and the second leading cause of cancer-related death. The current routine diagnostic approach employs a combination of digital rectal examination (DRE) and measurement of serum level of prostate specific antigen (PSA) followed by histological examination of prostate biopsies. However, negative biopsy results have been reported for 70–80 % of the men in the United States who undergo prostate biopsy each year [1]. Considering the fact that in those men, cancer foci might have been missed due to sampling error, repeated biopsies for cases with elevated PSA level are an assuring option. Re-biopsies or increasing the number of biopsy cores have been shown to improve the diagnostic accuracy and reduce false negative results [2], but the procedures are costly and generate discomfort for patients. Therefore, biomarkers associated with high risk of presence of malignancy on histologically benign biopsies could provide an additional tool in identifying those patients who would truly benefit from a repeat biopsy or intensive follow-up.

Extensive research based on high-throughput gene expression profiling has aimed to identify new biomarkers in PCa tissues to better address the limitations of present diagnostic and prognostic approaches. Here we performed validation of diagnostic capabilities of quantitative measurement of alpha-methylacyl CoA racemase (*AMACR*) and androgen receptor (*AR*) transcripts by RT-PCR for PCa diagnosis.

AMACR enzyme is involved in peroxisomal beta-oxidation of branched-chain fatty acids and their derivatives [3]. In PCa *AMACR* is highly expressed at both mRNA and protein levels [4]. However, *AMACR* is also frequently expressed in prostatic intraepithelial neoplasia (PIN) [5] and variable expression may be found in benign prostatic glandular epithelium across all age groups [6]. Therefore, to resolve diagnostic challenges in clinical pathology AMACR staining is typically combined with a basal epithelial cell marker such as p63 or 34βE12 that are not present in PCa.

The growth and maintenance of prostate tissue is dependent on androgens produced in testes and adrenal glands [7] and the intracellular androgen receptor (*AR*) signaling plays a key role in the formation and development of PCa. Androgen-ablation therapy is one of the most common and successful treatments of PCa but with time the tumor frequently reaches an androgen-independent state. One mechanism for PCa to become castration resistant is due to the amplification and overexpression of *AR* gene enabling the cancer cells to grow with very low levels of androgen [8, 9]. Thus, overexpression of *AR* promotes the formation and progression of PCa as well as castration resistant PCa.

Overexpression of *AMACR* - at both mRNA and protein levels - has been reported in cancerous prostatic tissue when compared to benign prostatic hyperplasia (BPH) and normal prostate tissue [4, 10–14]. The aim of our study was to investigate the potential use of *AMACR* and *AR* mRNA expression levels to improve detection of PCa. We examined the mRNA levels of *AMACR* and *AR* in 157 prostate tissues by using internally standardized, truly quantitative reverse-transcription PCR (qRT-PCR) assays. The samples were collected from 79 cases of radical prostatectomies (RP) rapidly after the procedure both from the suspected tumor sites and from areas away from the tumor site. Cystoprostatectomy derived samples (CP) from 19 non-PCa patients or patients harboring incidental PCa were used as controls. All cystoprostatectomies were performed because of bladder cancer with no clinical suspicion of PCa. Based on the initial, *AMACR*-related findings of these experiments, we also set out to perform a preliminary, systematic evaluation of whole prostate cross-sections from three PCa patients to determine if samples from areas outside the pathologically determined tumor lesions could be equally informative of the presence of cancer. *AMACR* expression in these cross-sections was examined on both mRNA and protein levels by qRT-PCR and immunohistochemistry, respectively, and compared to the tissue morphology.

Methods

Radical prostatectomy and cystoprostatectomy samples

The study protocol was approved by the Ethics Committee of the Hospital District of Southwest Finland and it was in accordance with the Helsinki Declaration of 1975, as revised in 1996, with written informed consent obtained from each participant.

In total, 157 prostate tissue samples were examined. The cohort consisted 79 RP patients (Table 1) from

Table 1 Patients characteristics

Number of patients	79	
Age at surgery (years) Average (min,max)	61.5 (48, 71)	
Preoperative serum PSA Average (min,max)	8.4 (1.4, 30)	
Pathological T-category	Number of samples (percentage)	
	pT2	33 (42 %)
	pT3 and pT4	41 (52 %)
	Unknown	5 (6 %)
Pathological Gleason score		
	≤6	45 (57 %)
	7	18 (23 %)
	≥8	12 (15 %)
	Unknown	4 (5 %)

whom 138 tissue samples containing 69 histologically benign samples (RP-Be) and 69 cancerous samples (RP-PCa) were obtained after radical prostatectomies in Turku University Hospital in Turku, Finland for clinically localized PCa. (Table 2 represents clinicopathological data for 138 samples obtained from 79 radical prostatectomy specimens). Two tissue samples were collected from each prostate: one from an area suspected to contain cancer and one from a macroscopically normal area as a control [15]. Pathological examination revealed that for some patients both samples had been taken from either benign or cancerous areas. For 59 prostates we examined both samples (for 30/59 prostates one of the samples had been taken from a benign area and the other from a cancerous area; for 15/59 both samples were from a cancerous area; and for 14/59 both samples were from a benign area), and for 9 and 11 prostates, we only had access to one sample per prostate, similarly taken either from the cancerous or control area, respectively. The samples were collected immediately after the removal of the organ and stored in quanidine isothiocyanate buffer [15]. The final content of the samples (benign or cancerous) was determined from hematoxylin-eosin (HE) stained frozen sections obtained next to the fresh frozen tissue samples.

Additionally, 19 histologically benign prostatic tissue samples were obtained from patients who underwent cystoprostatectomy due to bladder cancer without clinical evidence of PCa in Skåne University Hospital in Malmö, Sweden. At the time of histological evaluation, seven cases showed no evidence of PCa (CP-Be) while 12 had incidental PCa (CP-PCa)).

Prostate cross-section samples

Single whole prostate cross-sections were obtained from three patients with localized PCa who underwent RP in Turku University Hospital in Turku, Finland. The cohort and sample collection has been previously reported [16]. Briefly, a 2 mm horizontal mid-plane tissue slice covering the entire gland was obtained from each prostate for the experiment. To be able to have a unique coordinate code for each piece of tissue, the prostate slice was fixed on a Styrofoam plate with a 5 × 5 mm grid guide on it. To avoid cross-contamination, sterile blades were used to cut the prostate slices further into 5 × 5 × 2 mm pieces. Based on the size of the prostate gland, 48, 62 and 44 pieces of tissue were obtained from prostates A, B and C, respectively. The samples were stored in RNAlater (Qiagen) at −20 °C until RNA extraction.

For histological examination, from each specimen, the tissue adjacent to the slice used for mRNA measurements were fixed in formalin and embedded in macro paraffin blocks (FFPE). The FFPE blocks covering the superior and inferior side of the cross-section were cut to 5 μm sections and HE-stained.

Table 2 Clinicopathological data for 138 samples obtained from 79 radical prostatectomy specimens

	Number of samples (percentage)
Pathological T-category	
pT2	57 (41 %)
pT3 and pT4	72 (52 %)
Unknown	9 (7 %)
Pathological Gleason score	
≤6	81 (58 %)
7	27 (20 %)
≥8	22 (16 %)
Unknown	8 (6 %)

RNA isolation and reverse transcription

Total RNA was extracted from the tissues and reverse transcribed to cDNA as previously described [15]. During the extraction, a known amount of RNA of artificially mutated *KLK3* gene called mmPSA [17] was added to samples as internal standard after the cell lysis.

Real-time PCR

A previously described concept utilizing target-specific oligonucleotide probes and time-resolved fluorometry were used to detect the accumulation of *AMACR* and *AR* transcripts [18, 19]. Oligonucleotide primers and probes (Table 3) were purchased from Thermo (Germany). All samples were run in triplicate in a reaction volume of 25 μl containing 2.5 μl of template cDNA using a previously described temperature profile [19] and external DNA standards [15].

Immunohistochemistry

For cross-section studies, histological macrosections of 5 μm in thickness were cut from the FFPE blocks of each prostate (A,B and C), next to the HE-stained sections. Paraffin was removed with xylene and the sections were rehydrated with series of alcohol. Antigen retrieval was carried out by microwaving the slides in Target Retrieval solution (Dako) at pH 9 for 7 min. The tissue sections were incubated for one hour with rabbit monoclonal AMACR (P504S) antibody (1:200, clone 13H4, Zeta Corporation). The primary antibody was detected with EnVision + Dual Link System-HRP (Dako) and visualized with DAB+ chromogen solution (Dako). The slides were observed by an experienced uropathologist using a Leica DM3000 light microscope equipped with Leica DFC 420 digital camera and Leica Application Suite version 2.5.0 R1 (Leica Microsystems, Wetzlar).

Table 3 The oligonucleotides used in this study

Oligonucleotide	Sequence (5′ to 3′)	Position[a]	Lanthanide chelate label or quencher molecule
AMACR forward primer	TTGTCAGGTGTTCTCTCAAA	481–500	
AMACR reverse primer	CTTCCACCATATTTGCATC	637–655	
AMACR reporter probe	C[b]TGAATCTCCTGGCTGACTTTGCTGG	535–560	9d-α gal-Eu^{III}
AMACR quencher probe	TCAGCCAGGAGATTCAG[c]	535–551	Dabcyl
AR forward primer	GCTGAAGGGAAACAGAAGTAC	328–348	
AR reverse primer	CTCTCCTTCCTCCTGTAGTTTC	480–501	
AR reporter probe	T[b]TGTCGTCTTCGGAAATGTTATGAAGCAGG	408–437	9d-α gal-Eu^{III}
AR quencher probe	AACATTTCCGAAGACGACAA[c]	408–427	Dabcyl

[a]gene bank accession numbers NM_014324 and NM_001011645 were used for *AMACR* and *AR* nucleotide sequences, respectively
[b]internally amino-modified C6-base for labeling with Eu chelate
[c]quencher molecule

Data analysis

The obtained mRNA levels were normalized to total RNA amount and the previously determined internal RNA standard levels. Samples were considered as positive only when all three replicates were positive and above the lowest detection limit of the assay. To calculate the expression levels of *AMACR* or *AR* in relation to *KLK3* (the gene encoding PSA), the mRNA copy numbers were divided by previously determined *KLK3* mRNA levels [20].

Linear regression models were created to test whether the type of sample (RP-BE, RP-PCa, CP-Be, CP-PCa) was associated with the log-transformed expression levels of *AR*, *AMACR*, *KLK3*, *AR/KLK*3 or *AMACR/KLK3*. Mann–Whitney *U* test was used to evaluate whether there were statistically significant differences in the gene expression levels between any two of the groups. A significance level of $p = 0.05$ was used.

For the systematic study of cross-sections, the histology of tissue samples used for mRNA expression measurements was defined by dividing the digital images of HE-stained tissue slides into equal amount of regions with the cross-sections used in mRNA experiments. Each sample piece was given coordinates on two axes (one axis got values from A to K and the other axis from 1 to 10). Based on histopathological examination, the samples were categorized into three groups: carcinoma ($n = 35$), if one or both adjacent HE-stained sections revealed adenocarcinoma at that location; histologically benign tissue ($n = 112$), if that is what both HE-stained sections contained; and PIN ($n = 7$), if one or both HE-stained sections contained PIN lesions but no carcinoma.

Results

AMACR, AR and *KLK3* mRNA expression in RP and CP samples

For the PCa patients, the median, minimum and maximum age and preoperative PSA level in serum were 63 (48 and 71) years and 6.95 (1.4 and 30) ng/ml, respectively. Detailed clinicopathological data of the patients are shown in Table 1.

The limit of detection for the *AMACR* assay was 10 copies/μl of template DNA and 1 copy/μl of template DNA for the *AR* and *KLK3* assays. *AMACR* mRNA was detected in all RP-Be, RP-PCa and CP-PCa samples but only in 2 out of 7 CP-Be tissue samples (Fig. 1a). All tissue samples were found to contain detectable levels of *AR* and *KLK3* transcripts. Table 4 represents the mRNA expression level of target genes in different group of samples.

Compared to the 19 CP samples, the median *AMACR* expression level was 126 times higher in the RP-Be samples ($p < 0.0001$) and 195 times higher in the RP-PCa samples ($p < 0.0001$) (Fig. 1). When the median *AMACR* expression level in the RP-PCa samples was compared to the mean value of the two *AMACR* positive CP-Be samples there was a 682-fold difference ($p < 0.0001$). There was no statistically significant difference in *AMACR* mRNA levels between the RP-PCa and RP-Be groups. Comparison of AMACR expression level by paired *t*-test between cancerous and benign samples for 30 patients who had two matched samples resulted in insignificant difference ($P > 0.05$). However, the *AMACR* to *KLK3* mRNA ratio was 5.3 times higher in the RP-PCa than in the RP-Be group ($p = 0.012$).

In comparison to all of the 19 CP samples, the median level of *AR* expression was 6.4 times higher in the RP-Be samples ($p < 0.0001$) and 6.6 times higher in the RP-PCa samples ($p = 0.0004$) (Fig. 1). The greatest difference in median levels of *AR* expression was found between the RP-PCa samples and the CP-Be samples (11.5-fold, $p = 0.004$). No statistically significant differences were seen in *AR* or *KLK3* expression, nor in *AR*/*KLK3* mRNA ratio between the RP-PCa and RP-Be samples.

The mRNA levels of the target genes were not associated with Gleason grade in the RP samples, but the

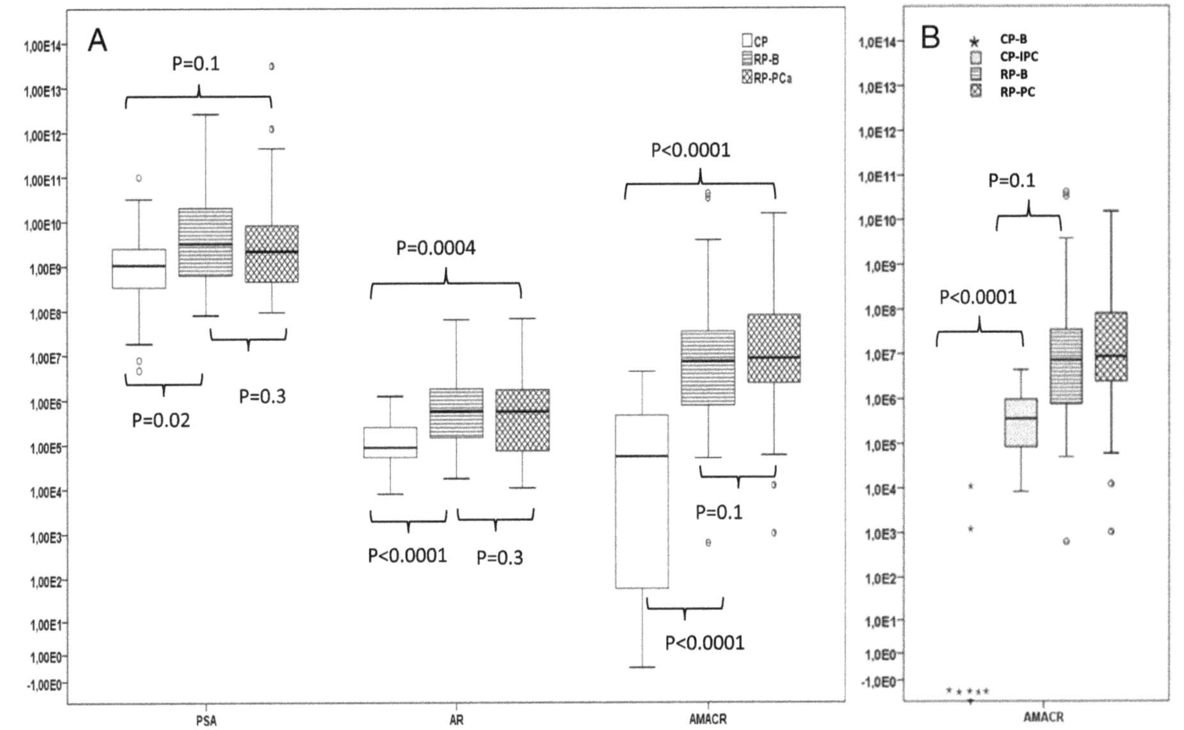

Fig. 1 **a** *KLK3*, *AR* and *AMACR* mRNA levels in cystoprostatectomy (CP) samples (with and without incidental PCa), histologically benign radical prostatectomy (RP-Be) samples and cancerous radical prostatectomy (RP-PCa) samples. **b** *AMACR* mRNA levels in CP samples without incidental PCa (CP-Be), CP samples with incidental PCa (CP-PCa), RP-Be and RP-PCa samples. The top whisker represents highest case within 1.5 times IQR. The top line of the box represents the 3rd quartile, the line in the middle of the box represents the median, the bottom line of the box represents 1st quartile and bottom whisker represents the lowest case within 1.5 times IQR. Open circles represent the outlier values

expression levels of target genes were statistically significantly higher in samples from men with either stage pT3 or pT4 tumors ($n = 72$) than in samples from men with PCa classified as pT2 ($n = 57$) (*AMACR*, $p = 0.006$; *AR*, $p = 0.005$ and *KLK3*, $p = 0.004$).

Based on Pearson's correlation coefficient, there was a strong correlation ($r = 0.86$) between *AR* and *AMACR* expression levels when samples from all groups were combined. Furthermore there was no strong correlation between *AMACR* or *AR* and serum PSA ($R = 0.46$ and $R = 0.18$, respectively).

The receiver operating characteristic (ROC) curve analyses for *AMACR, AR* and *KLK3* mRNA expression for evaluating the diagnostic potency and discrimination power of the target genes between all RP samples and CP samples produced area under the curve (AUC) values of 0.94, 0.74 and 0.61, respectively. The ROC curve analyses for *AMACR*, *AR* and *KLK3*mRNA expression for evaluating the correlation of the expression level with histology between RP-PCa and CP samples produced AUC values of 0.923, 0.717 and 0.58, respectively (Fig. 2a). Corresponding AUC values for RP-Be specimens were 0.89, 0.77 and 0.64, respectively (Fig. 2b).

Systematic analysis of *AMACR* mRNA and protein expression in prostate tissue cross-sections

AMACR mRNA was universally expressed in all tissue pieces covering the whole cross-section of prostates A, B and C included in the analysis. As a comparison, all

Table 4 The mRNA expression level (copies/µg of total RNA) of target genes in different group of samples

	Expression level (copies/µg of total RNA)			
Target genes	CP-Be ($n = 7$)	CP-PCa ($n = 12$)	RP-Be ($n = 69$)	RP-PCa ($n = 69$)
KLK3	1×10^9 (4.6×10^6, 3.2×10^{10})	1.2×10^9(7.8×10^6, 9.9×10^{10})	3.2×10^9(7.8×10^7,2.6×10^{12})	2.1×10^9(9.9×10^7,3.1×10^{13})
AMACR	0 (0, 2.7×10^4)	3.5×10^5(8.1×10^3,4.2×10^6)	7×10^6(6.2×10^2,4.1×10^{10})	8.3×10^6(1×10^3,1.5×10^{10})
AR	5.1×10^4 (7.8×10^3, $1,2 \times 10^6$)	1×10^5(4.4×10^4,1.1×10^6)	5.6×10^5(1.7×10^4,6.2×10^7)	5.5×10^5(1×10^4,6.5×10^7)

Data are presented as median (min, max). CP-Be represents cystoprostatectomy samples with no evidence of PCa, CP-PCa represents cystoprostatectomy samples with incidental PCa, RP-Be represent histologically benign samples from radical prostatectomy specimens and RP-PCa represents cancerous samples from radical prostatectomy specimens

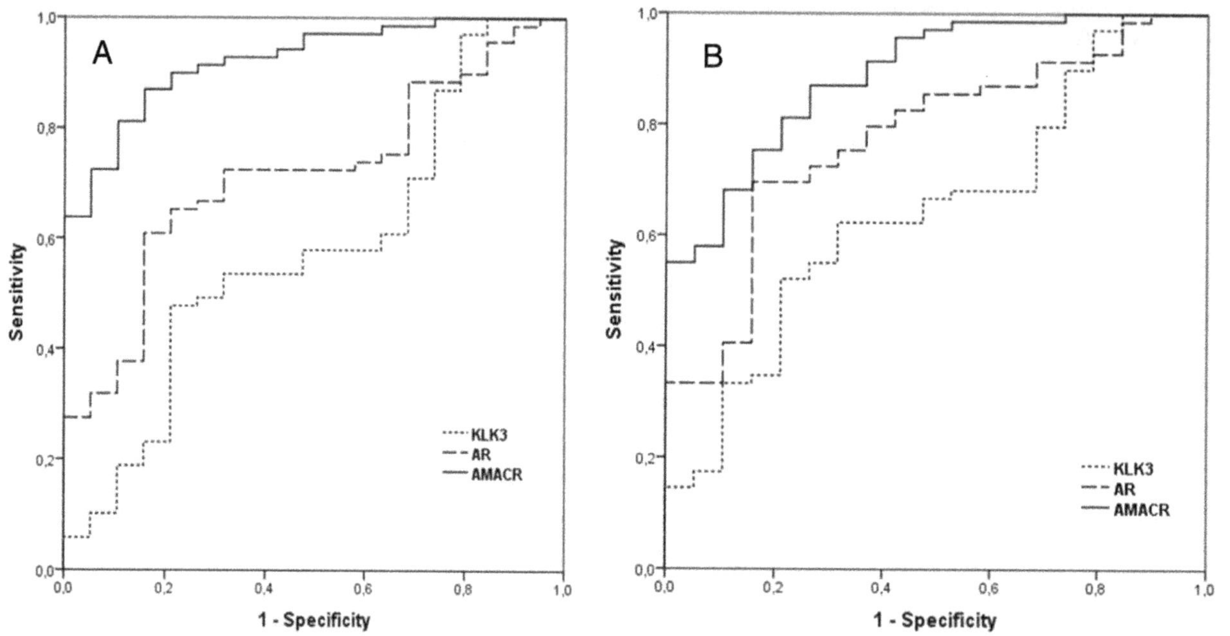

Fig. 2 ROC curve analyses for *KLK3, AR* and *AMACR* mRNA expression. **a** ROC curve analysis for RP-PCa and CP tissues. AUC values are 0.58, 0.717 and 0.923 for *KLK3, AR* and *AMACR* mRNA levels, respectively. **b** ROC curve analysis for RP-Be and CP tissues. AUC values are 0.64, 0.77 and 0.89 for *KLK3, AR* and *AMACR* mRNA levels, respectively

measured values from the cross-section samples were above the highest expression level seen in CP-Be samples (Fig. 3). There was a significant, 1.9-fold difference ($p < 0.001$) in median *AMACR* mRNA levels between carcinoma samples ($n = 35$) and histologically benign ($n = 112$) samples. There was no significant difference between PIN samples ($n = 7$) and either carcinoma or histologically benign samples.

In the immunohistochemical analysis (Fig. 4), AMACR protein was detected in all of the three prostate cross-

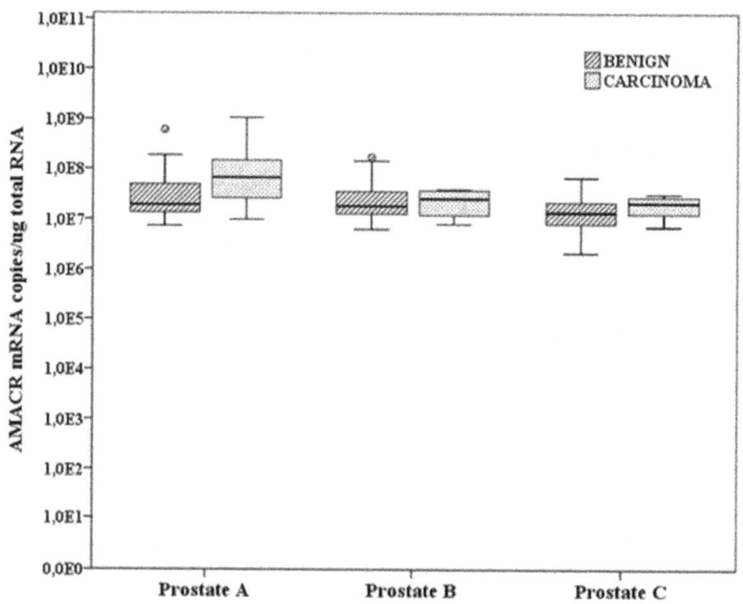

Fig. 3 *AMACR* mRNA expression levels in histologically benign and cancerous (carcinoma) samples from three prostate cross-sections obtained from three patients with localized PCa who underwent RP. The 10/25/50/75/90th percentiles are marked in the figures. Open circles represent the outlier values

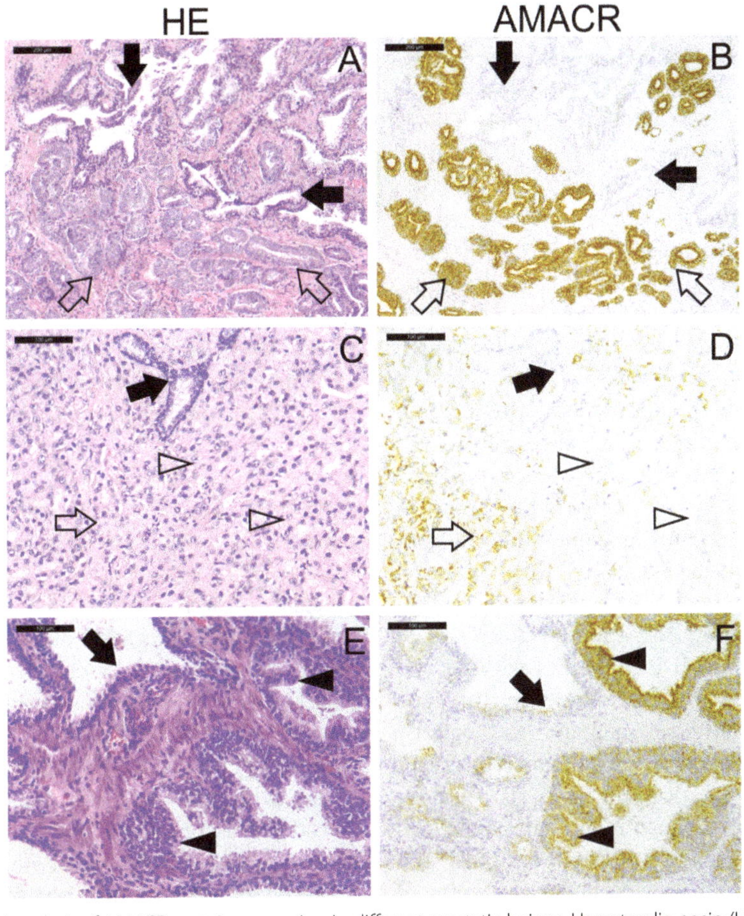

Fig. 4 Immunohistochemical analysis of AMACR protein expression in different prostatic lesions. Hematoxylin-eosin (HE) and AMACR staining from the same region of interest are shown. **a**, **b** Typical acinar Gleason 3 + 4 adenocarcinoma stains strongly for AMACR (*open arrow*) while the normal glands are AMACR negative (*filled arrow*). **c**, **d** Gleason 4 + 5 adenocarcinoma shows focal positive staining for AMACR (*open arrow*) while some of the poorly differentiated carcinoma glands (*open arrowhead*) and normal glands (*filled arrow*) are AMACR negative. **e**, **f**: High grade PIN lesion shows positive AMACR staining (*filled arrowhead*) while morphologically normal glands show weak or no AMACR staining (*filled arrow*). Scale bar 200 μm (**a-b**), 100 μm (**c-f**)

sections. More specifically, AMACR staining was positive in 100 % of areas that contained carcinoma in both superior and inferior sides of cross-sections from prostate B and C. However on the superior side of prostate A, AMACR staining was positive in 96 % of the carcinoma areas while some Gleason 4 + 5 carcinoma foci were found virtually AMACR negative (Fig. 4c-d). Strong positive AMACR staining was constantly observed in prostatic intraepithelial neoplasia (PIN) lesions (Fig. 4e-f). While the great majority of normal prostatic glands were AMACR negative, we occasionally observed some weak AMACR staining in morphologically benign glands especially adjacent to carcinoma lesions. However, the staining in such glands was virtually significantly weaker when compared to that seen in carcinoma and PIN lesion. These results suggest that AMACR mRNA is globally expressed in cancerous prostates while AMACR protein is most abundant in carcinoma and PIN lesions.

Discussion

Each year a large number of the men undergo repeat biopsy due to elevated PSA level. Repeat biopsy results have demonstrated high rates of false negative results of initial prostate biopsy (10 % to 30 %) [21, 22]. The biopsy procedure is expensive and carries several risks and discomfort for the patients. Therefore, finding reliable molecular markers that would enable early and accurate diagnosis of PCa is of importance.

Numerous studies based on the measurement of mRNA and/or protein expression have reported the upregulation of a variety of markers in PCa such as *AMACR* and *AR*. Based on several previous immunohistochemistry studies, AMACR is used as a routine tissue biomarker to support the diagnosis of prostate cancer [4, 12, 23, 24] and especially useful for detection of small carcinoma foci in needle biopsies when combined with basal cell marker such as keratin 5/6 or p63 [12]. Furthermore, AMACR immunocytochemistry and microscopic evaluation of cells captured from post-DRE urine has been applied for detection of PCa [25]. However, there are relatively few studies on *AMACR* or *AR* mRNA expression levels in prostate cancer tissue [26, 27]. Against this background, we measured the mRNA expression levels of *AMACR* and *AR* in 157 malignant and histologically benign prostate tissues with qRT-PCR assays.

We observed an overexpression of both *AMACR* and *AR* mRNA in not only cancerous, but also in histologically benign tissue from prostates with clinically significant carcinomas when they were compared to prostates without tumor or harboring only incidental lesions. Both mRNAs were also positively associated with advanced pathologic stage. The detected overexpression in cancerous tissues was 682-fold for *AMACR* mRNA and 11.5-fold for *AR* mRNA compared to prostates without any evidence of cancer. However, no differences in gene expression were seen when cancerous and histologically benign tissues from PCa patients were compared, except for *AMACR/KLK3* mRNA ratio. This supports the finding in a previous study by Laxman et al. that *AMACR* as a single marker does not have sufficient sensitivity and specificity and that it could provide better detection of PCa only in a multiplex setting [28].

Finding abnormal *AMACR* levels in benign tissues motivated us to examine the alteration in *AMACR* mRNA levels and protein expression in a systematic way in cross-sections of whole cancerous prostates. On the protein level, expression of AMACR is sometimes detected in benign biopsies from patients with PCa, as well as in normal glands that were in closer proximity to a carcinoma foci [5]. Similar results we obtained in the present study (Fig. 4). The phenomenon of increased biomarker expression in histologically benign tissue in itself can be due to cancer field effect [29, 30]. Field cancerization or field effect which was suggested by Slaughter et al. in 1953 [31] has an extended definition nowadays and it defines as any molecular abnormalities in tissues that appear histologically benign [32]. We found that in contrast to the carcinoma-free CP specimens where *AMACR* expression was rare, *AMACR* mRNA was detectable in all benign, carcinoma and PIN samples obtained from the three studied prostate cross sections with highest levels in carcinoma samples. As expected, AMACR staining was detected in the carcinoma areas, but not in all of them, and additionally, it was seen in some of the benign and PIN areas. As expected, AMACR staining was strongly positive in the great majority (but not all) carcinoma and PIN lesions. In additionally, we occasionally observed variable AMACR positivity in morphologically benign glands either adjacent to or separated from the cancerous foci showing that AMACR expression is not specific for PCa. Accordingly, measurement of the AMACR protein in urine samples by ELISA has not been able to discriminate between BPH and PCa better than serum PSA suggesting that AMACR may also be expressed under reactive conditions such as hyperplasia

In addition to the naturally occurring variable expression in benign glands [5], the difference between mRNA and protein level may be at least partly due to sensitivity limitations and differences in antibodies and detection systems [10, 13, 23]. Another possibility is the fact that the experimental set-up used here is unable to specifically account for the tissue shrinkage during fixation, which may affect the accuracy in defining the exact sample areas that correspond to the sample pieces in mRNA measurements and thereby affect especially the data obtained from samples adjacent to carcinoma foci. In this study we used samples from men with Caucasian ethnicity, but previously lower sensitivity and specificity of AMACR for the diagnosis of PCa has been reported for example in Japanese patients [33]. The involvement of AMACR in peroxisomal beta-oxidation of branched-chain fatty acids and the differences in diet habits between western and Japanese men could be considered as one explanation but extra validation using patient cohorts from different ethnic origins are needed to fully understand the differences in AMACR expression in the future. Nevertheless, the combined mRNA and protein data from the cross-sections could suggest that qRT-PCR assays are more sensitive than immunohistochemistry to reveal potential carcinoma lesions, because in accordance with our results for carcinoma samples in immunohistochemical analysis, it has been reported that some small foci of prostate cancers can be negative for AMACR staining [34]. One limitation of this study was using fresh frozen material while FFPE material is used in routine practice. The positive aspect of using fresh frozen, rapidly processed and stored in RNA stabilization reagent is that it clearly approaches the in-vivo situation. Using FFPE samples for gene expression studies are challenging due to RNA degradation and modification during the embedding and fixation. Gene expression analysis of AMACR and AR in FFPE samples using novel technologies such as nCounter (NanoString® Technologies, USA) could be considered as further validation in future.

Conclusion

Similar expression of AMACR transcripts in all of the RP-Be and RP-PCa samples suggests that AMACR expression is increased also in the histologically benign areas of cancerous prostates. This could potentially indicate a global overexpression of AMACR as was detected in the preliminary yet systematic cross-section study here. Hence, it could be deduced that patients with false negative biopsies (i.e., lesion missed in the biopsies) might benefit from an AMACR mRNA measurement with a qRT-PCR assay when assessing their cancer risk. Although this study was limited in the number of control tissue samples from PCa-free patients, but these data poses interesting options for further studies. In the future, this assay could also be applied to different sample matrices such as urine samples in order to move towards developing a noninvasive assay.

Abbreviations

AMACR: alpha-methylacyl CoA racemase; AR: androgen receptor; CP: cystoprostatectomy; CP-Be: benign cystoprostatectomy samples; CP-PCa: cystoprostatectomy samples with incidental PCa; CRPC: castration resistant prostate cancer; BPH: benign prostatic hyperplasia; HE: hematoxylin-eosin; KLK3: kallikrein-related peptidase 3; PCa: prostate cancer; PIN: prostatic intraepithelial neoplasia; PSA: prostate specific antigen; qRT-PCR: quantitative reverse transcription polymerase chain reactions; RP: radical prostatectomies; RP-Be: histologically benign radical prostatectomy samples; RP-PCa: cancerous radical prostatectomy samples.

Competing interests

The authors declare that they have no competing interests

Authors' contributions

SA: As first author designed and developed the RT-PCR assays and analyzed the results and wrote the first draft of manuscript. R-MV: Helped as co-supervisor and performed some of the analysis specially for staining part also helped to draft the manuscript. NTO: Carried out the AMACR protein staining and RT-PCR for cross sections and analyzed the results. EAV: Helped in statistical analyses. AB: Provided the Cystoprostatectomy samples and provided the clinicopathological data for these samples. PJB: Provided the radical prostatectomy samples and helped to draft the manuscript. PT: Provided the clinicopathological data for radical prostatectomy samples and supervised the AMACR staining part. KP: As supervisor, participated in study design and coordination and helped to draft the manuscript. All authors read and approved the final manuscript.

Acknowledgments

Funding is acknowledged from Marie Curie (FP-7) Prostate Research Organizations-Network of Early Stage Training (PRO-NEST Project reference: 238278).

Author details

[1]Division of Biotechnology, University of Turku, Tykistökatu 6A 6th floor, 20520 Turku, Finland. [2]Department of Epidemiology and Biostatistics, Memorial Sloan-Kettering Cancer Center, New York, NY, USA. [3]Department of Clinical Sciences, Division of Urological Cancers, Lund University, Skåne University Hospital, Malmö, Sweden. [4]Department of Urology, Turku University Hospital, Turku, Finland. [5]Department of Pathology, University of Turku and Turku University Hospital, Turku, Finland.

References

1. Shariat SF, Roehrborn CG. Using biopsy to detect prostate cancer. Rev Urol. 2008;10(4):262–80.
2. de la Taille A, Antiphon P, Salomon L, Cherfan M, Porcher R, Hoznek A, Saint F, Vordos D, Cicco A, Yiou R et al. Prospective evaluation of a 21-sample needle biopsy procedure designed to improve the prostate cancer detection rate. Urology. 2003;61(6):1181–6.
3. Ferdinandusse S, Denis S, IJlst L, Dacremont G, Waterham HR, Wanders RJ. Subcellular localization and physiological role of alpha-methylacyl-CoA racemase. J Lipid Res. 2000;41(11):1890–6.
4. Rubin MA, Zhou M, Dhanasekaran SM, Varambally S, Barrette TR, Sanda MG, Pienta KJ, Ghosh D Chinnaiyan AM. alpha-methylacyl coenzyme A racemase as a tissue biomarker for prostate cancer. JAMA. 2002;287(13):1662–70.
5. Ananthanarayanan V, Deaton RJ, Yang XJ, Pins MR, Gann PH. Alpha-methylacyl-CoA racemase (AMACR) expression in normal prostatic glands and high-grade prostatic intraepithelial neoplasia (HGPIN): association with diagnosis of prostate cancer. Prostate. 2005;63(4):341–6.
6. Gologan A, Bastacky S, McHale T, Yu J, Cai C, Monzon-Bordonaba F, Dhir R. Age-associated changes in alpha-methyl CoA racemase (AMACR) expression in nonneoplastic prostatic tissues. Am J Surg Pathol. 2005;29(11):1435–41.
7. Andersson S, Berman DM, Jenkins EP, Russell DW. Deletion of steroid 5 alpha-reductase 2 gene in male pseudohermaphroditism. Nature. 1991; 354(6349):159–61.
8. Koivisto P, Kononen J, Palmberg C, Tammela T, Hyytinen E, Isola J, Trapman J, Cleutjens K, Noordzij A, Visakorpi T et al. Androgen receptor gene amplification: a possible molecular mechanism for androgen deprivation therapy failure in prostate cancer. Cancer Res. 1997;57(2):314–9.
9. Bubendorf L, Kononen J, Koivisto P, Schraml P, Moch H, Gasser TC, Willi N, Mihatsch MJ, Sauter G, Kallioniemi OP. Survey of gene amplifications during prostate cancer progression by high throughput fluorescence in situ hybridization on tissue microarrays. Cancer Res. 1999;59(4):803–6.
10. Luo J, Zha S, Gage WR, Dunn TA, Hicks JL, Bennett CJ,Ewing CM, Platz EA, Ferdinandusse S, Wanders RJ et al. Alpha-methylacyl-CoA racemase: a new molecular marker for prostate cancer. Cancer Res. 2002;62(8):2220–6.
11. Neves AF, Araujo TG, Biase WK, Meola J, Alcantara TM, Freitas DG, Goulart LR. Combined analysis of multiple mRNA markers by RT-PCR assay for prostate cancer diagnosis. Clin Biochem. 2008;41(14–15):1191–8.
12. Jiang Z, Wu CL, Woda BA, Dresser K, Xu J, Fanger GR, Yang XJ. P504S/alpha-methylacyl-CoA racemase: a useful marker for diagnosis of small foci of prostatic carcinoma on needle biopsy. Am J Surg Pathol. 2002;26(9):1169–74.
13. Beach R, Gown AM, De Peralta-Venturina MN, Folpe AL, Yaziji H, Salles PG, Grignon DJ, Fanger GR, Amin MB. P504S immunohistochemical detection in 405 prostatic specimens including 376 18-gauge needle biopsies. Am J Surg Pathol. 2002;26(12):1588–96.
14. Visakorpi T, Hyytinen E, Koivisto P, Tanner M, Keinanen R, Palmberg C, Palotie A, Tammela T, Isola J, Kallioniemi OP. In vivo amplification of the androgen receptor gene and progression of human prostate cancer. Nat Genet. 1995;9(4):401–6.
15. Vaananen RM, Rissanen M, Kauko O, Junnila S, Vaisanen V, Nurmi J, Pettersson K. Quantitative real-time RT-PCR assay for PCA3. Clin Biochem. 2008;41(1–2):103–8.
16. Riina-Minna Väänänen, Natalia Tong Ochoa, Peter J Boström, Pekka Taimen, Kim Pettersson. Altered PCA3 and TMPRSS2-ERG expression in histologically benign regions of cancerous prostates: a systematic, quantitative mRNA analysis in five prostates. BMC Urol. 2015;15:88. doi: 10.1186/s12894-015-0077-7
17. Nurmi J, Lilja H, Ylikoski A. Time-resolved fluorometry in end-point and real-time PCR quantification of nucleic acids. Luminescence. 2000;15(6):381–8.
18. Rissanen M, Helo P, Vaananen RM, Wahlroos V, Lilja H, Nurmi M, Pettersson K, Nurmi JI. Novel homogenous time-resolved fluorometric RT-PCR assays for quantification of PSA and hK2 mRNAs in blood. Clin Biochem. 2007; 40(1–2):111–8.
19. Alinezhad S, Vaananen RM, Lehmusvuori A, Karhunen U, Soukka T, Kahkonen E, Taimen P, Alanen K, Pettersson K. Lanthanide chelate complementation and hydrolysis enhanced luminescent chelate in real-time reverse transcription polymerase chain reaction assays for KLK3 transcripts. Anal Biochem. 2014;444:1–7.
20. Vaananen RM, Lilja H, Cronin A, Kauko L, Rissanen M, Kauko O, Kekki H, Vidback S, Nurmi M, Alanen K et al. Association of transcript levels of 10 established or candidate-biomarker gene targets with cancerous versus non-cancerous prostate tissue from radical prostatectomy specimens. \Clin Biochem. 2013;46(7–8):670–4.
21. Patel AR, Jones JS, Rabets J, DeOreo G, Zippe CD. Parasagittal biopsies add minimal information in repeat saturation prostate biopsy. Urology. 2004; 63(1):87–9.
22. Stewart CS, Leibovich BC, Weaver AL, Lieber MM. Prostate cancer diagnosis using a saturation needle biopsy technique after previous negative sextant biopsies. J Urology. 2001;166(1):86–91.
23. Jiang Z, Woda BA, Rock KL, Xu Y, Savas L, Khan A, Pihan G, Cai F, Babcook JS, Rathanaswami P et al. P504S: a new molecular marker for the detection of prostate carcinoma. Am J Surg Pathol. 2001;25(11):1397–404.

24. Kristiansen G. [Immunohistochemical algorithms in prostate diagnostics: what's new?]. Pathologe. 2009;30 Suppl 2:146–53.
25. Nickens KP, Ali A, Scoggin T, Tan SH, Ravindranath L, McLeod DG, Dobi A, Tacha D, Sesterhenn IA, Srivastava S et al. Prostate cancer marker panel with single cell sensitivity in urine. Prostate. 2015;75(9):969–75.
26. Kumar-Sinha C, Shah RB, Laxman B, Tomlins SA, Harwood J, Schmitz W, Conzelmann E, Sanda MG, Wei JT, Rubin MA et al. Elevated alpha-methylacyl-CoA racemase enzymatic activity in prostate cancer. Am J Pathol. 2004;164(3):787–93.
27. Ouyang B, Leung YK, Wang V, Chung E, Levin L, Bracken B, Cheng L, Ho SM. alpha-Methylacyl-CoA racemase spliced variants and their expression in normal and malignant prostate tissues. Urology. 2011;77(1):249. e241-247.
28. Laxman B, Morris DS, Yu J, Siddiqui J, Cao J, Mehra R, Lonigro RJ, Tsodikov A, Wei JT, Tomlins SA et all. A first-generation multiplex biomarker analysis of urine for the early detection of prostate cancer. Cancer Res. 2008;68(3): 645–9.
29. Ogden GR, Cowpe JG, Green MW. Evidence of field change in oral cancer. Br J Oral Maxillofac Surg. 1990;28(6):390–2.
30. Popa I, Fradet Y, Beaudry G, Hovington H, Tetu B. Identification of PCA3 (DD3) in prostatic carcinoma by in situ hybridization. Mod Pathol. 2007; 20(11):1121–7.
31. Slaughter DP, Southwick HW, Smejkal W. Field cancerization in oral stratified squamous epithelium; clinical implications of multicentric origin. Cancer. 1953;6(5):963–8.
32. Hockel M, Dornhofer N. The hydra phenomenon of cancer: why tumors recur locally after microscopically complete resection. Cancer Res. 2005; 65(8):2997–3002.
33. Yamada H, Tsuzuki T, Maeda N, Yamauchi Y, Yoshida S, Ishida R, Nishikimi T, Yokoi K, Kobayashi H. Alpha methylacyl-CoA racemase (AMACR) in prostate adenocarcinomas from Japanese patients: Is AMACR a "race"-dependent marker? Prostate. 2013;73(1):54–9.
34. Magi-Galluzzi C, Luo J, Isaacs WB, Hicks JL, de Marzo AM, Epstein JI. Alpha-methylacyl-CoA racemase: a variably sensitive immunohistochemical marker for the diagnosis of small prostate cancer foci on needle biopsy. Am J Surg Pathol. 2003;27(8):1128–33.

Permissions

All chapters in this book were first published in UROLOGY, by BioMed Central; hereby published with permission under the Creative Commons Attribution License or equivalent. Every chapter published in this book has been scrutinized by our experts. Their significance has been extensively debated. The topics covered herein carry significant findings which will fuel the growth of the discipline. They may even be implemented as practical applications or may be referred to as a beginning point for another development.

The contributors of this book come from diverse backgrounds, making this book a truly international effort. This book will bring forth new frontiers with its revolutionizing research information and detailed analysis of the nascent developments around the world.

We would like to thank all the contributing authors for lending their expertise to make the book truly unique. They have played a crucial role in the development of this book. Without their invaluable contributions this book wouldn't have been possible. They have made vital efforts to compile up to date information on the varied aspects of this subject to make this book a valuable addition to the collection of many professionals and students.

This book was conceptualized with the vision of imparting up-to-date information and advanced data in this field. To ensure the same, a matchless editorial board was set up. Every individual on the board went through rigorous rounds of assessment to prove their worth. After which they invested a large part of their time researching and compiling the most relevant data for our readers.

The editorial board has been involved in producing this book since its inception. They have spent rigorous hours researching and exploring the diverse topics which have resulted in the successful publishing of this book. They have passed on their knowledge of decades through this book. To expedite this challenging task, the publisher supported the team at every step. A small team of assistant editors was also appointed to further simplify the editing procedure and attain best results for the readers.

Apart from the editorial board, the designing team has also invested a significant amount of their time in understanding the subject and creating the most relevant covers. They scrutinized every image to scout for the most suitable representation of the subject and create an appropriate cover for the book.

The publishing team has been an ardent support to the editorial, designing and production team. Their endless efforts to recruit the best for this project, has resulted in the accomplishment of this book. They are a veteran in the field of academics and their pool of knowledge is as vast as their experience in printing. Their expertise and guidance has proved useful at every step. Their uncompromising quality standards have made this book an exceptional effort. Their encouragement from time to time has been an inspiration for everyone.

The publisher and the editorial board hope that this book will prove to be a valuable piece of knowledge for researchers, students, practitioners and scholars across the globe.

List of Contributors

Tobias Engel Ayer Botrel and Otávio Clark
Evidencias Scientific Credibility, Campinas, São Paulo, Brazil
Comitê Brasileiro de Estudos em Uro-Oncologia (CoBEU), São Paulo, Brazil

Rodolfo Borges dos Reis, Antônio Carlos Lima Pompeo, Ubirajara Ferreiara, Marcus Vinicius Sadi and Francisco Flávio Horta Bretas
Comitê Brasileiro de Estudos em Uro-Oncologia (CoBEU), São Paulo, Brazil

Josef Hoefler
Department of Mathematics, Technische Universitaet Muenchen, Boltzmannstr 3, Garching 85748, Germany

Donna P. Ankerst
Department of Mathematics, Technische Universitaet Muenchen, Boltzmannstr 3, Garching 85748, Germany
Department of Urology, University of Texas Health Science Center at San Antonio, 7703 Floyd Curl Dr, San Antonio, TX 78229, USA
Department of Epidemiology and Biostatistics, University of Texas Health Science Center at San Antonio, 7703 Floyd Curl Dr, San Antonio, TX 78229, USA

Michael Liss, David Zapata and Ian M. Thompson
Department of Urology, University of Texas Health Science Center at San Antonio, 7703 Floyd Curl Dr, San Antonio, TX 78229, USA

Robin J. Leach
Department of Urology, University of Texas Health Science Center at San Antonio, 7703 Floyd Curl Dr, San Antonio, TX 78229, USA
Department of Cellular and Structural Biology, University of Texas Health Science Center at San Antonio, 7703 Floyd Curl Dr, San Antonio, TX 78229, USA

Satoru Taguchi, Hiroshi Fukuhara, Takeshi Azuma, Motofumi Suzuki, Tetsuya Fujimura, Tohru Nakagawa, Akira Ishikawa, Haruki Kume, Yasuhiko Igawa and Yukio Homma
Department of Urology, Graduate School of Medicine, The University of Tokyo, 7-3-1 Hongo, Bunkyo-ku, Tokyo 113-8655, Japan

Vahakn B Shahinian
Department of Internal Medicine, University of Michigan, 1415 Washington Heights, Room 3627, SPH I, Ann Arbor, MI 48109-2029, USA

Yong-Fang Kuo
Department of Internal Medicine, University of Texas Medical Branch, Galveston, TX, USA
Sealy Center on Aging, University of Texas Medical Branch, Galveston, TX, USA
Department of Preventive Medicine and Community Health, University of Texas Medical Branch, Galveston, TX, USA

Jae Heon Kim
Department of Urology, Soonchunhyang University Hospital, Soonchunhyang University College of Medicine, Seoul, Republic of Korea

Ji Sung Shim, Hoon Choi, Jae Hyun Bae and Jae Young Park
Department of Urology, Korea University Ansan Hospital, Ansan, Republic of Korea
Department of Urology, Korea University College of Medicine, Seoul, Republic of Korea

Du Geon Moon, Jeong Gu Lee and Je Jong Kim
Department of Urology, Korea University College of Medicine, Seoul, Republic of Korea

Philippe Tuppin, Solène Samson, Anne Fagot-Campagna, François Alla, Fred Paccaud, Jean-Christophe Thalabard, Eric Vicaut, Michel Vidaud and Bertrand Millat
National general health insurance scheme (Caisse Nationale d'Assurance Maladie des Travailleurs Salariés, CNAMTS), Paris, France

Bertrand Lukacs
Department of Urology, Tenon Hospital, Assistance Publique- Hôpitaux de Paris, 4 Rue de la Chine, 75020 Paris, France

P. G. Konan, C. C. Vodi, A. H. Dekou, A. Fofana, E. E. Gowé and K. Manzan
Service d'Urologie, CHU de Cocody, Abidjan, Ivory Coast, Africa

Kuniyasu Muraoka, Shuichi Morizane, Masashi Honda, Takehiro Sejima and Atsushi Takenaka
Division of Urology, Department of Surgery, Tottori University Faculty of Medicine, Yonago 683-8504, Japan

Nobuyuki Hinata
Department of Urology, Kobe University Graduate School of Medicine, Kobe, Japan

Gen Murakami
Division of Internal Medicine, Iwamizawa Kojin-kai Hospital, Iwamizawa, Japan

Ashutosh K Tewari
Department of Urology, Mount Sinai Hospital, New York, NY, USA

Dimitrios Hatzichristou
Centre for Sexual and Reproductive Health and 1st Department of Urology, Aristotle University of Thessaloniki, Thessaloniki, Greece

Gianluca d'Anzeo and Andrea Rossi
Medical Advisor Urology, Eli Lilly Italy S.p.A., Via A. Gramsci 731/733, 50019 Sesto Fiorentino, FI, Italy.

Hartmut Porst
Private Practice of Urology and Andrology, Hamburg, Germany

Jacques Buvat
Centre d'Etude et de Traitement de la Pathologie de l'Appa reil Reproducteur et de la Psychosomatique (CETPARP), Lille, France

Carsten Henneges and Hartwig Büttner
Lilly Deutschland GmbH, Bad Homburg, Germany

Karim Hamidi
Eli Lilly and Company, Neuilly sur Seine, France

Frank Friedersdorff, Seven Johannes Aghdassi, Ahmed Magheli, Maximilian Richter, Carsten Stephan, Jonas Busch, Kurt Miller and T Florian Fuller
Department of Urology, Charité University Hospital, Charitéplatz 1, 10117 Berlin, Germany

Dirk Boehmer
Department of Radiation Oncology, Charité University Hospital, Berlin, Germany

Daksha Trivedi and Michael Kirby
Centre for Research in Primary and Community Care, University of Hertfordshire, Hatfield, UK

David M Wellsted and Jade B Collard
Centre for Lifespan and Chronic Illness Research, University of Hertfordshire, Hatfield, UK

Jayoung Kim
Departments of Surgery and Biomedical Sciences, Cedars-Sinai Medical Center, 8700 Beverly Blvd., Davis Room 5071, Los Angeles, CA 90048, USA
Departments of Medicine, University of California, Los Angeles, CA, USA
Department of Surgery, Harvard Medical School, Boston, MA, USA

Seok Joong Yun and Wun-Jae Kim
Department of Urology, Chungbuk National University College of Medicine, 62 Kaeshin-dong, Heungduk-gu, Cheongju 361-763, Republic of Korea

Stephanie Sauer, Tobias Gassenmaier, Andreas S Kunz, Thorsten A Bley, Detlef Klein and Bernhard Petritsch
University Hospital Würzburg, Institute of Diagnostic and Interventional Radiology, Oberdürrbacher Str. 6, 97080 Würzburg, Germany

Jan P Goltz
University Hospital Schleswig-Holstein, Campus Lübeck, Clinic for Radiology and Nuclear Medicine, Ratzeburger Allee 160, 23538 Lübeck, Germany

Zhengyan Tang
Department of Urology, Xiangya Hospital of Central South University, Changsha, Hunan 410013, China

Dongjie Li and Xiaobo Zhang
Department of Geriatric Urology, Xiangya Hospital of Central South University, Changsha, Hunan 410013, China

Lu Yi
Department of Urology, The Second Xiangya Hospital of Central South University, Changsha, Hunan, China

Xiangsheng Zhu
Department of The Andrology, Central Hospital of Xiangtan, Xiangtan, Hunan, China

Xiangyang Zeng
Department of Urology, The First People's Hospital of Chenzhou, Chenzhou, Hunan, China

Yuxin Tang
Department of Urology, The Third Xiangya Hospital of Central South University, Changsha, Hunan, China

Takashige Abe, Ryuji Matsumoto, Sachiyo Murai, Naoto Miyajima, Kunihiko Tsuchiya, Satoru Maruyama and Nobuo Shinohara
Department of Urology, Hokkaido University Graduate School of Medicine, North-15, West-7, North Ward, Sapporo 060-8638, Japan

Fumi Kato, Taisuke Harada and Kohsuke Kudo
Department of Diagnostic and Interventional Radiology, Hokkaido University Hospital, Sapporo, Japan

Hiromi Fujita
Department of Surgical Pathology, Hokkaido University Hospital, Sapporo, Japan

Teoman Cem Kadioglu
Department of Urology, Istanbul School of Medicine, University of Istanbul, 34365 Istanbul, Turkey

Peter D Temple-Smith
Department of Obstetrics and Gynaecology, Monash Medical Centre, Melbourne, Australia

Graeme Southwick
Melbourne Institute of Plastic Surgery, Melbourne, Victoria, Australia

Nandu D. Dantanarayana
University of Sydney, Discipline of Surgery, Sydney, Australia

Andrew Brooks and Manish I. Patel
University of Sydney, Discipline of Surgery, Sydney, Australia
Department of Urology, Westmead Hospital, Sydney, Australia

Tania Hossack and Howard Lau
Department of Urology, Westmead Hospital, Sydney, Australia

Paul Cozzi
St George Hospital, Sydney, Australia

Warick Delprado
Douglass Hanley Moir Pathology, Sydney, Australia

Xiaotian Wang and Yongsheng Song
Department of Urology, Shengjing Hospital of China Medical University, 36 Saohao Road, Shenyang, Liaoning, China

Zimu Gong and Wei Yan
Department of Hematology, Shengjing Hospital of China Medical University, Shenyang, China

Shawn Xiang Li
Department of Hematology, Shengjing Hospital of China Medical University, Shenyang, China
International College, China Medical University, Shenyang, China

Zoran Krstanoski
Department of Urology, General Hospital Slovenj Gradec, Gosposvetska 1, 2380 Slovenj Gradec, Slovenia

Nadja Kokalj Vokac and Andreja Zagorac
Laboratory of Medical Genetics, University Medical Centre Maribor, Maribor, Slovenia

Boris Pospihalj
Division of Gynecology, Department of Gynecological Pathology and Cytology, University Medical Center Ljubljana, Ljubljana, Slovenia

Miha Munda
Institute for Anatomy, Histology and Embryology, Medical Faculty, University of Maribor, Maribor, Slovenia

Saso Dzeroski
Jozef Stefan Institute, Ljubljana, Slovenia

Rastko Golouh
Institute of Pathology, Medical Faculty University of Maribor, Maribor, Slovenia

Daniar K. Osmonov, Alexey V. Aksenov, David Trick, Carsten M. Naumann, Moritz F. Hamann, Amr Abou Faddan and Klaus-Peter Jünemann
Department of Urology and Pediatric Urology, University Hospital Schleswig-Holstein, Campus Kiel, Arnold-Heller Strasse 3, Haus 18, D-24105 Kiel, Germany

A. W. Postema, M. J. V. Scheltema, C. K. Mannaerts, T. Idzenga and J. J. M. C. H. De la Rosette
Department of Urology, AMC University Hospital, Amsterdam, The Netherlands

H. Wijkstra
Department of Urology, AMC University Hospital, Amsterdam, The Netherlands.
Department of Electrical Engineering, Eindhoven University of Technology, Eindhoven, The Netherlands

R. J. G. Van Sloun M. Mischi
Department of Electrical Engineering, Eindhoven University of Technology, Eindhoven, The Netherlands

M. R. E. Engelbrecht
Department of Radiology, AMC University Hospital, Amsterdam, The Netherlands

Masahiko Nakayama, Hisanori Kobayashi, Tomihiro Takahara and Kazutake Yoshizawa
Medical Affairs Division, Janssen Pharmaceutical K.K., 5-2, Nishi-kanda, 3-Chome, Chiyoda-ku, Tokyo 101-0065, Japan

Ryo Oyama and Keiichiro Imanaka
Research and Development Division, Janssen Pharmaceutical K.K., 5-2, Nishi-kanda, 3-Chome, Chiyoda-ku, Tokyo 101-0065, Japan

Myong Kim, Cheryn Song and Hanjong Ahn
Department of Urology, Asan Medical Center, University of Ulsan College of Medicine, 88 Olympic-Ro 43 Gil Songpa-Gu, Seoul 05505, Republic of Korea

Se Un Jeong and Yong Mee Cho
Department of Pathology, Asan Medical Center, University of Ulsan College of Medicine, Seoul 05505, Republic of Korea

Jae Yoon Ro
Department of Pathology and Genomic Medicine, Houston Methodist Hospital, Weill Medical College of Cornell University, Houston, TX 10065, USA

Aram Kim
Department of Urology, Konkuk University Medical Center, Konkuk University School of Medicine, Seoul 05030, Republic of Korea

Ping Meng, Geng Zhang, Yan-zhu Wang, Yu-ming Jing, Wei-jun Qin and Jian-lin Yuan
Department of Urology, Xijing Hospital, Fourth Military Medical University, Xi'an, Shaanxi, China

Qing-chuan Dong
Department of Urology Surgery, Peoples' Hospital of Shaanxi Province, Xi'an, Shaanxi, China

Guang-guo Tan
Department of Pharmaceutical Analysis, School of Pharmacy, Fourth Military Medical University, Xi'an, Shaanxi, China

Wei-hong Wen
Department of Immunology, Fourth Military MedicalUniversity, Xi'an, Shaanxi, China

He Wang
Department of Urology, Tangdu Hospital, The Fourth Military Medical University, Xi'an, Shaanxi, China

Chen Wang
State Key Laboratory of NBC Protection for Civilian, Beijing, China

Liancheng Fan, Baijun Dong, Chenfei Chi, Yanqing Wang, Yiming Gong, Jianjun Sha, Jiahua Pan, Xun Shangguan, Yiran Huang, Lixin Zhou and Wei Xue
Department of Urology, School of Medicine, Renji Hospital, Shanghai Jiao Tong University, Shanghai 200127, China

Kerri T. Barnes
Department of Urology, University of Iowa, 200 Hawkins Dr., 3 RCP, Iowa City, IA 52242-1089, USA

Amit Gupta
Department of Urology, University of Iowa, 200 Hawkins Dr., 3 RCP, Iowa City, IA 52242-1089, USA
Department of Epidemiology, University of Iowa, Iowa City, IA, USA

Bradley D. McDowell and Anna Button
Holden Comprehensive Cancer Center, University of Iowa, Iowa City, IA, USA

Charles F. Lynch
Holden Comprehensive Cancer Center, University of Iowa, Iowa City, IA, USA
Department of Epidemiology, University of Iowa, Iowa City, IA, USA

Brian J. Smith
Department of Biostatistics, University of Iowa, Iowa City, IA, USA

Saeid Alinezhad, Riina-Minna Väänänen, Natalia Tong Ochoa and Kim Pettersson
Division of Biotechnology, University of Turku, Tykistökatu 6A 6th floor, 20520 Turku, Finland

Emily A. Vertosick
Department of Epidemiology and Biostatistics, Memorial Sloan-Kettering Cancer Center, New York, NY, USA

Anders Bjartell
Department of Clinical Sciences, Division of Urological Cancers, Lund University, Skåne University Hospital, Malmö, Sweden

Peter J Boström
Department of Urology, Turku University Hospital, Turku, Finland

Pekka Taimen
Department of Pathology, University of Turku and Turku University Hospital, Turku, Finland

Index

www.ingramcontent.com/pod-product-compliance
Lightning Source LLC
LaVergne TN
LVHW080652210926
848485LV00003B/365

* 9 7 8 1 6 3 2 4 2 9 6 2 9 *